Practicing Medicine in the Third World

1967–2010

AF701909

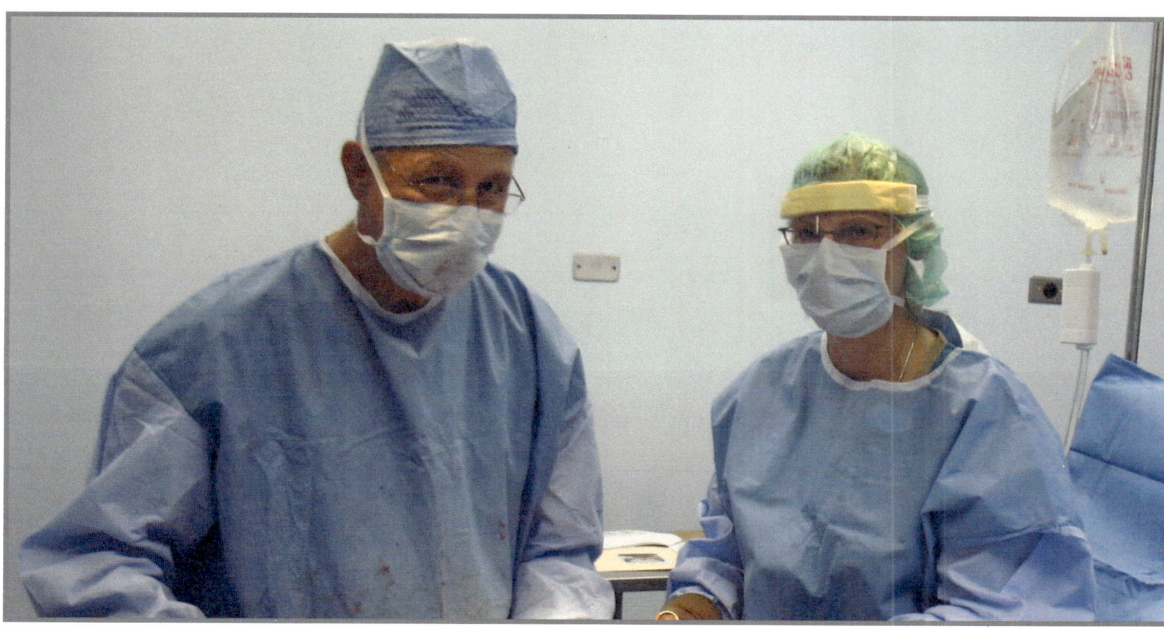

Ronald Sandler, MD

Copyrighted Material

Practicing Medicine in the Third World 1967–2010

Copyright © 2020 by Ron Sandler. All Rights Reserved.

No part of this publication may be reproduced, stored in a retrieval system or transmitted, in any form or by any means—electronic, mechanical, photocopying, recording or otherwise—without prior written permission from the publisher, except for the inclusion of brief quotations in a review.

For information about this title or to order other books and/or electronic media, contact the publisher:
Ron Sandler
rbhs@mac.com

ISBN: 978-1-7349417-0-8

Printed in the United States of America

Cover and Interior design: 1106 Design

My purpose in creating this document is to leave a written log of the foreign travels experienced by Rita and me over a 29-year period, plus my time spent in Bolivia with the Peace Corps from 1967 to 1969.

I wish to express my deep gratitude to my oldest daughter, Laura, for her painstaking and caring editing of this manuscript.

I would also like to acknowledge Professor Mark Montgomery of Grinnell College, who prodded me into recording my experiences in writing.

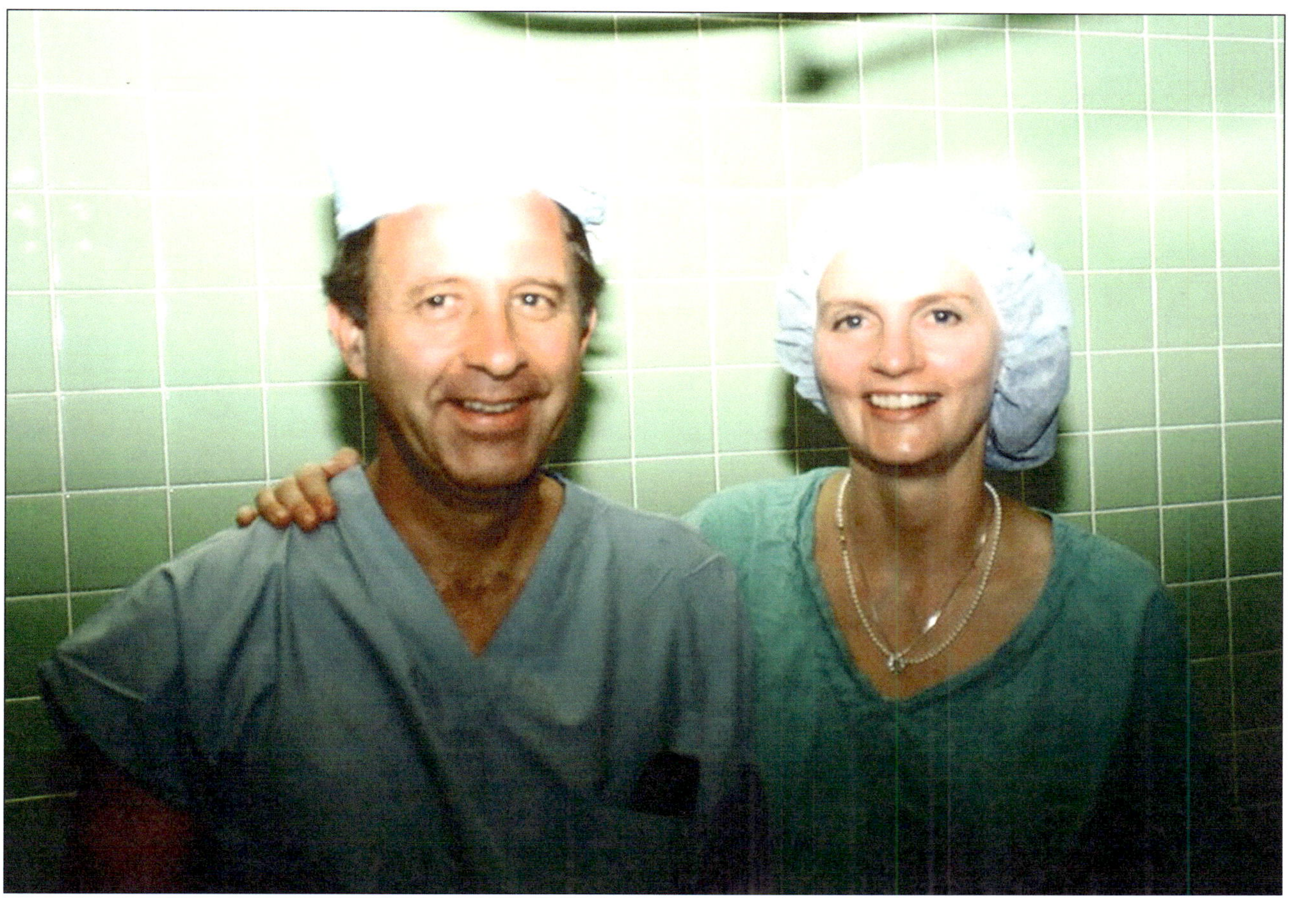

Bolivia

My interest in Third World medicine began during my undergraduate years at Grinnell College, when I read a series of books by Dr. Thomas Dooley and by/about Dr. Albert Schweitzer. Dr. Dooley recounted his experiences providing healthcare in rural Laos in the late '50s. The passion for his work, the satisfaction he received aiding those who would otherwise go untreated was obvious in his description of his experiences. Unfortunately, his work was cut short when he succumbed to malignant melanoma at the age of 36. Dr. Schweitzer was a famous healer/philosopher who operated a rural hospital in Gabon, Africa. He presented his work more in ethical terms — that doing this work (treating the poor) was a moral obligation. Both authors inspired me to someday copy their efforts if I was ever in a position to do so.

The passion for his work, the satisfaction he received aiding those who would otherwise go untreated, was obvious in his description of his experiences.

While in medical school, during my third year, I encountered a patient who was back in the US for a few weeks before returning as a missionary to Riberalta, Bolivia, with the Wyclif Bible translators. I inquired about summer opportunities for medical students in her area. She was unaware of any but mentioned a Methodist Hospital in La Paz and that, perhaps, they could accommodate me. I corresponded with the mission board and was accepted for an externship during the summer of 1965. I, with my younger brother, David, spent 6 weeks working in the Clinica Americana in LaPaz. The American physicians were very capable, treating many conditions rarely encountered in the United States, e.g., parasitic diseases, advanced and untreated tumors, as well as untreated congenital abnormalities, and doing so without the latest technologies. The experience whetted my appetite to continue pursuing further opportunities in Third World medicine.

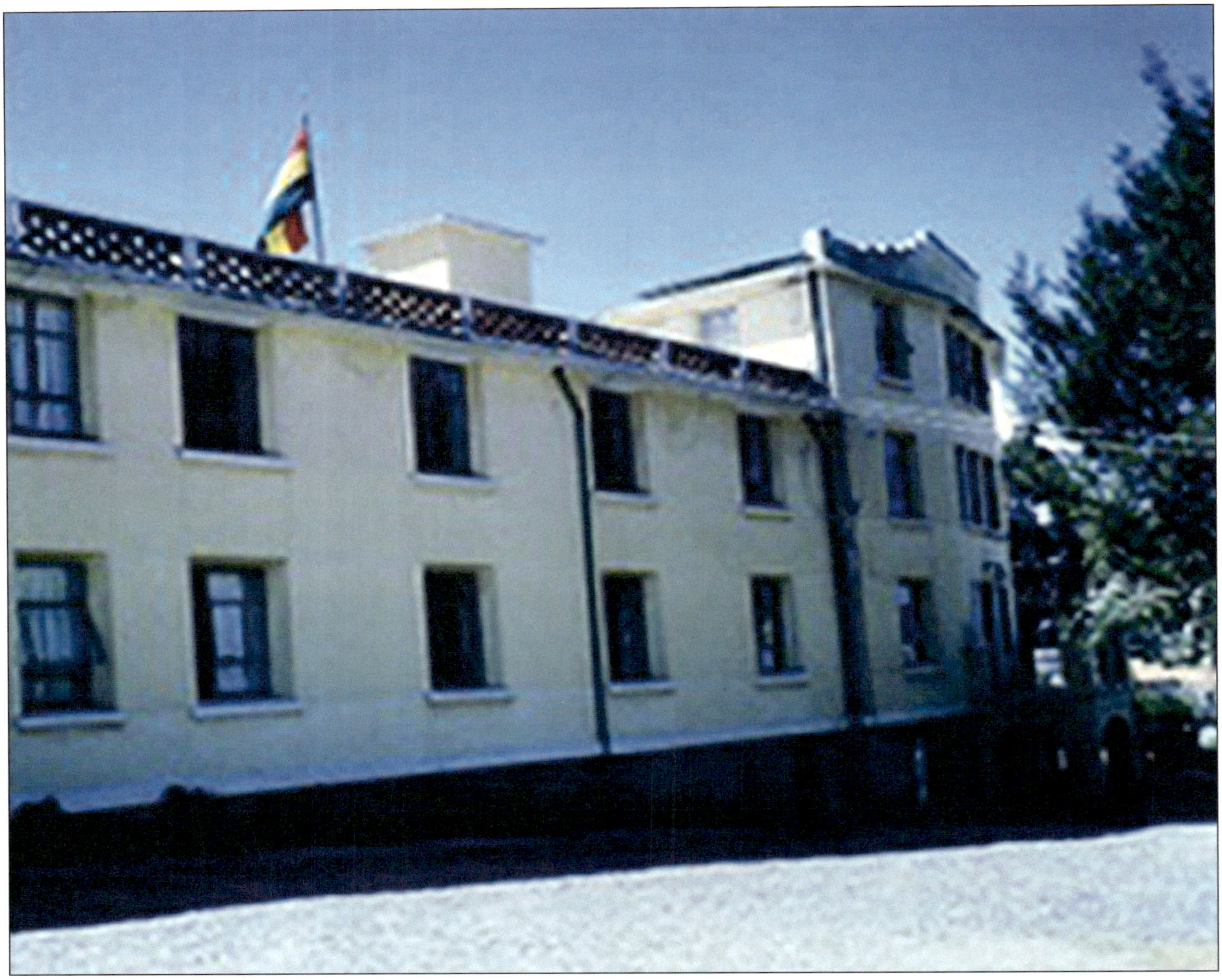

Clinica Americana 1965

My internship was in Portland, Oregon, from 1966 to 1967 at the peak of the Vietnam war. After internship, we were compelled to serve our country by getting drafted into the armed forces, obtaining a deferment to pursue specialty training and then enter service, or join the Public Health Service and provide medical care to their constituents, Indian reservations, or the Peace Corps to care for the volunteers. I applied for the latter and as part of the selection process was flown to Washington, DC, put up in a one-star hotel and interviewed by the Deputy Director. During our discussion, he inquired as to where I would like to go if selected, and when I replied, "Bolivia," he laughed and said "You're in," the implication being that no one wished to go to Bolivia. I was indeed chosen in the spring of '67. The Service provided private Spanish tutoring during my last few months of training. Then, in July, my then-wife, Janis, and two small children, ages one and three, drove across the country to Washington, DC, where we were housed in a hotel room for one month and received intensive Spanish-language instruction. After two weeks of hotel life, it became apparent the situation was too difficult for the children, so my wife took them to her parents in St. Louis, while I completed the program. In addition to language training, we received a short course in tropical medicine and even had a course on jeep driving, as one of the previous physicians spent two years driving in first gear since he was unable to drive a manual transmission. It turned out that he was the doctor I was replacing. In town, he was referred to as *Dr. Primero* (first) as you could hear the vehicle whining from blocks away as he drove to and from the office each day.

I developed a tremendous respect for the Peace Corps Volunteers.

In the late summer of '67, Janis and our two young children headed for Santa Cruz, Bolivia, to spend the next two years. My primary responsibility was caring for young, healthy volunteers, but my most-often-used talent was that of listener and, at times, counselor. As people who have lived for extended periods of time in a foreign land can attest, life can sometimes be challenging, away from friends and family, speaking a different language, and, for the volunteers, living as locals in often-difficult conditions. I developed a tremendous respect for the Peace Corps Volunteers. They commit two years of their life living in all manner of crude (by US standards) and unusual environs. They are required to live, eat, and survive as the locals. It was often a difficult, challenging endeavor but one that provided lifelong rewards.

The opportunity for people from different countries and cultures to truly get to know and interact with Americans is an invaluable way for them to form realistic impressions of who we are and what we stand for. I believe this is a great asset for US diplomacy, and the volunteers receive an invaluable educational experience while making long-lasting friendships and, at times, spouses.

Most of my time was spent maintaining the health of the volunteers, evaluating their sites before arrival for safety, and then following up after they had been in residence for a few months to confirm that their experience was satisfactory and safe, doing periodic vaccinations and treating the occasional diarrhea, upper-respiratory symptoms, or localized infections. There was a great amount of free time, and I learned to survive without TV or radio. I read extensively and learned how to play Bridge. Each Sunday, after church, we would take the children to the main square in town and watch the sloths that lived in the trees in the city square. The locals were very protective of these creatures, making sure they did not gain access to the streets and traffic.

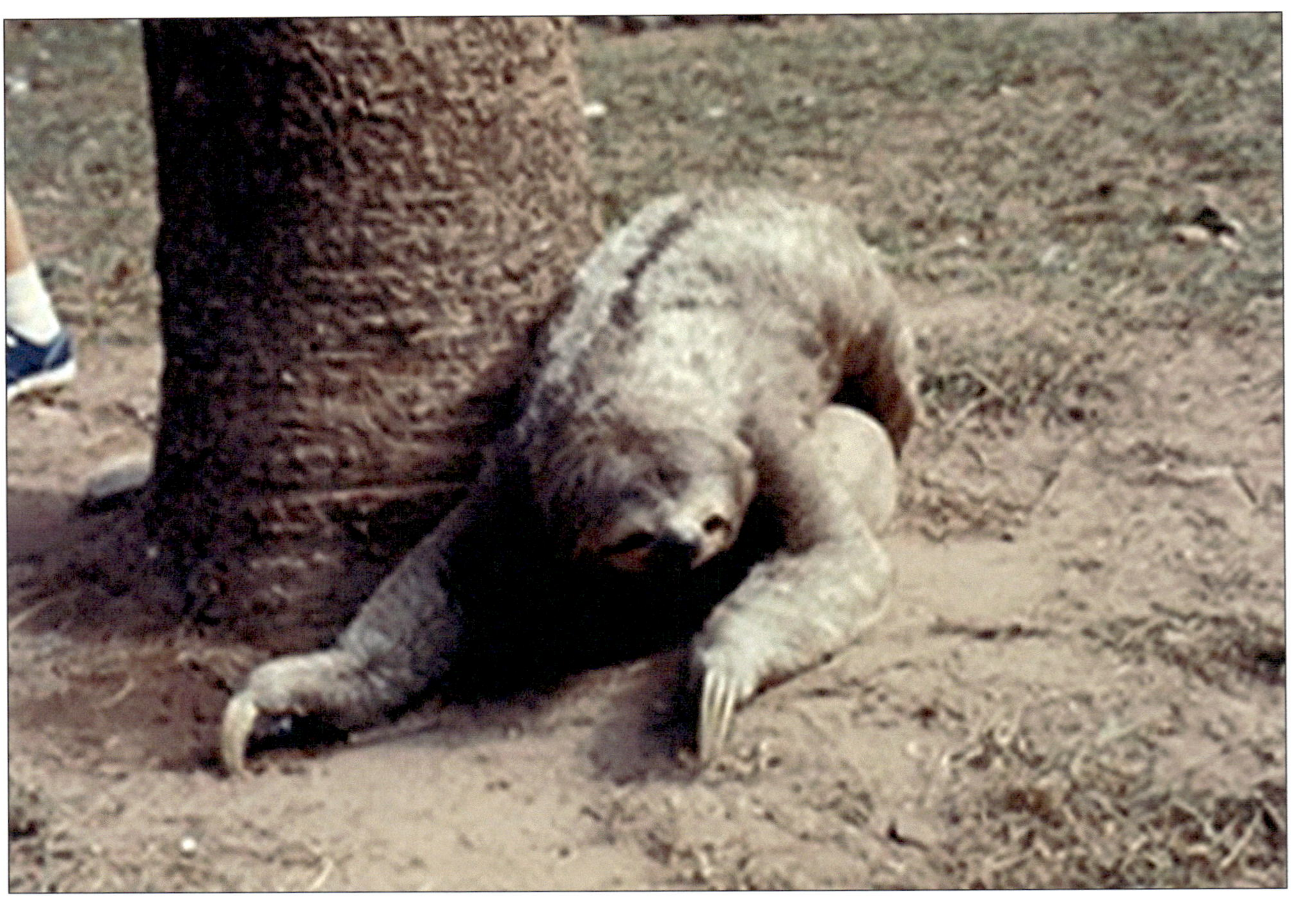

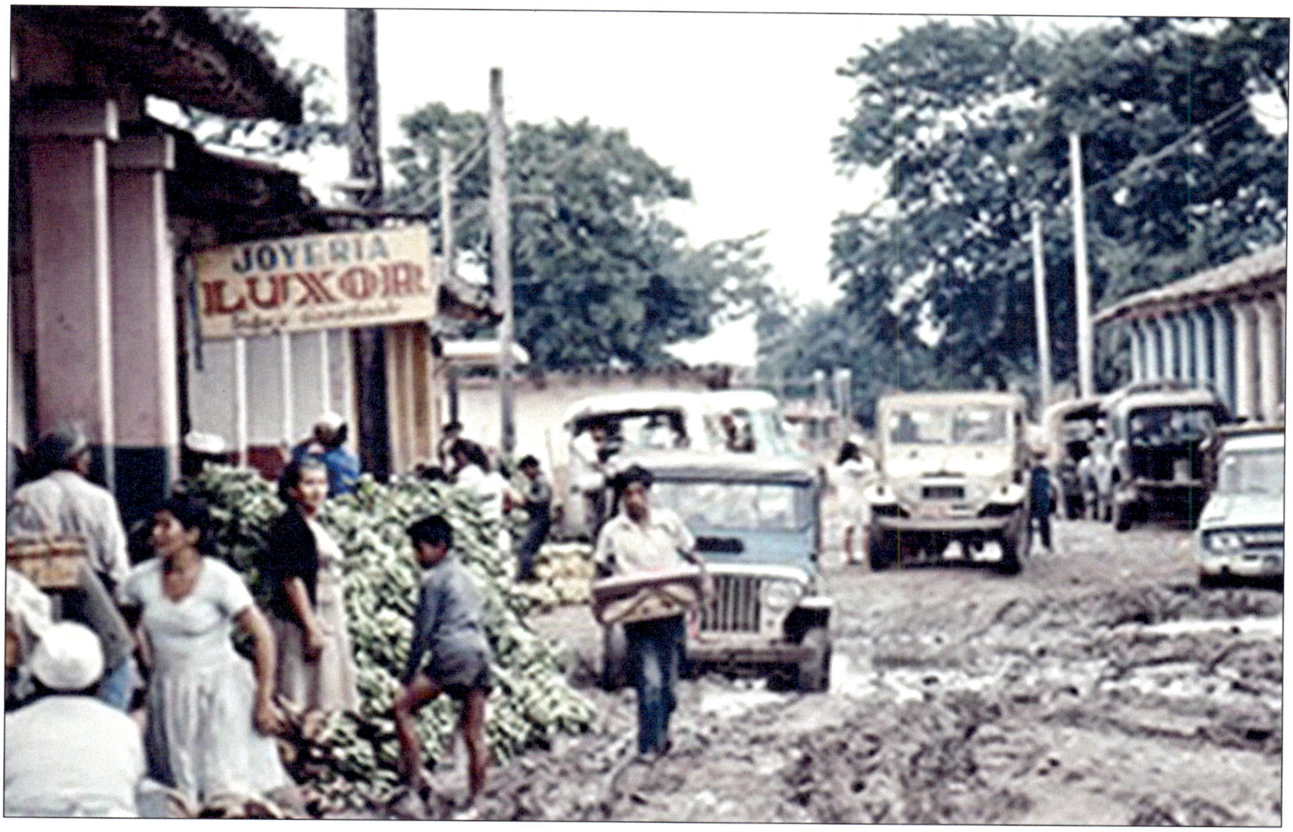

Santa Cruz after a rainfall

I also ran a weekly well-baby clinic for the locals, attempting to get the infants on a well-balanced diet by the age of 1 year, adding a different food group each month. Most of the children were fed nothing but breast milk for the first 2 years, with occasional addition of coffee and/or bread. The children were evaluated each month and their weights recorded to check their progress. I found it very difficult trying to change cultural dietary habits, but there were successes.

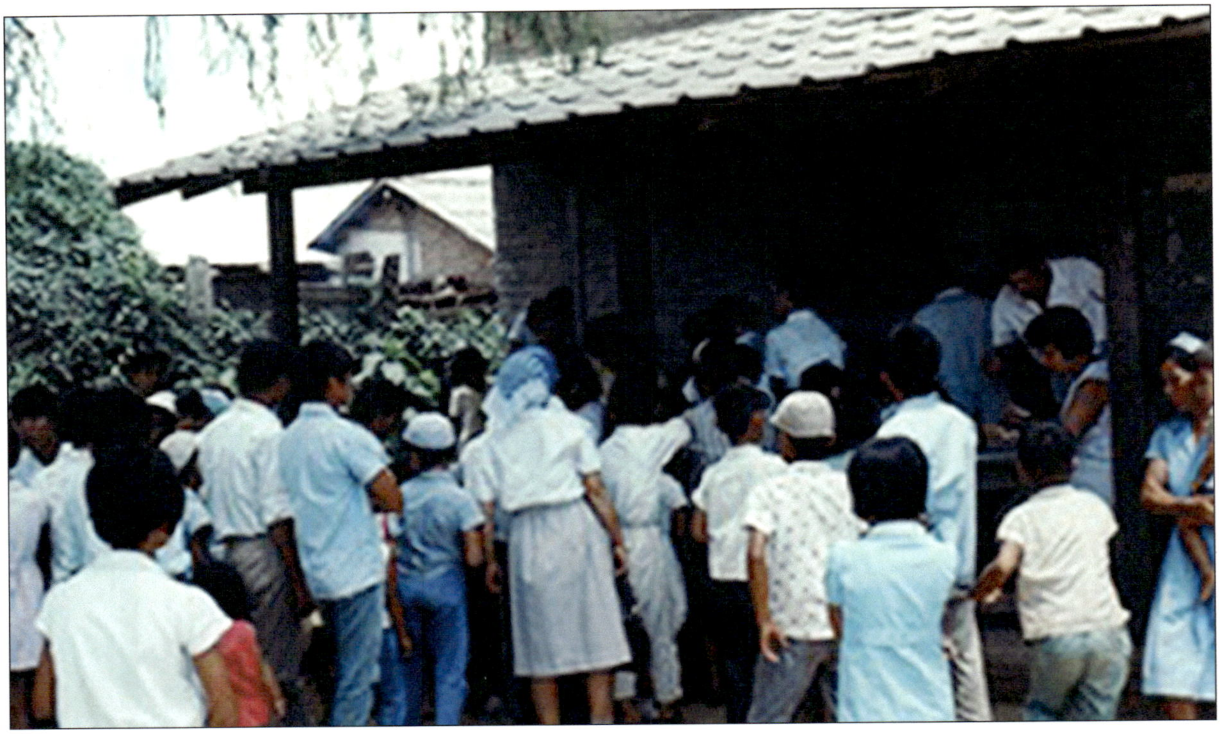

Patients waiting outside rural clinic

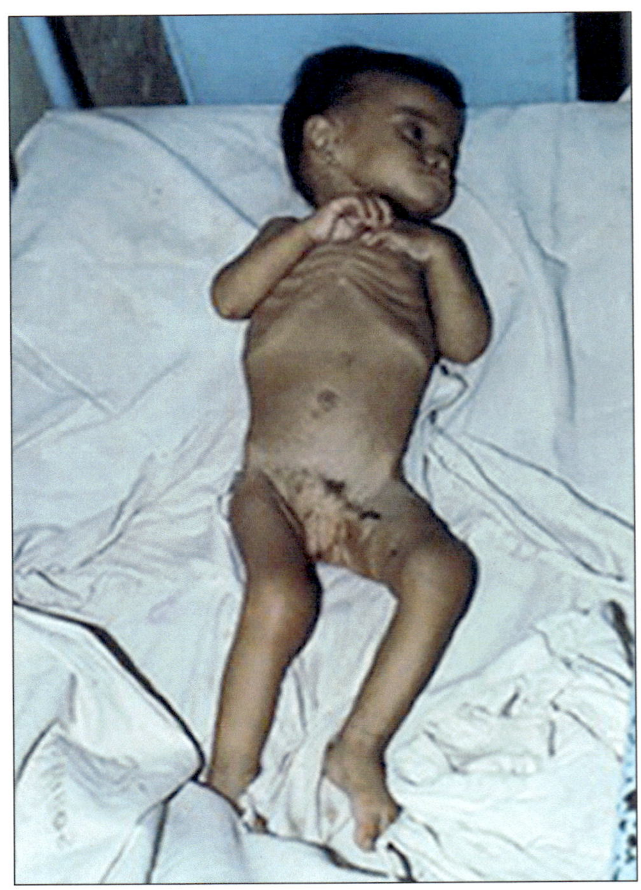

Malnourished child

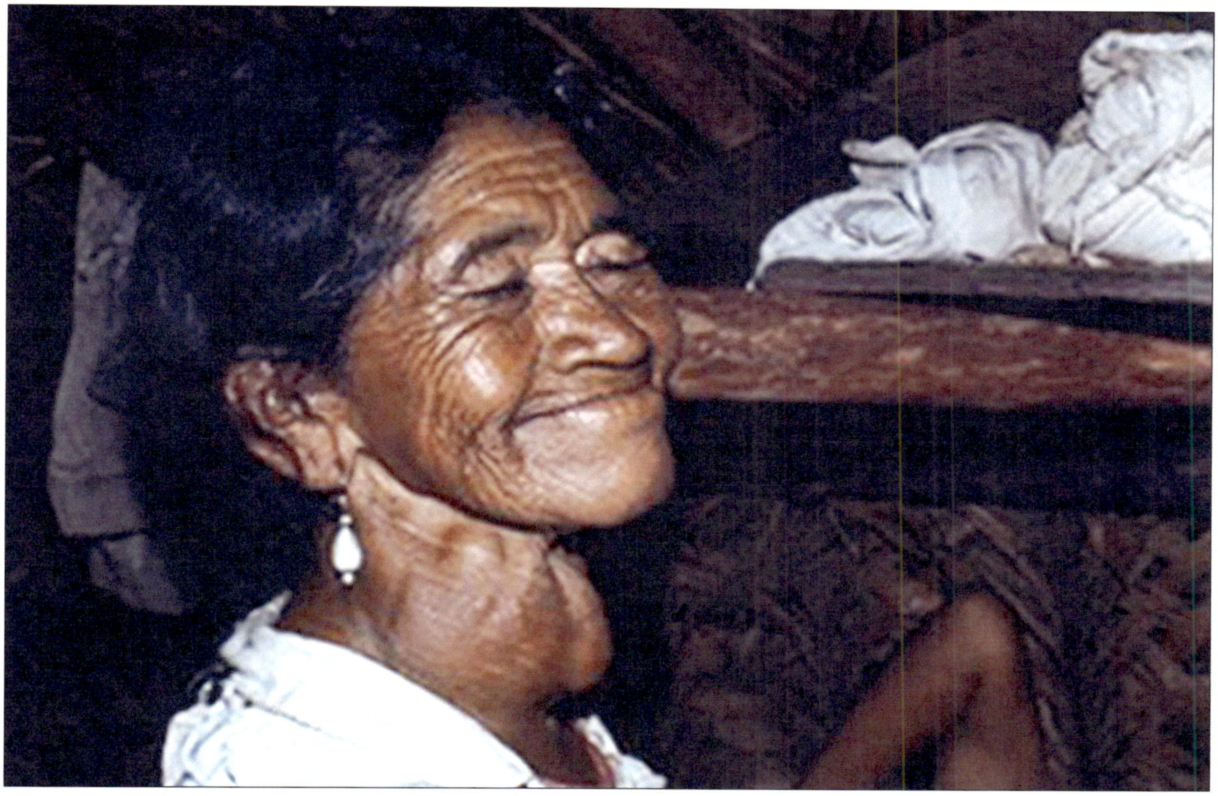

Woman with goiter

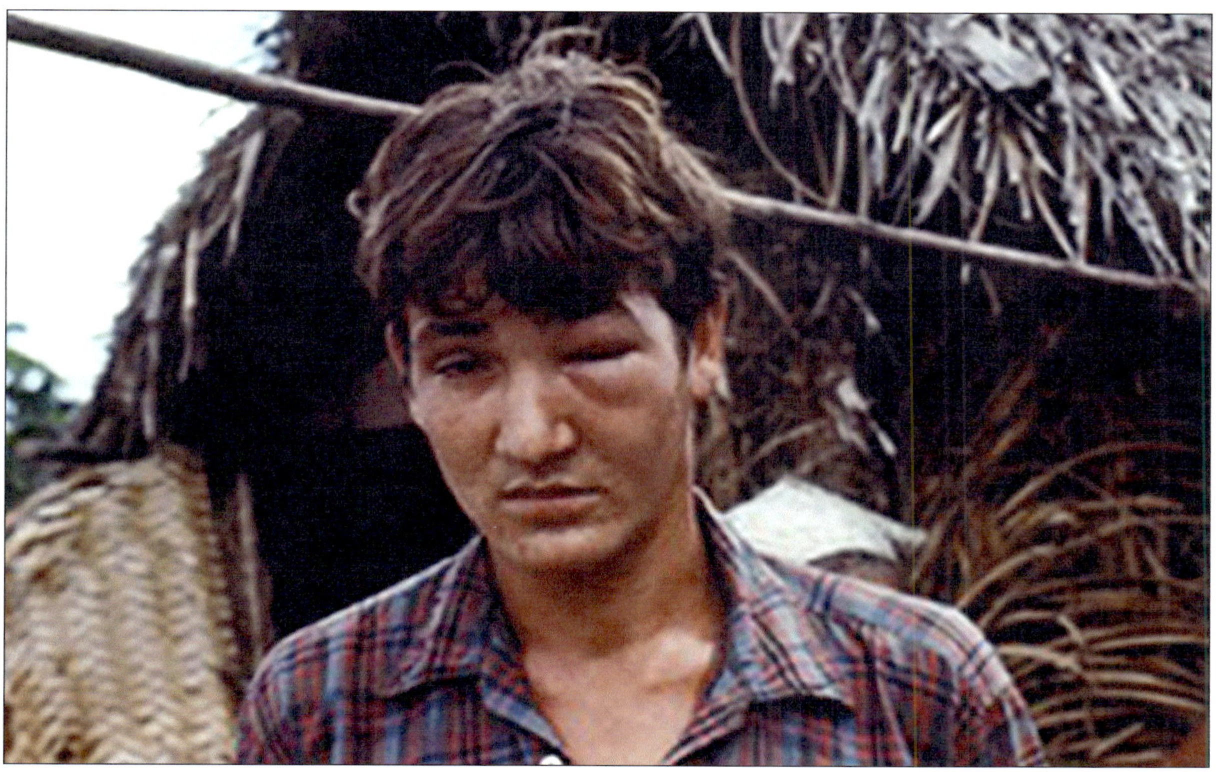

Chagas Disease, a potentially fatal parasitic disease

Since the volunteers as a group were quite healthy, I was seldom challenged medically, although one young lady presented with an alarming abnormality which required an emergency evacuation to the US. This volunteer had recently returned to Bolivia after undergoing spine surgery for a vascular abnormality on her spinal cord some six weeks previously. She did well for about 3 weeks before she began complaining of numbness and weakness in her legs. Her examination confirmed there was pressure on her spinal cord, a neurological emergency. By shortwave radio, I contacted the Neurosurgery Department at Georgetown University Medical Center, where she had received the initial surgery. They advised bringing her back to them as soon as possible. Boarding the plane that evening, she was having difficulty walking, and, during the flight, she lost bladder control. When we reached Washington, DC, that next day, I had to carry her off of the airplane. She did not return to Bolivia but came to see me almost 10 years later at my office in Mesa, Arizona. She was able to walk with lower extremity bracing and had returned to college after her surgery, graduated from dental school, and was on her way to practice in Oregon. I often wondered what had become of her, and I was pleased to see she had done so well.

Her examination confirmed there was pressure on her spinal cord, a neurological emergency.

Brazil

My Peace Corps tour ended in 1969, and I entered the orthopedic residency program at the University of Washington in Seattle. After completion in 1974, we moved to Mesa, Arizona, where I practiced for the next 26 years with Mezona Orthopedics.

In 1980, I read an article in our local newspaper about Esperanza, a Phoenix-based organization that was providing medical care to individuals in Santarem, Brazil, a city on the Amazon River approximately 500 miles inland from the mouth on the Atlantic Ocean, at the junction of the Amazon and Tapajos Rivers. The article ignited my interest in providing medical care to the underserved in the Third World. I contacted the organization and made my first trip in 1981, the first of five journeys we made to that site over the next 14 years.

The article ignited my interest in providing medical care to the underserved in the Third World.

Esperanza was founded by a Franciscan priest and physician, Father Luke Tupper. While practicing medicine in the Amazon, he realized the need for a surgical facility to treat the many abnormalities he was encountering. His brother, Jerry Tupper, a practicing lawyer in Phoenix, organized and spearheaded efforts that resulted in converting an old ferry boat into a hospital ship, which was subsequently transported to the Amazon. It was outfitted with an operating room, albeit an extremely small one, where orthopedic, plastic, and gyn surgeries were performed. The quarters were cramped, with air conditioning available only in the operating and recovery rooms. Surgery performed on the boat was often an adventure, not only because of the challenging pathology encountered, but because the large barges traveling up and down the Amazon would create wakes that caused the boat to rock back and forth.

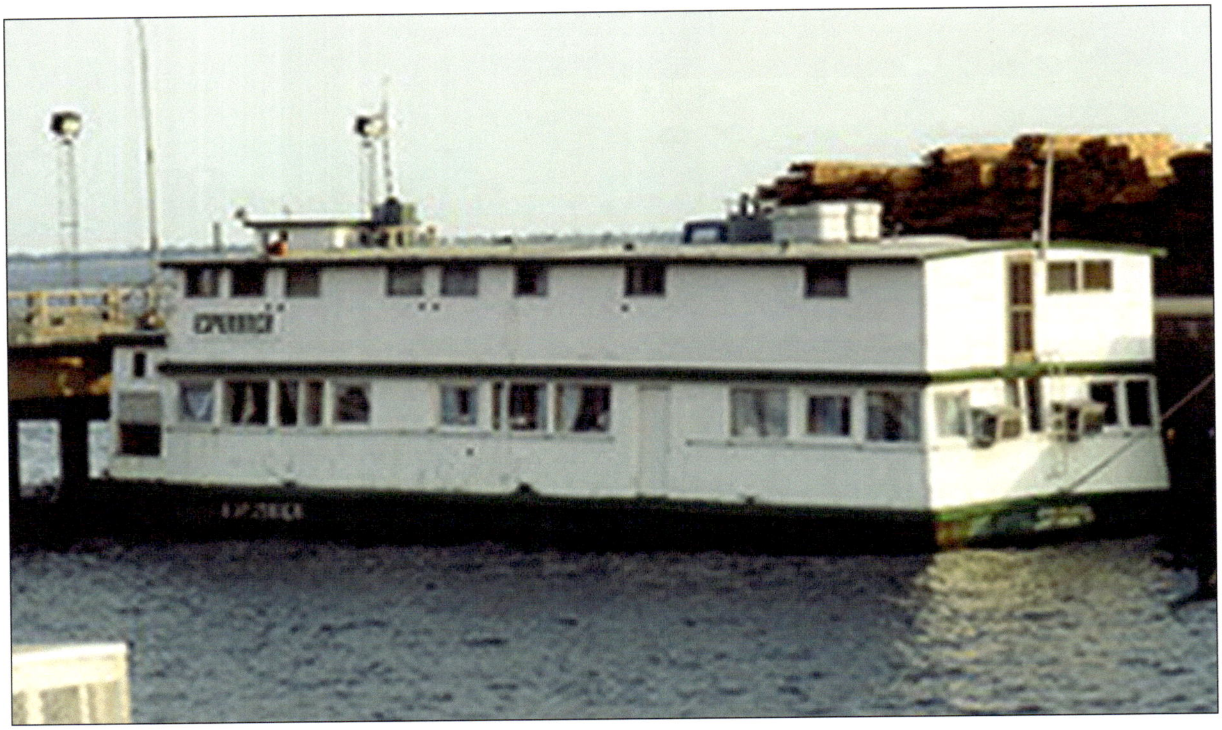

Hospital ship *Esperanza* with air conditioners at the rear of the ship

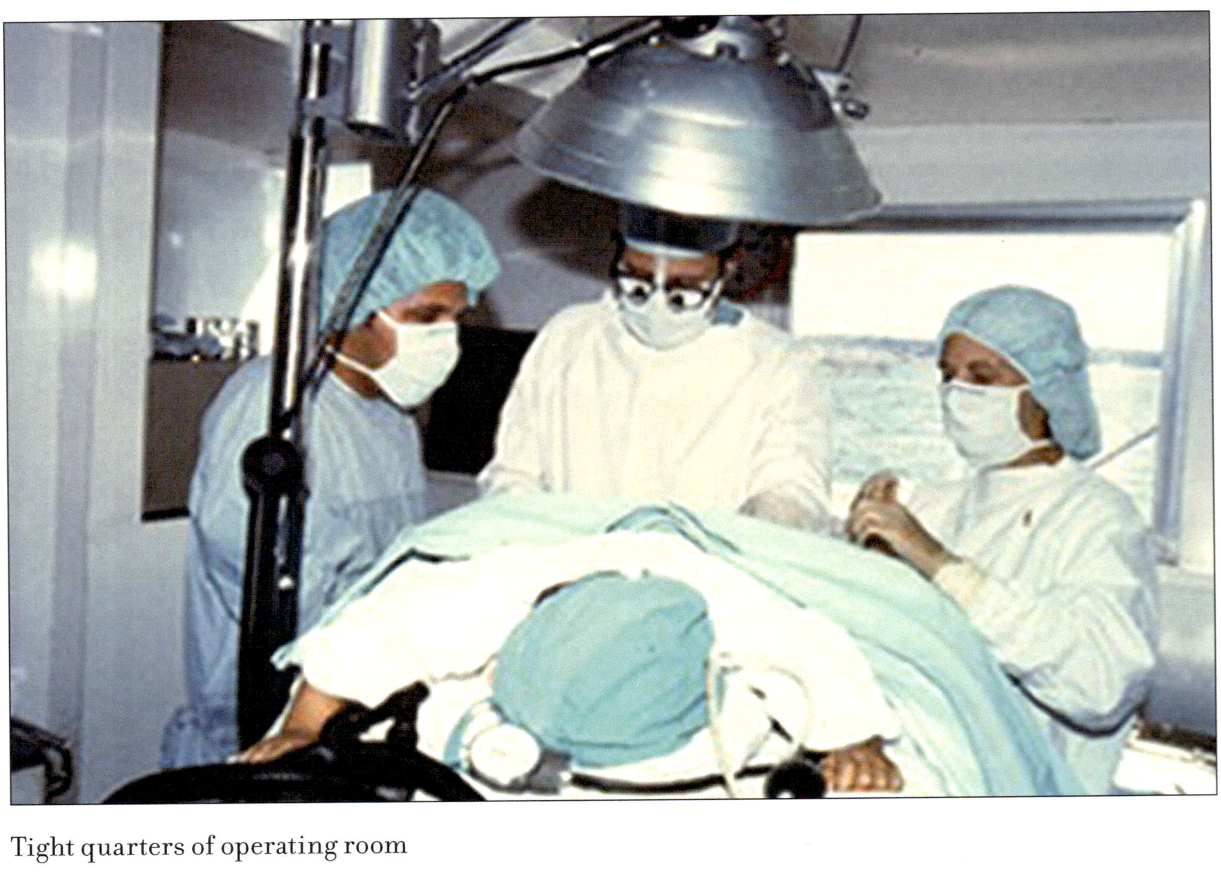

Tight quarters of operating room

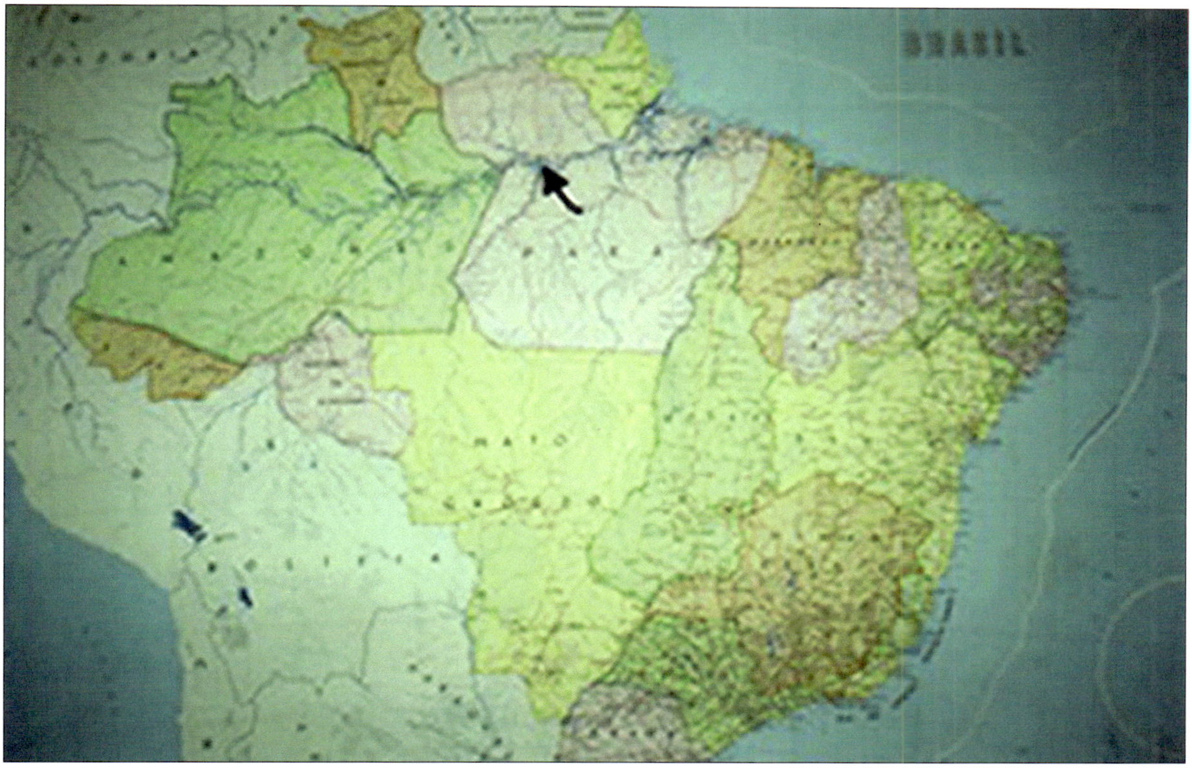

Santarem, Brazil, at junction of Amazon and Tapajos Rivers

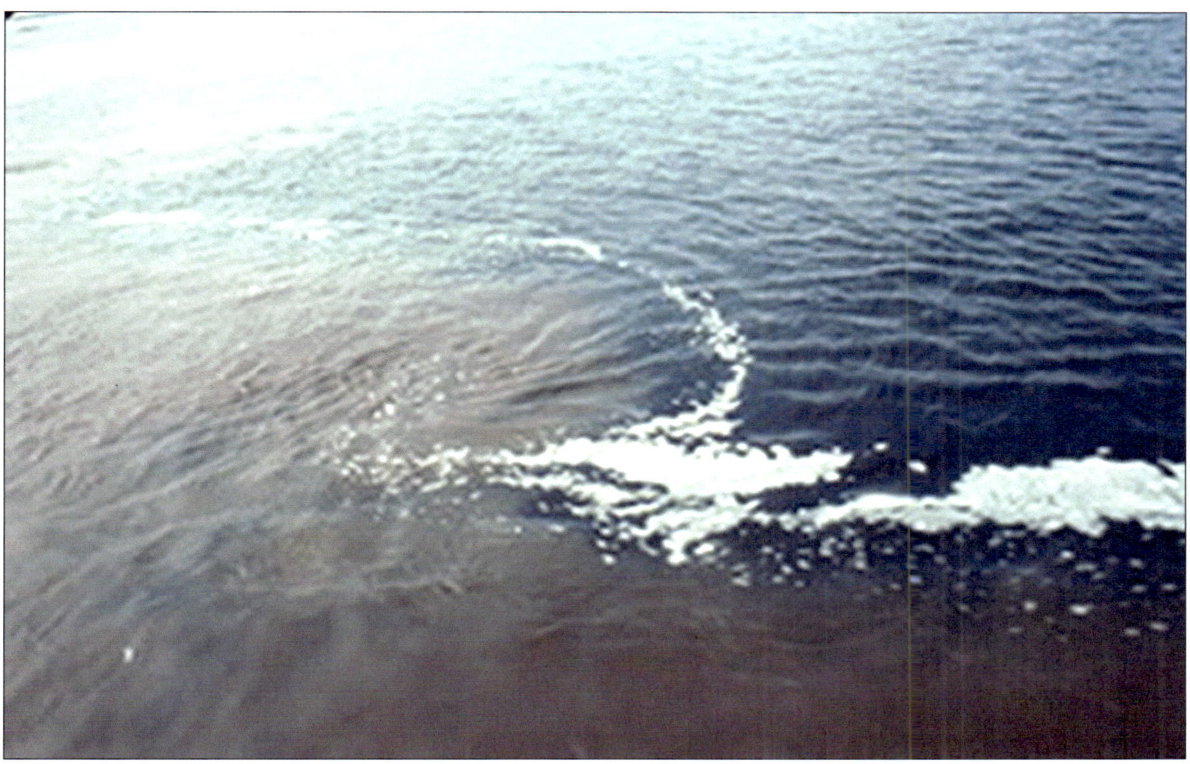

Muddy Amazon on left, Tapajos on right

An orthopedic team that consisted of a surgeon, anesthesiologist and 2–3 nurses would do surgery for stretches of 2–3 weeks at a time, with approximately 4 ortho teams performing throughout the year. At other times, plastic teams would treat primarily the untreated cleft lips and palates, and the gyn and general surgical teams worked at other times, with a different team arriving about every 6 weeks.

Upon arrival, usually early in the morning, from a 5–6 hour flight from Miami, we would rest for 2 or 3 hours, then begin seeing patients in the clinic and construct the operative schedule for the remainder of our stay. Surgery would commence the following day, and we would operate all day and sometimes into the night correcting abnormalities that would otherwise go untreated. Many of the patients traveled 2 to 3 days by boat to reach us and receive treatment.

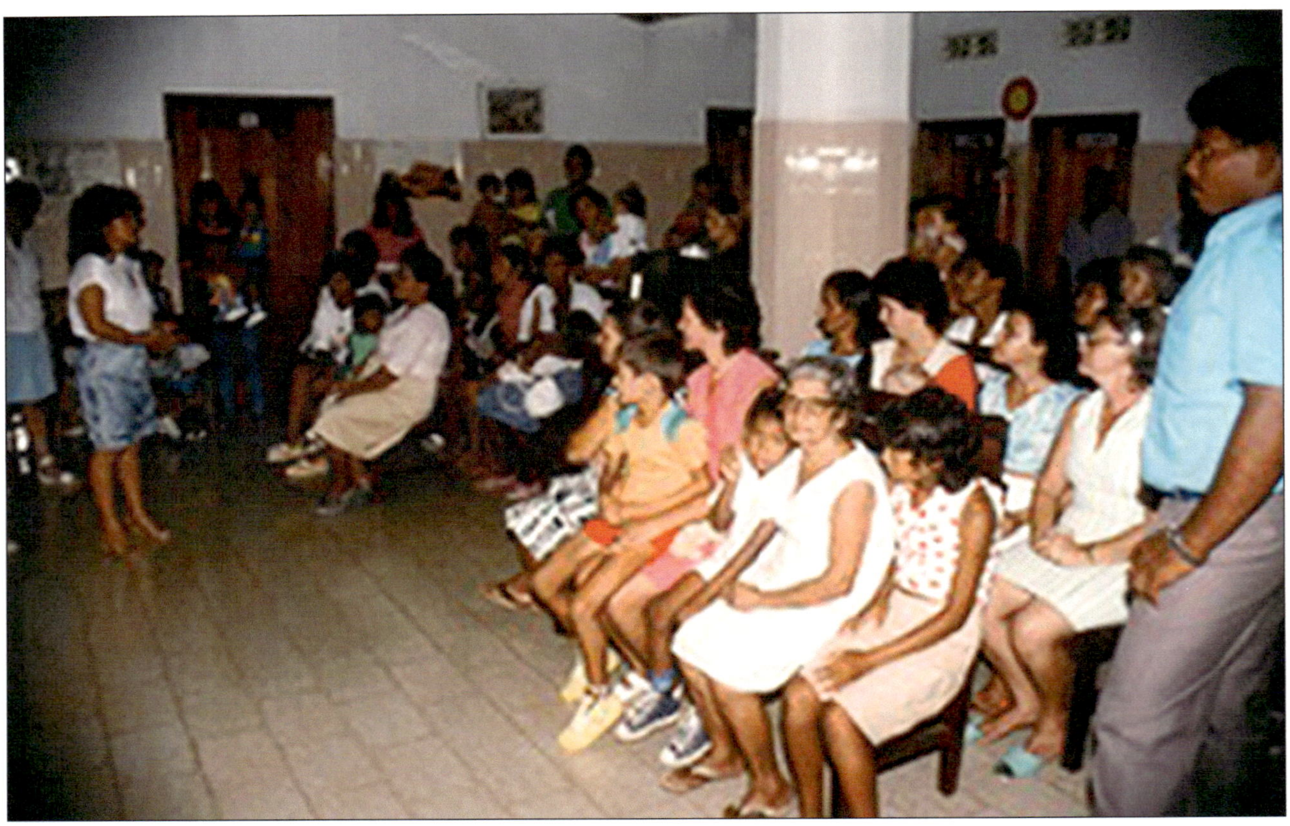

Patients waiting to be screened for surgery

Father Luke died tragically in a motorcycle accident in 1978, but his legacy lived on and thrived in the form of Esperanza. By the time of my first arrival, it was vibrant, efficient organization. They had a full-time Public Health Director, a general surgeon, and 2 local family physicians who treated patients year round. Their goal was not only to administer to the sick but also to improve the health of the community of Santarem and the outlying rural villages. They instituted projects to improve sanitation by proper waste disposal and stressing the importance of clean water. They also instituted a "barefoot doctor" program, which trained individuals from their local communities to diagnose and treat common conditions, like diarrhea and upper-respiratory conditions, which were responsible for a high rate of infant mortality in the region. To lend credibility to these "doctors," they were able to send patients to the hospital ship for treatment of conditions they were unable to manage. These were usually surgical problems that would otherwise go untreated. The most common orthopedic condition we encountered was the untreated clubfoot, although other maladies such as neglected infections, malunited fractures, unreduced dislocations, and polio residuals were also seen.

Their goal was not only to administer to the sick but also to improve the health of the community of Santarem and the outlying rural villages.

Post surgery, the patients remained on the boat for 1–3 days, depending on the procedure they had undergone. The children usually slept in hammocks with their mother, while the adults were in bunks in recovery rooms.

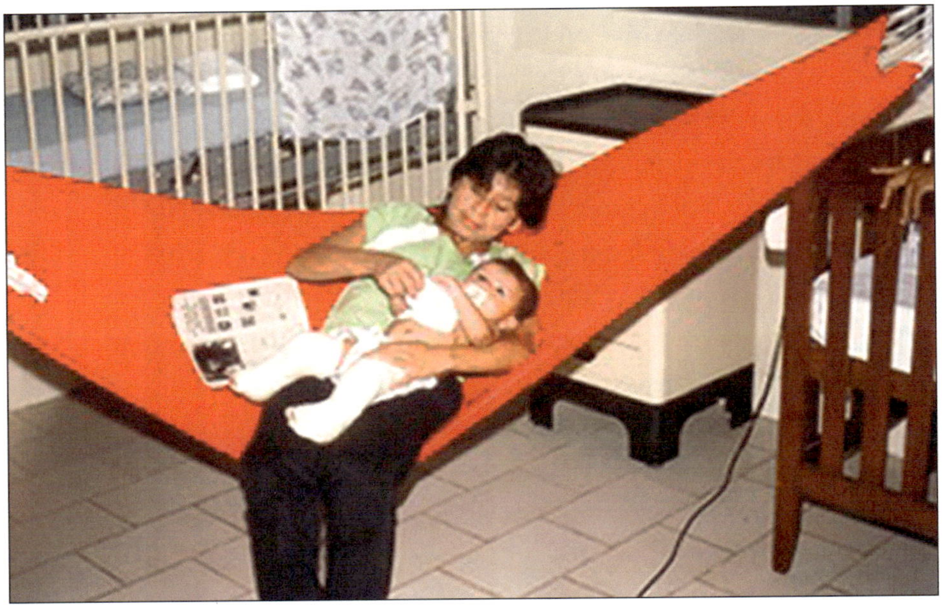

Cramped, hot, post-surgery rooms on the boat.

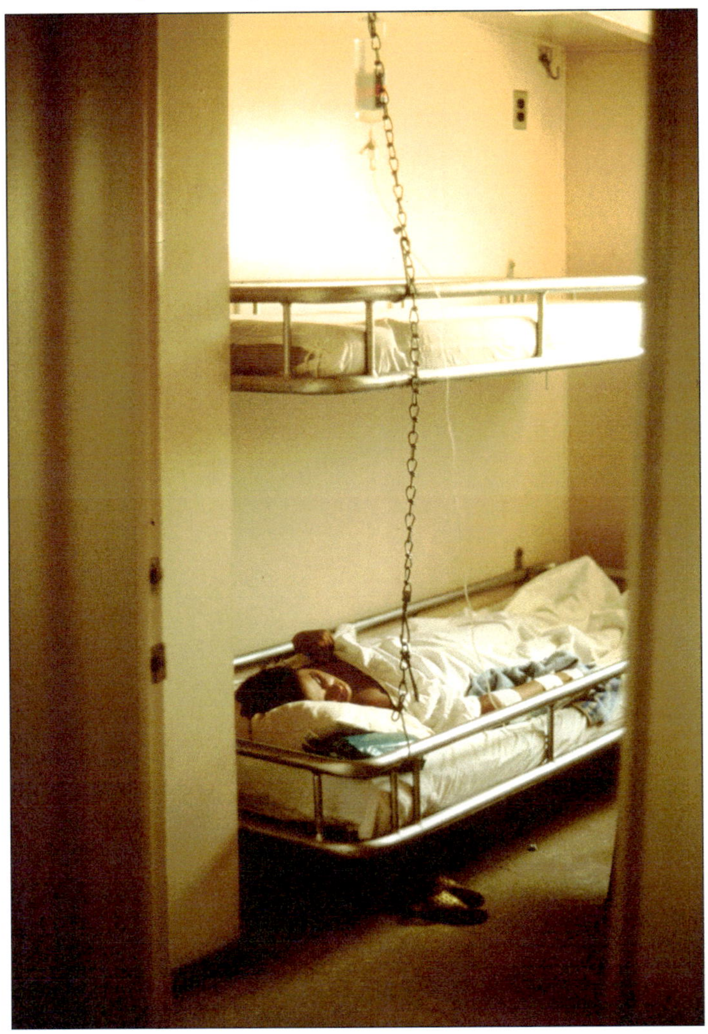

We brought many stuffed animals, balloons, and other toys to give to the children just prior to them entering the operating room. These were received with much enthusiasm and rarely left their sight during their stay.

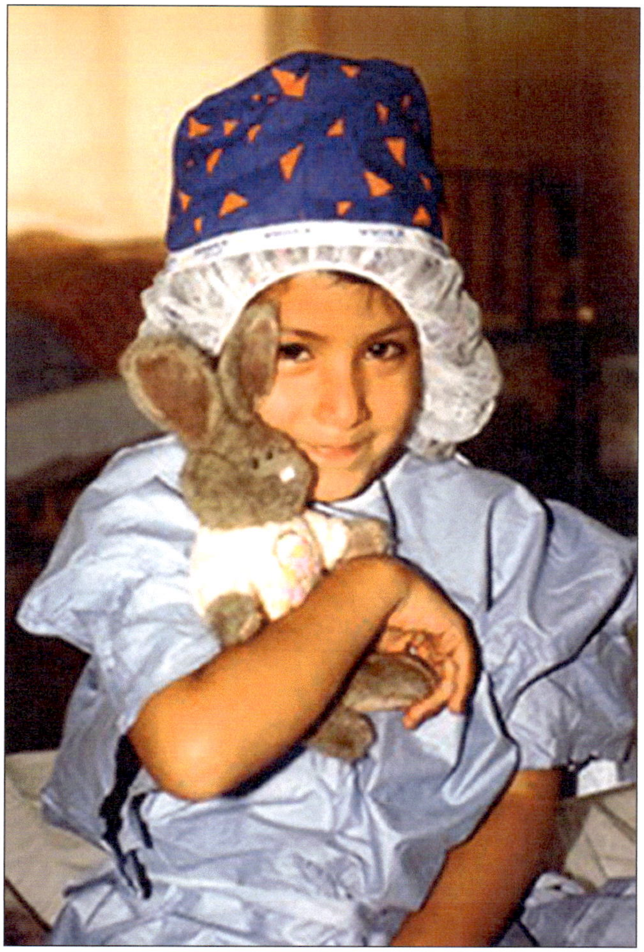

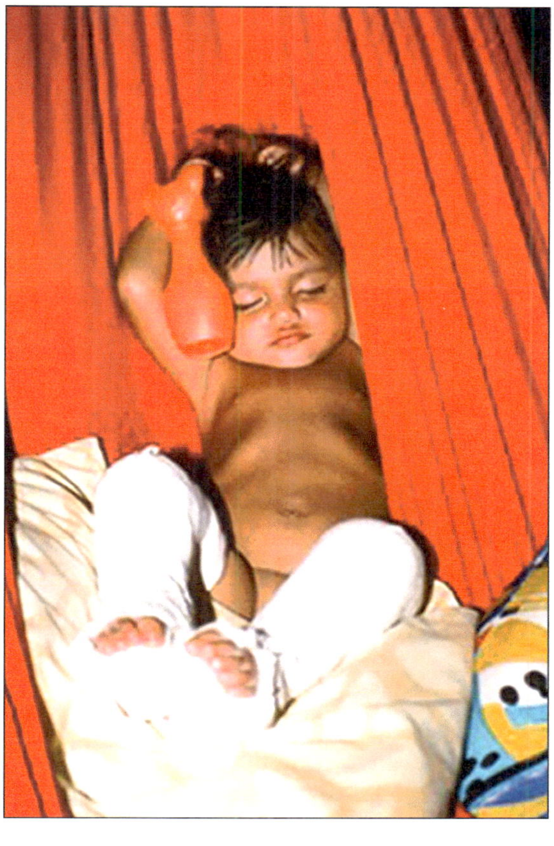

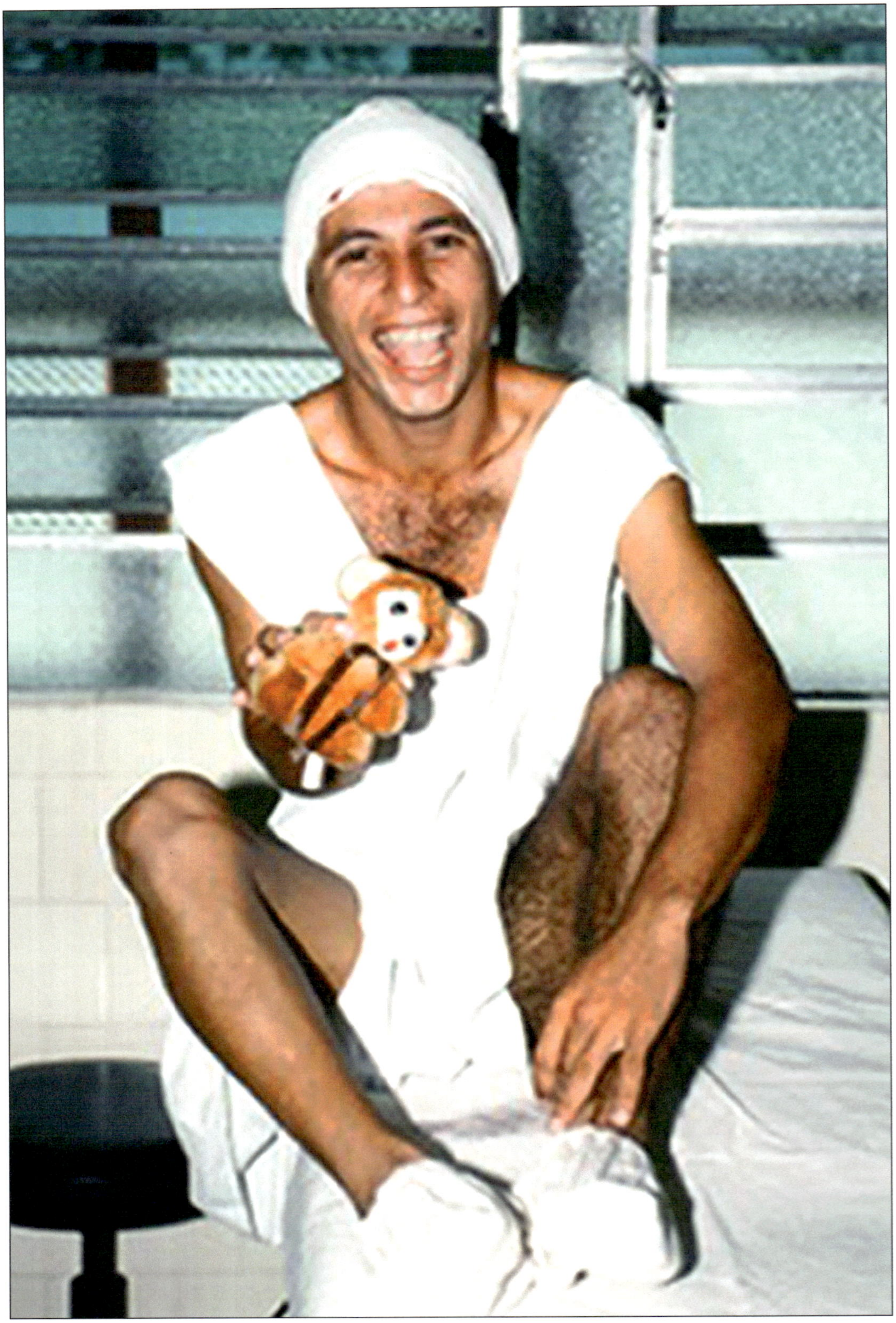

Even big kids loved the toys

An untreated clubfoot is a particularly cruel deformity in the Third World and a condition we almost never see in the United States, as most of these are treated at birth and corrected in the first few months of life, long before weight bearing is begun. If untreated, these individuals have severe limitations with ambulation as they walk on the outside of the foot, with the bottom portion being turned inward and sideways. This is a devastating deformity in an agrarian culture, as these individuals are unable to stand, walk, or work in the fields for hours at a time. We would operate on 4 or 5 of these deformities per day.

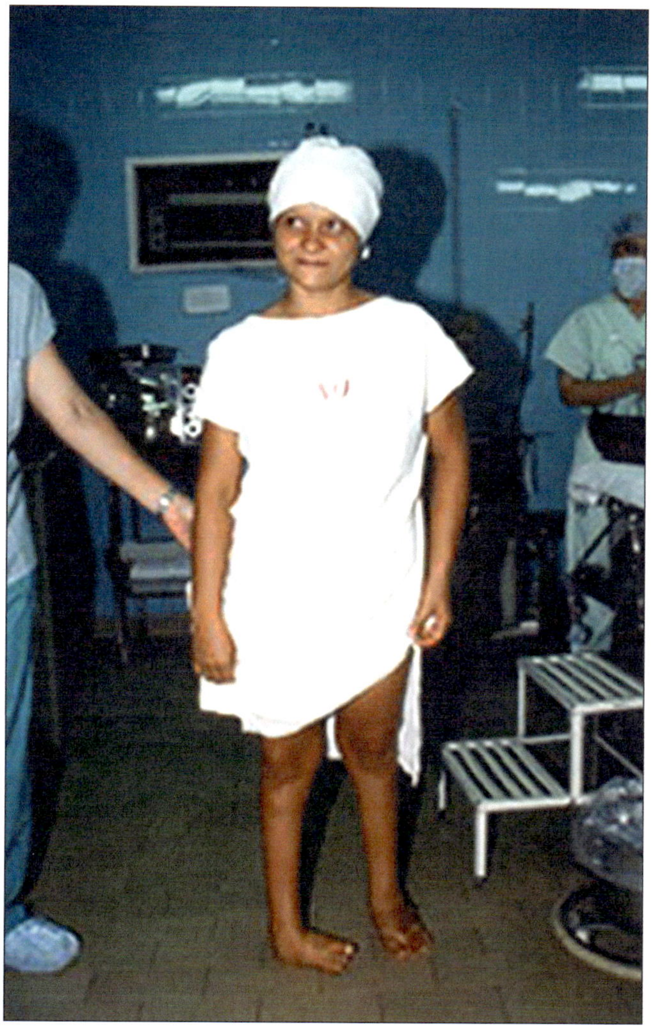

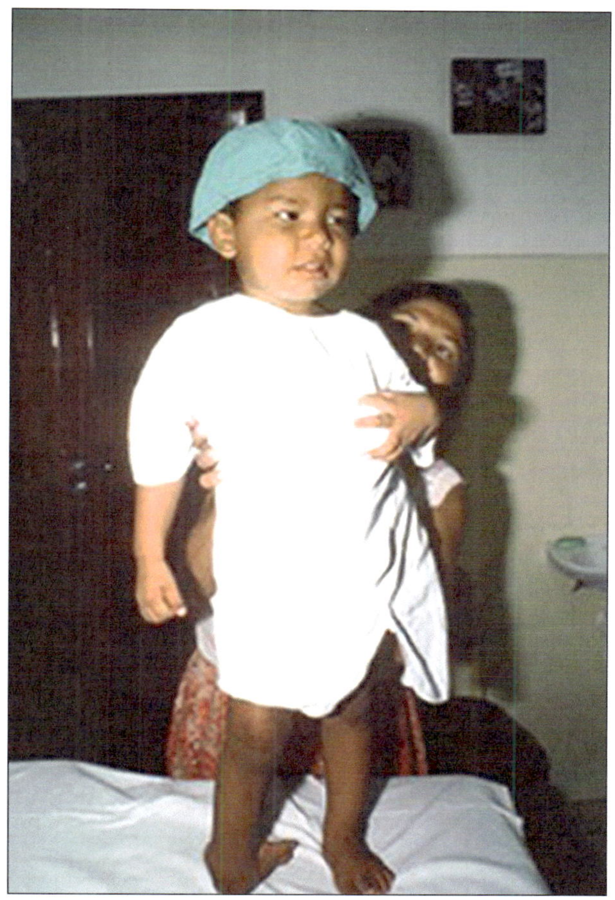

Today a relatively new casting technique, developed by Dr. Ignacio Ponsetti of the University of Iowa, is able to correct the vast majority of these deformities when treated early. There is now a Ponsetti Foundation that is training workers in the developing countries to cast these children and correct these deformities in their own environments, thus avoiding costly and technically demanding surgery.

During our first trip, we repaired more than 30 clubfeet, treated malunited fractures, removed an untreated bone tumor the size of a grapefruit from the knee region of a young woman, and 2 untreated elbow dislocations, which I had never encountered in the US, plus residual polio foot deformities. The work was exhausting and yet exhilarating, operating 10–12 hours per day. The gratitude and relief of the families was very rewarding.

Some examples of the patients we encountered during our visits:

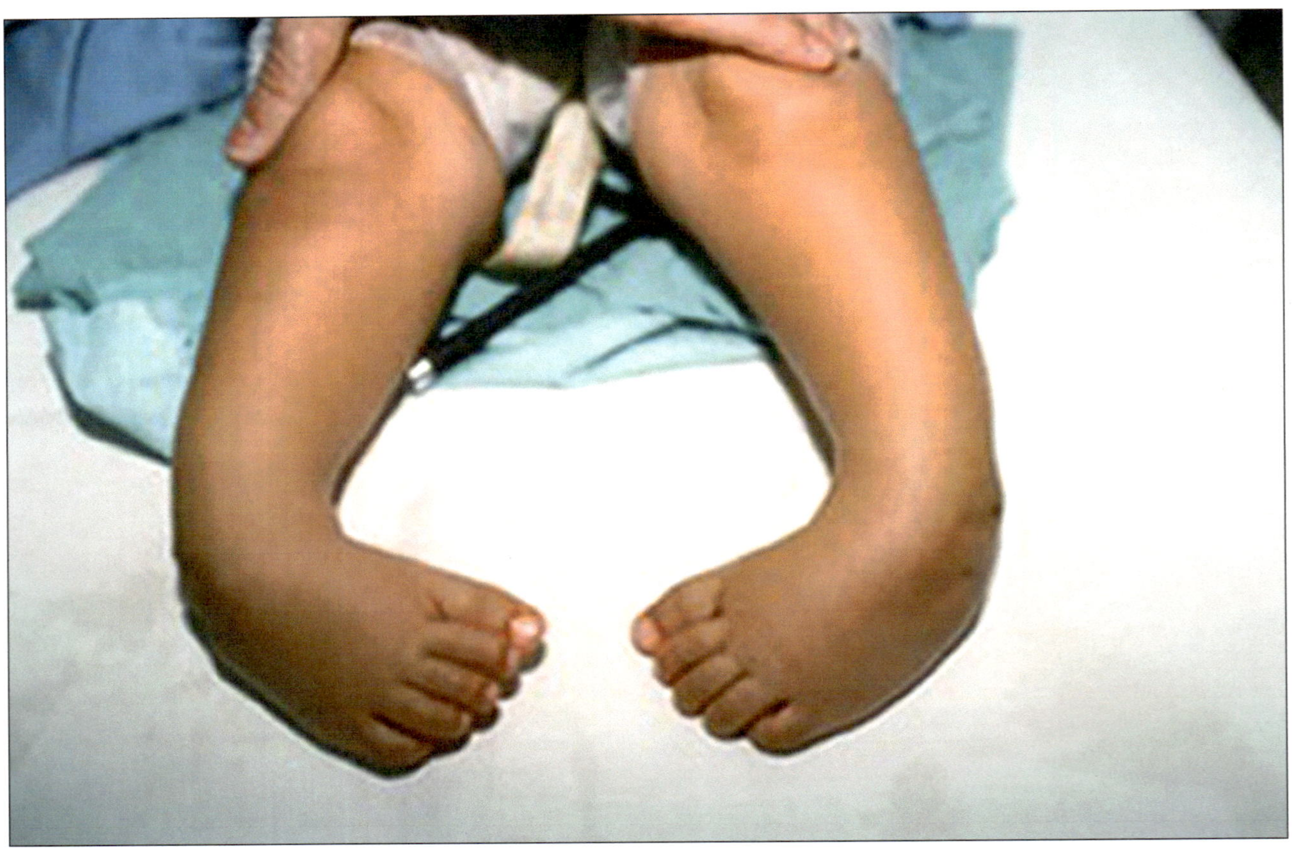

Pre-operative child with bilateral club feet

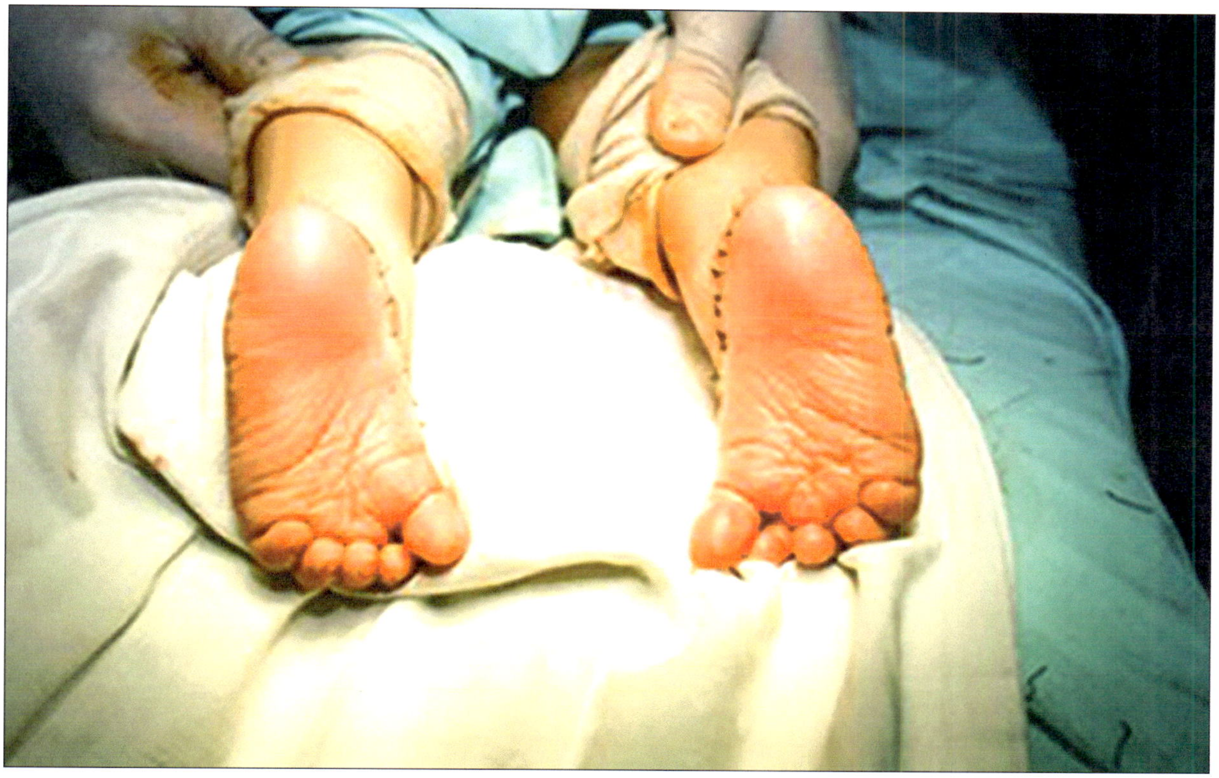

Post-op repair

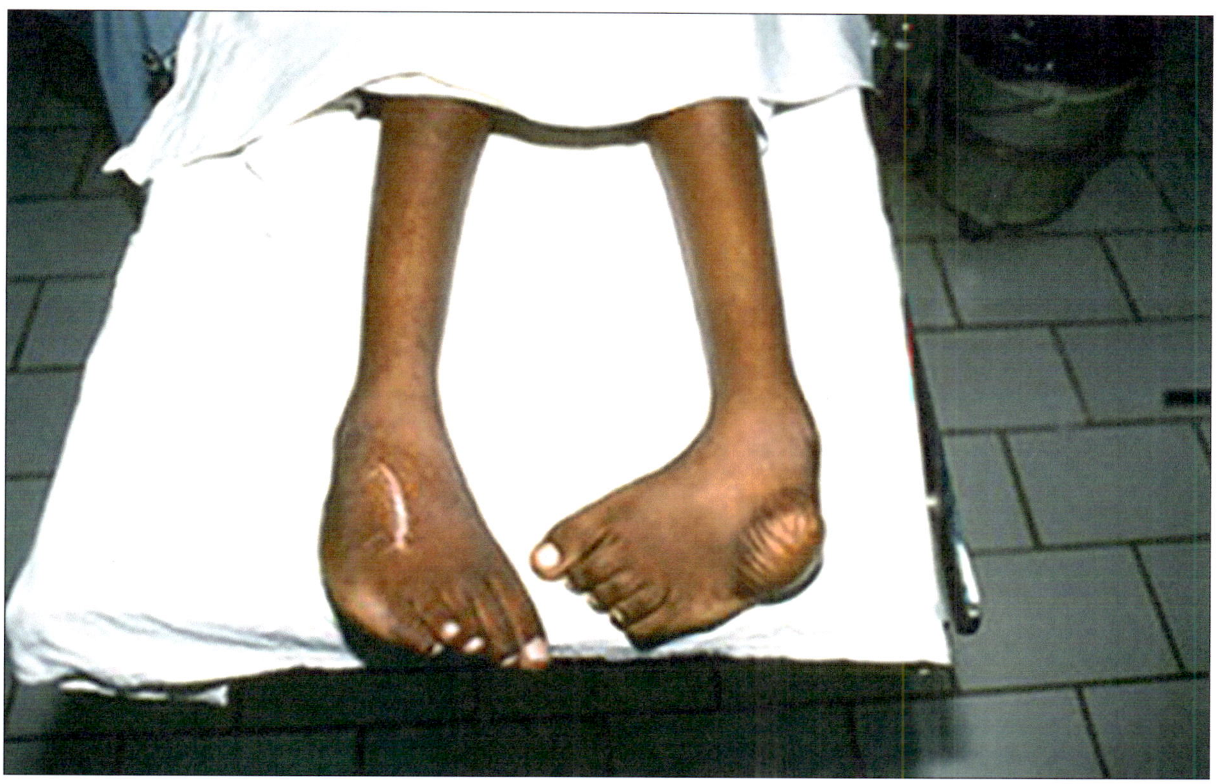

13-year-old with clubfoot

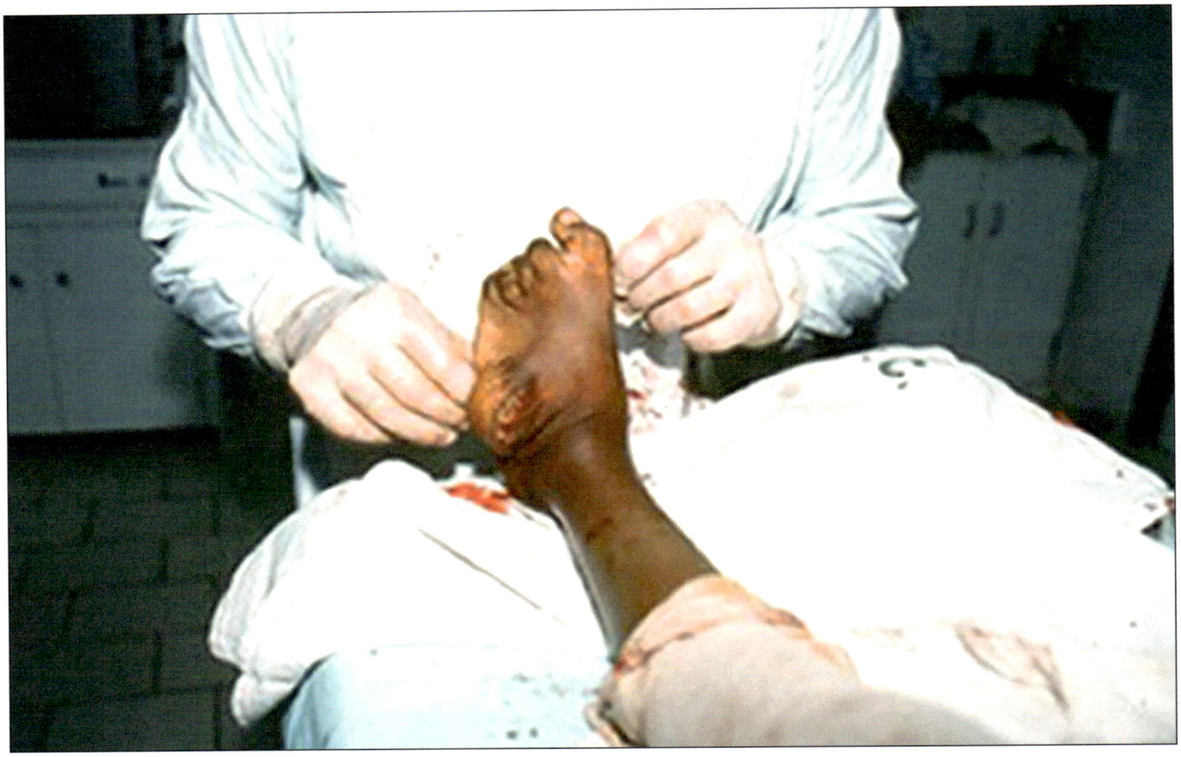

Post-op

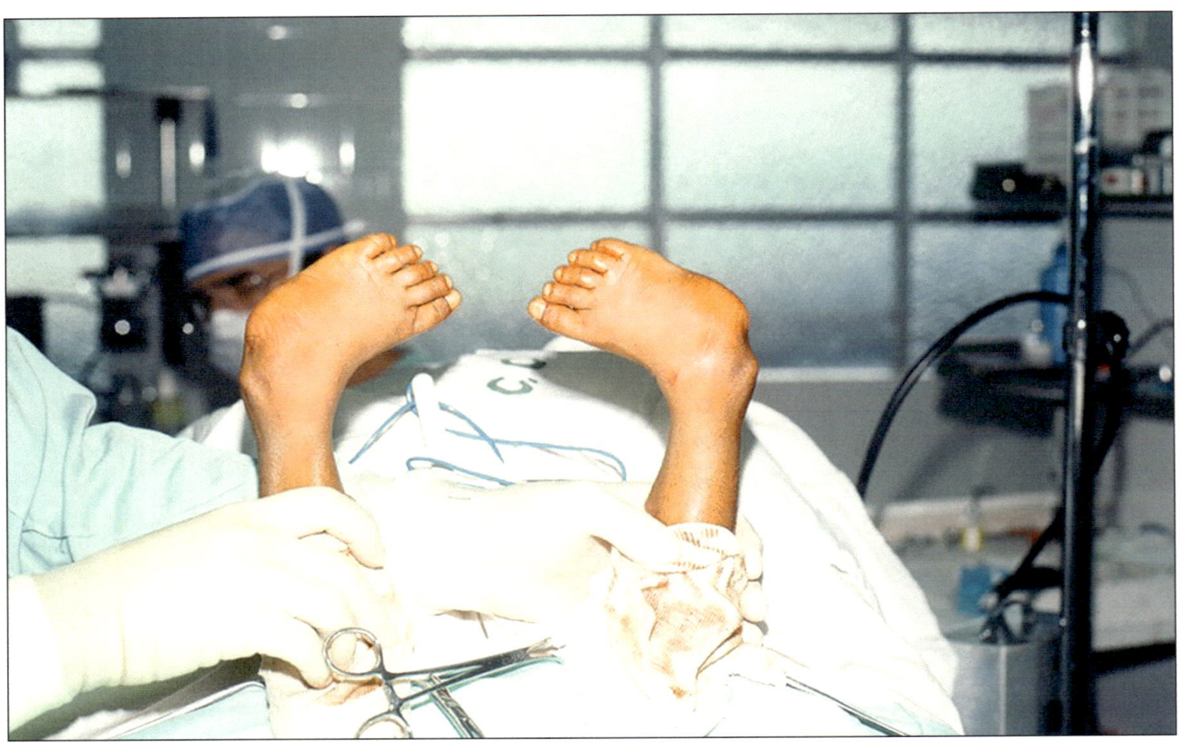

Adolescent young girl with uncorrected club feet. She was walking on the large masses seen on the outside of her feet.

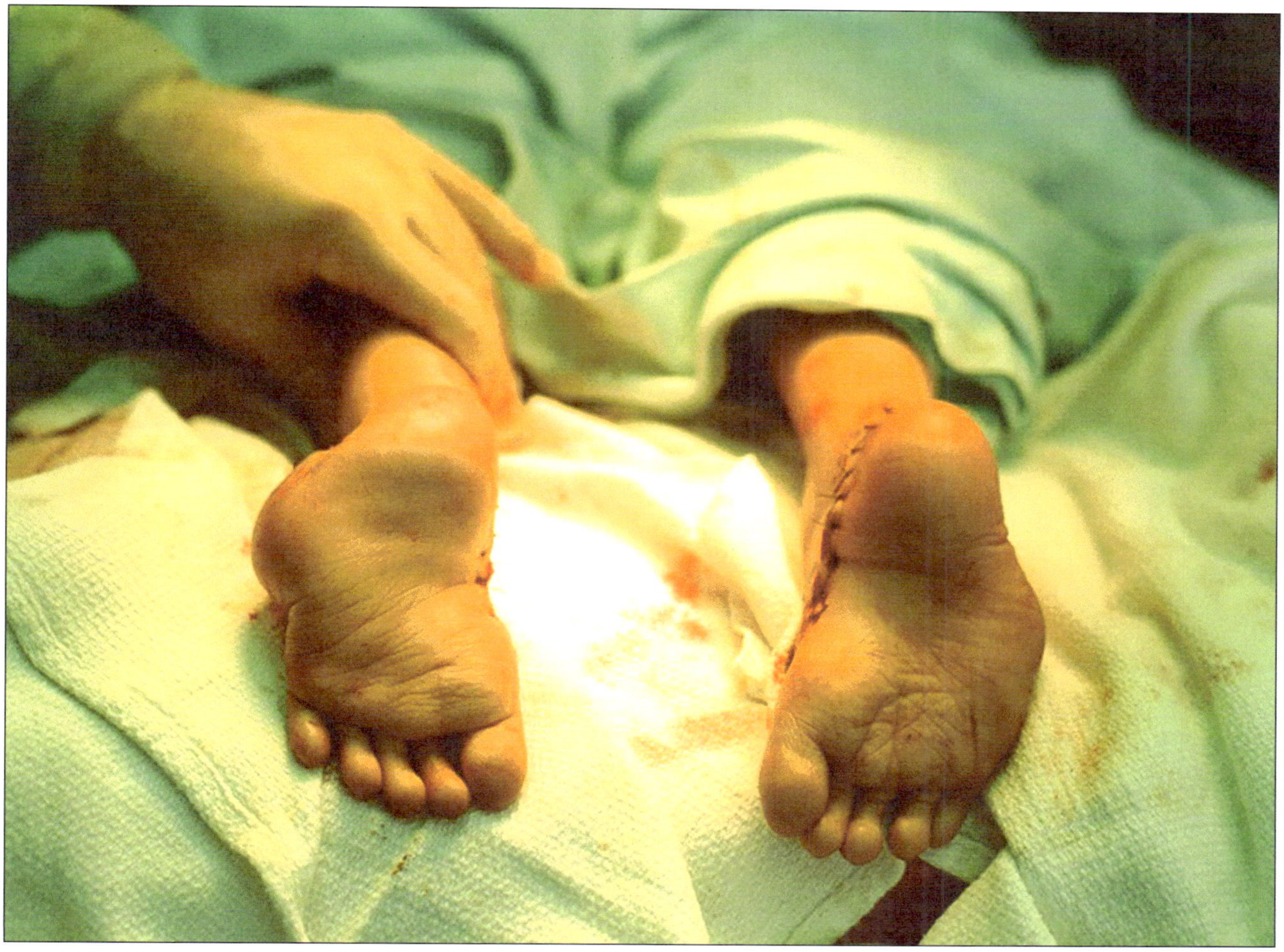

After surgical correction.

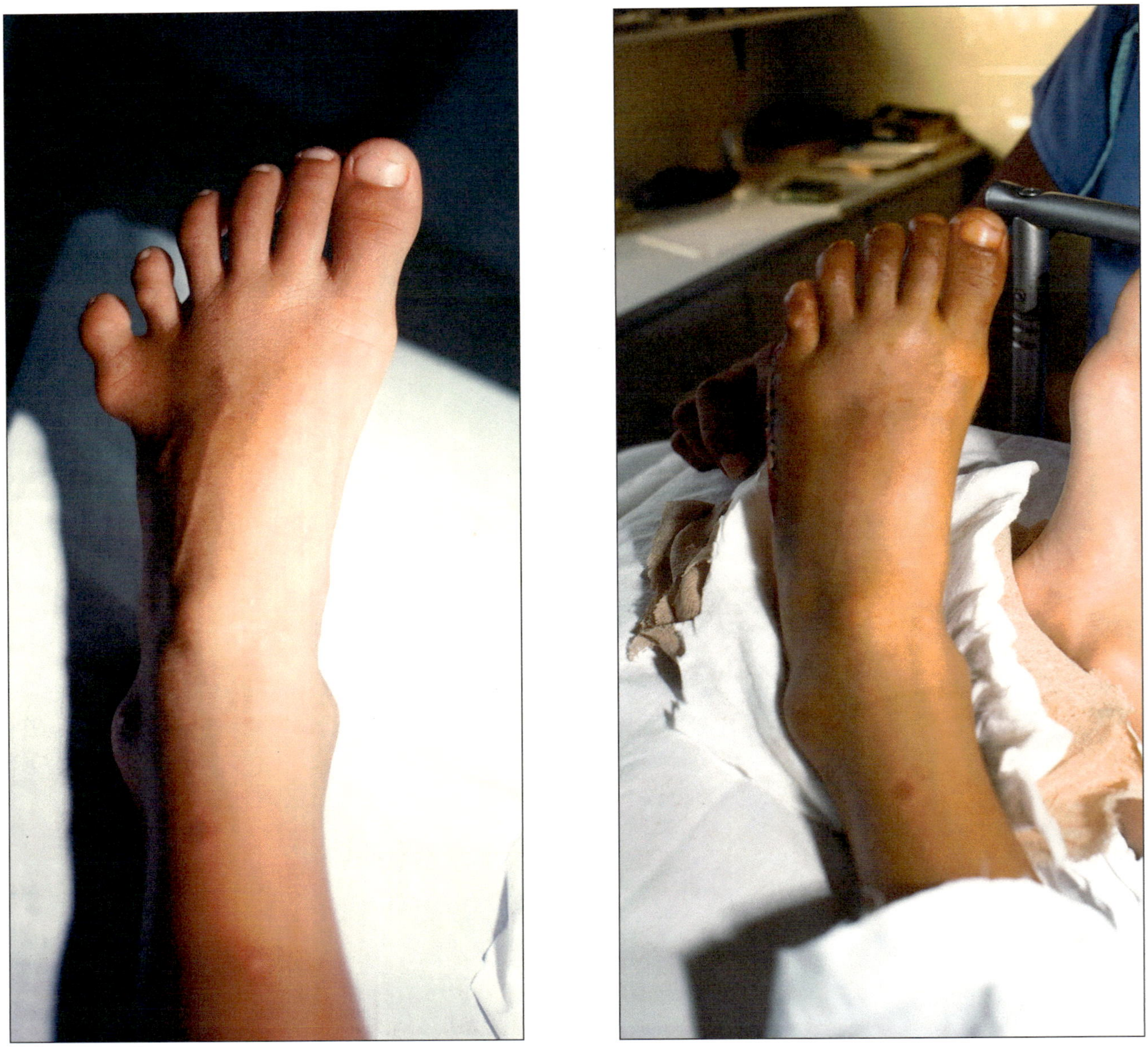

15 year old with extra 5th toe, before and after surgery

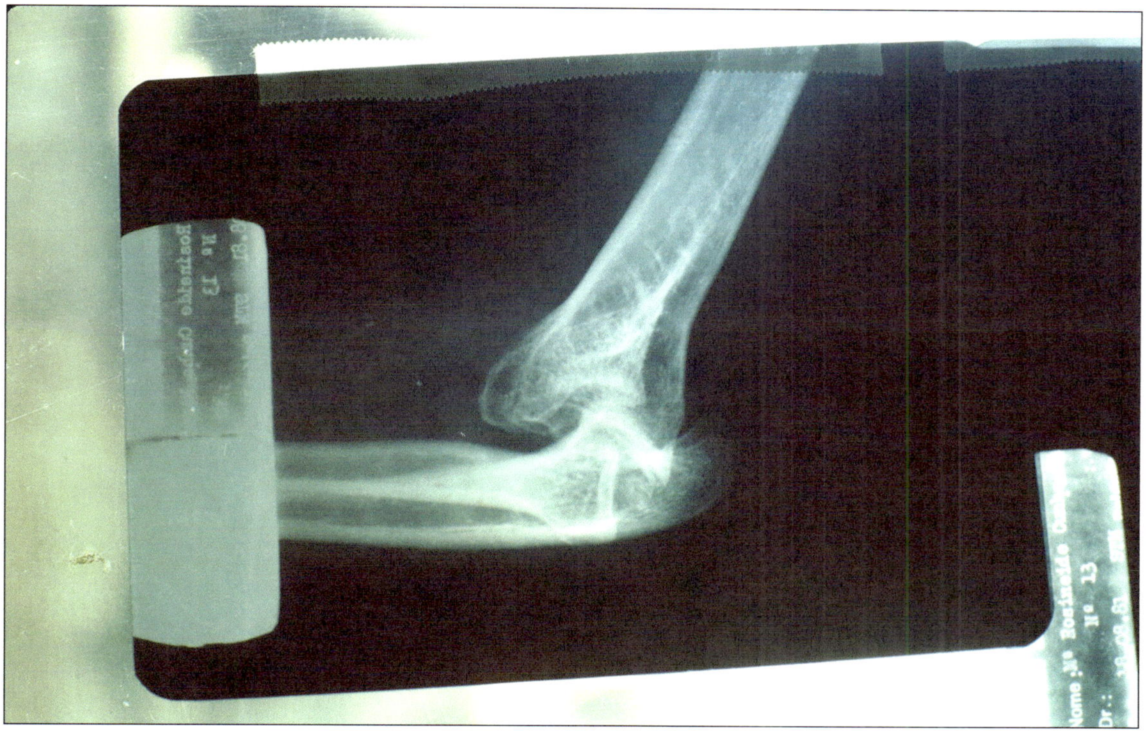

X-ray of 16 year old female with unreduced elbow dislocation and inability to bend elbow more than 90 degrees

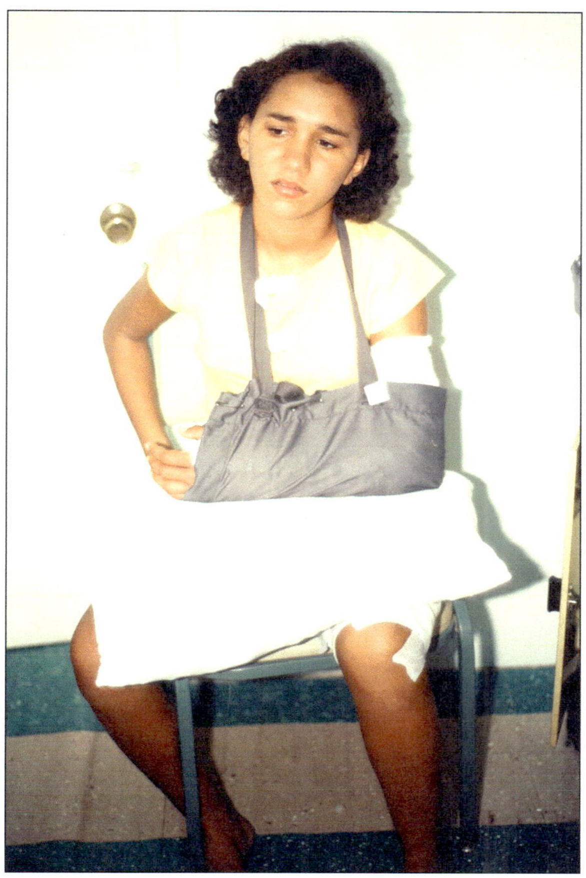

Post-op

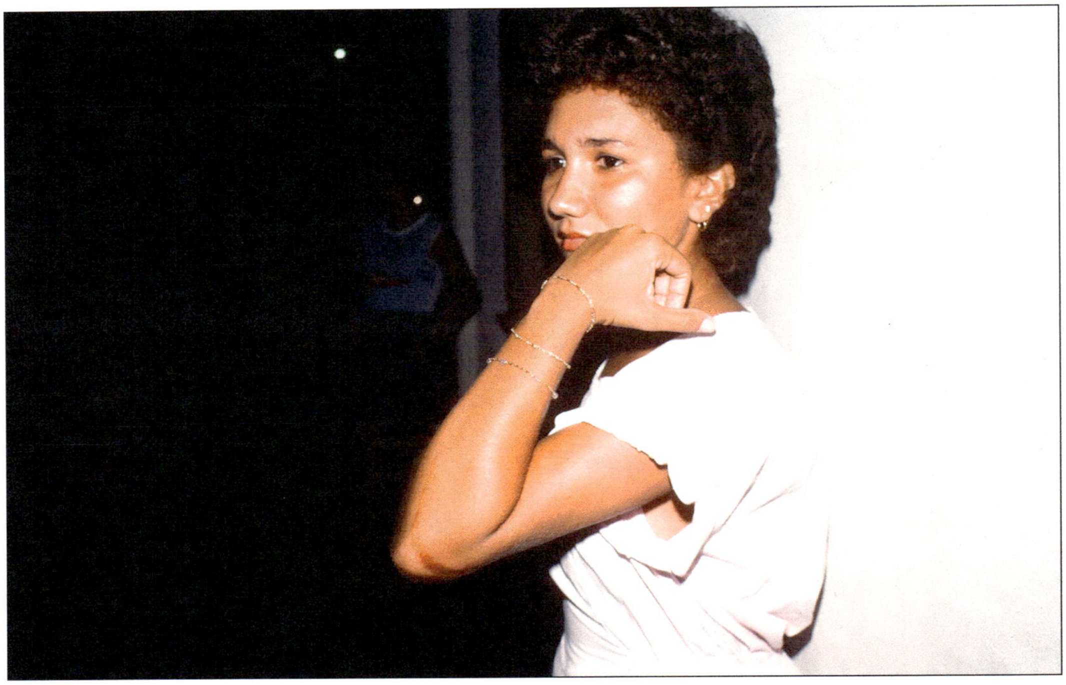

5 years later working as nursing assistance with full motion in elbow

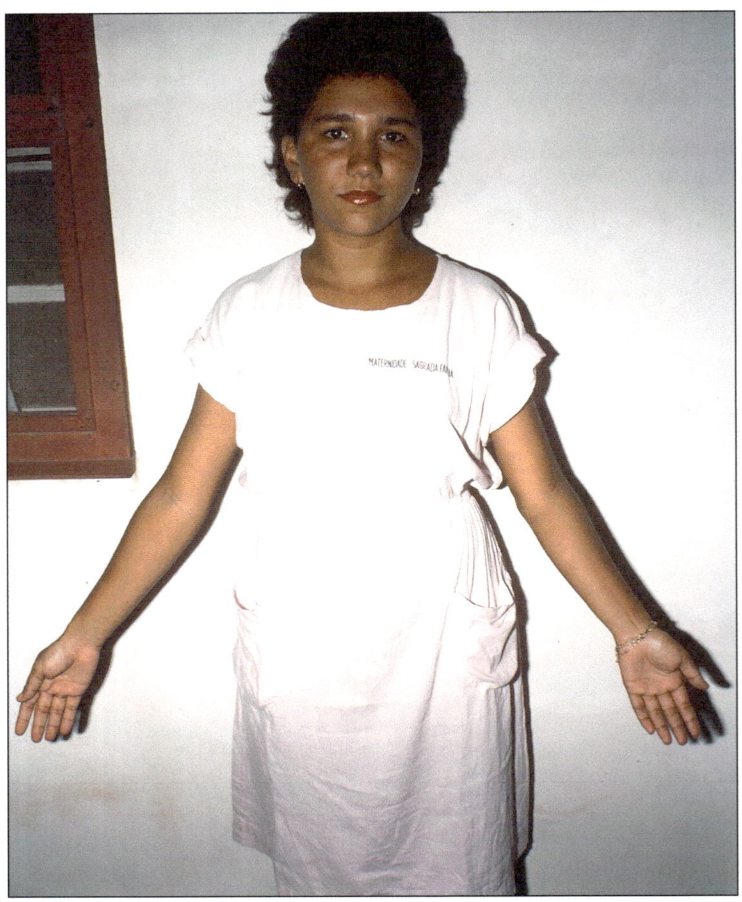

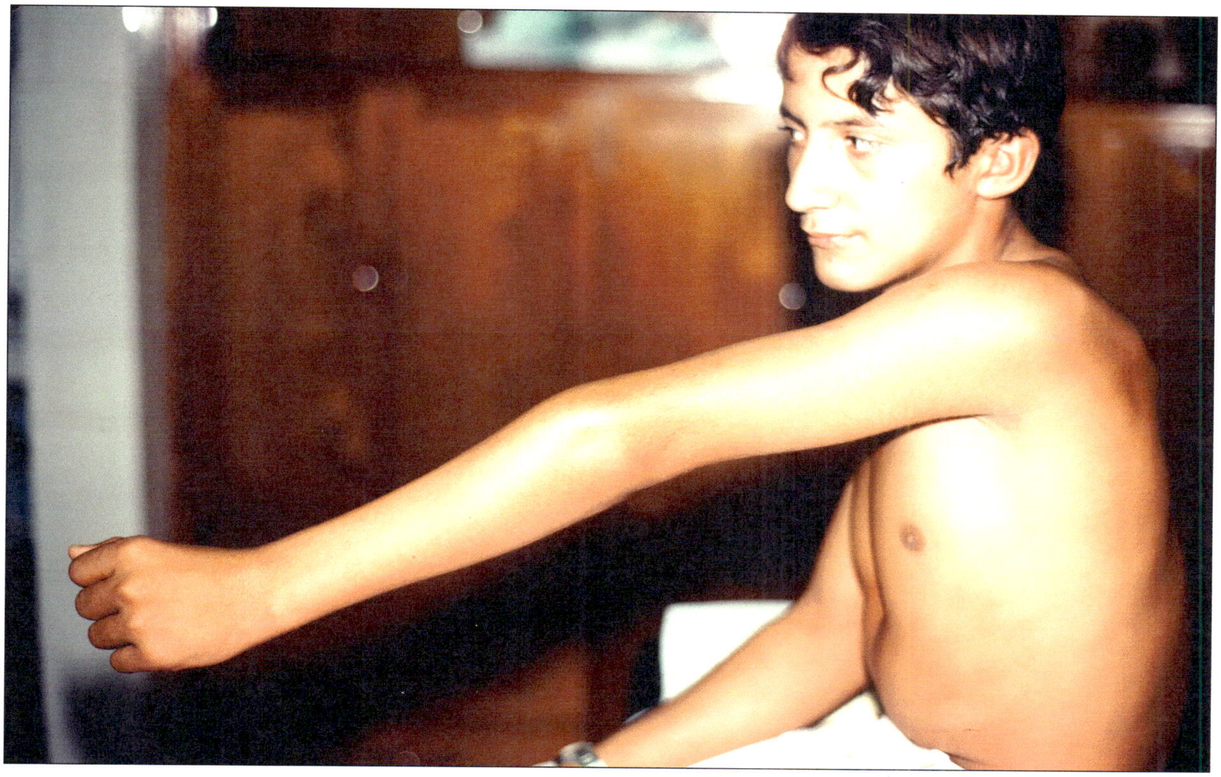

Teenager with unreduced elbow dislocation and no movement at elbow

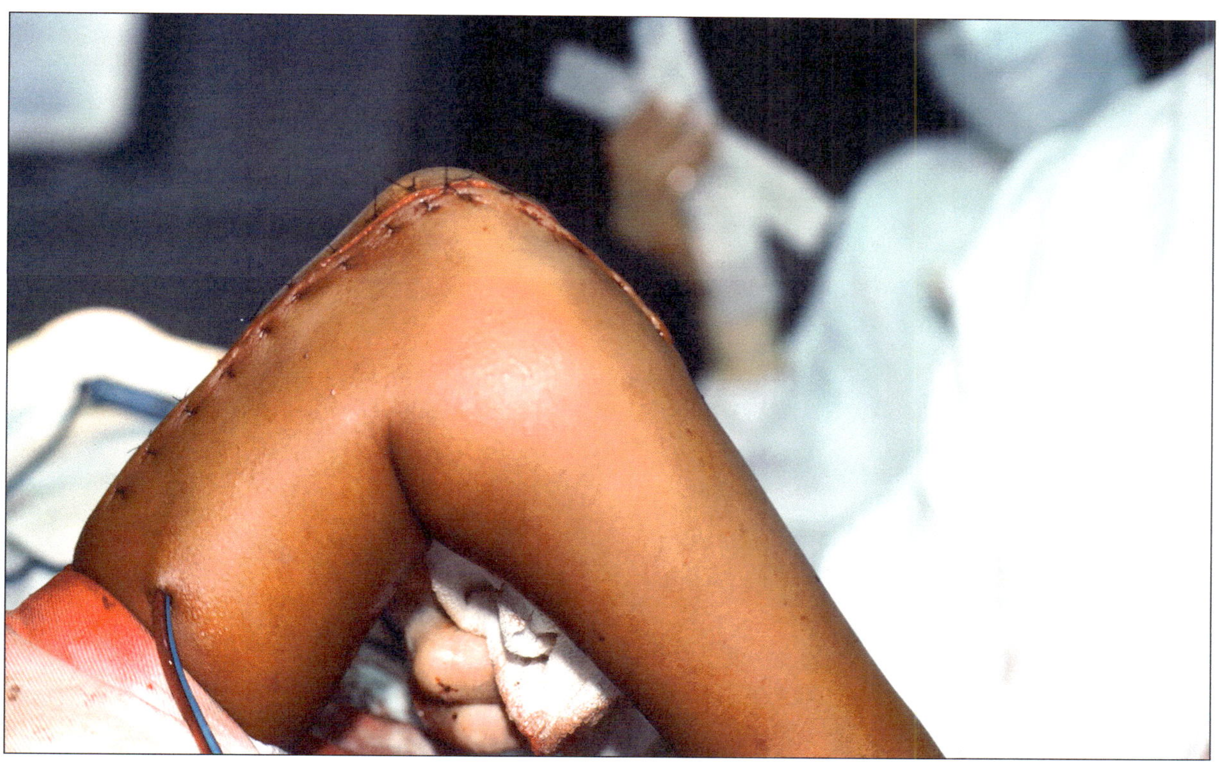

After surgery

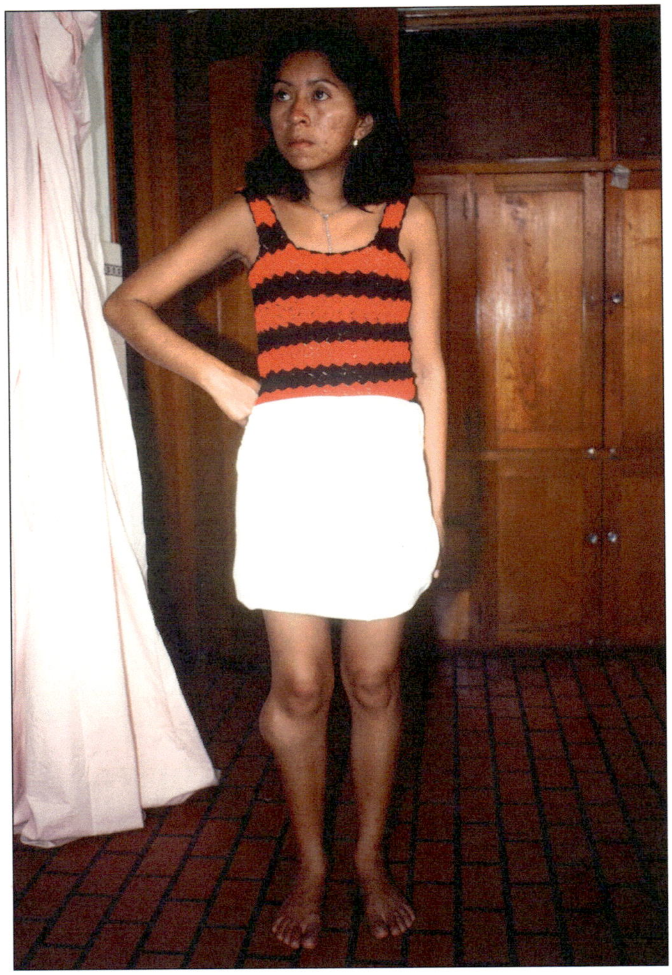

Young girl with large bone mass near right knee

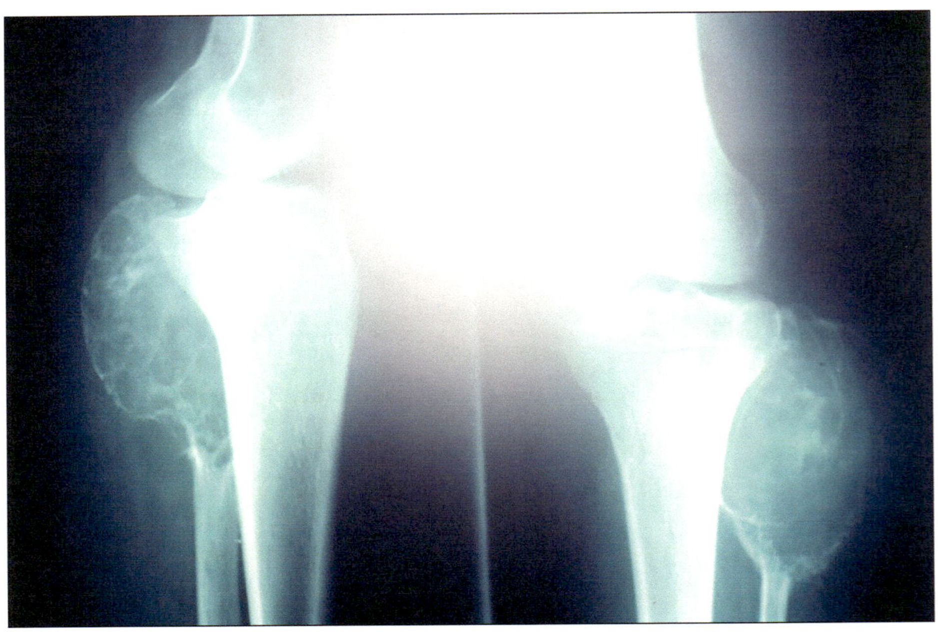

X-ray of mass at head of fibula

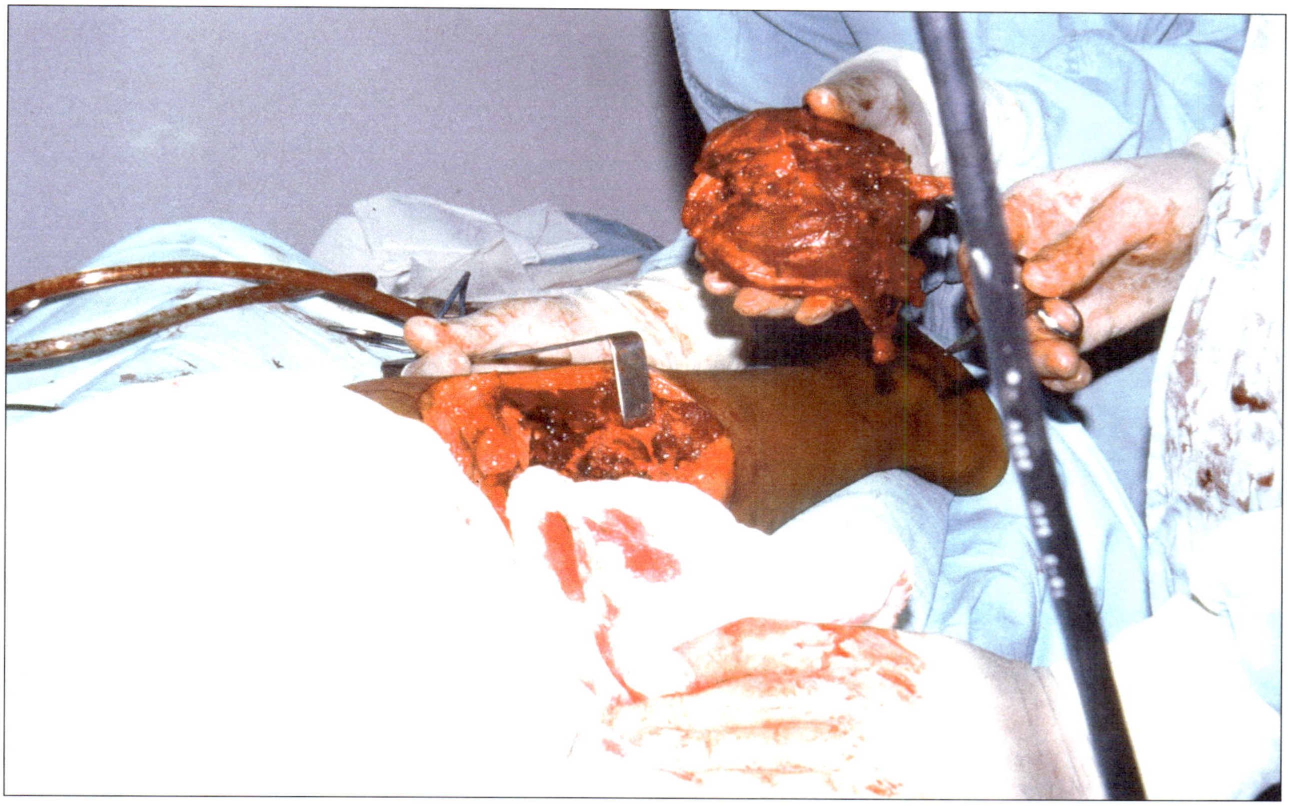

Mass removed at surgery

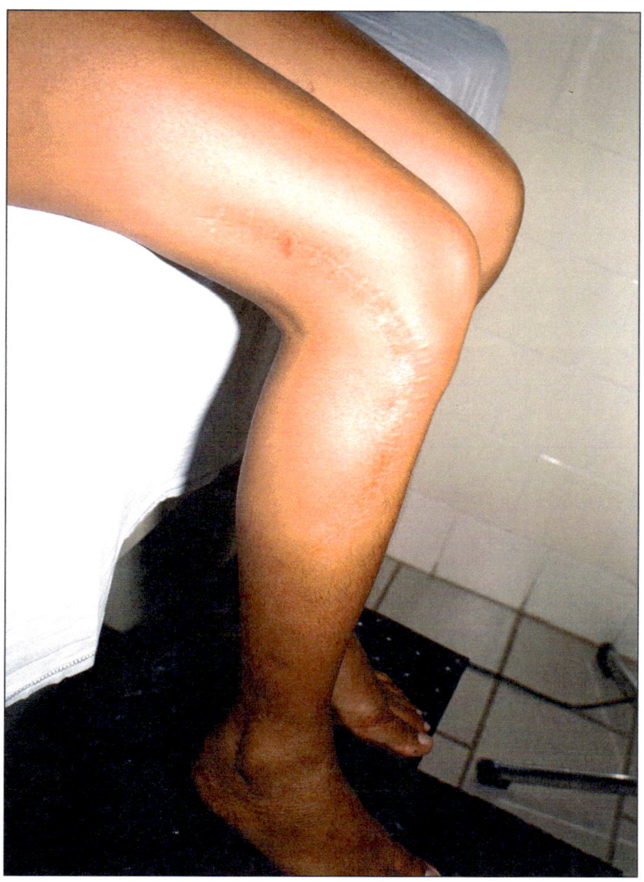

Patient's knee 5 years post removal

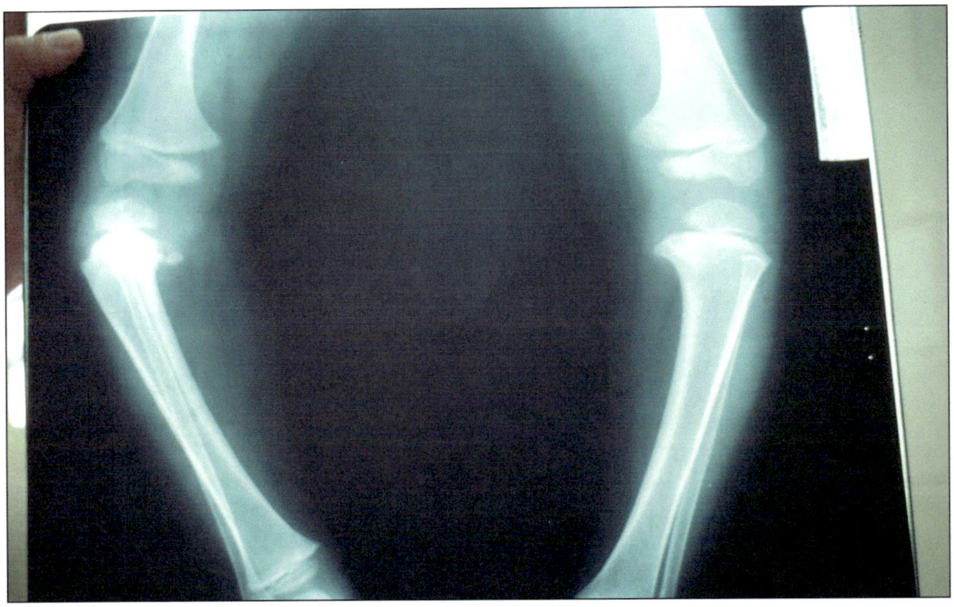

X-ray of toddler with severe bowing of lower legs

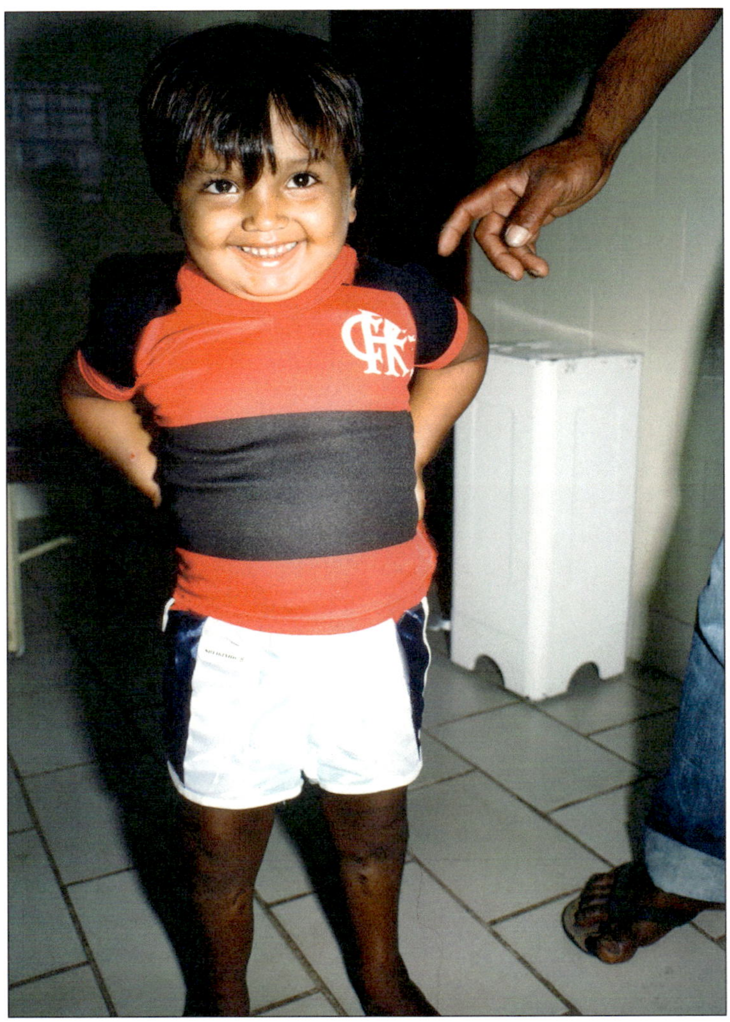

6 months
post correction

Man with malunited fracture of tibia, before and after surgical correct

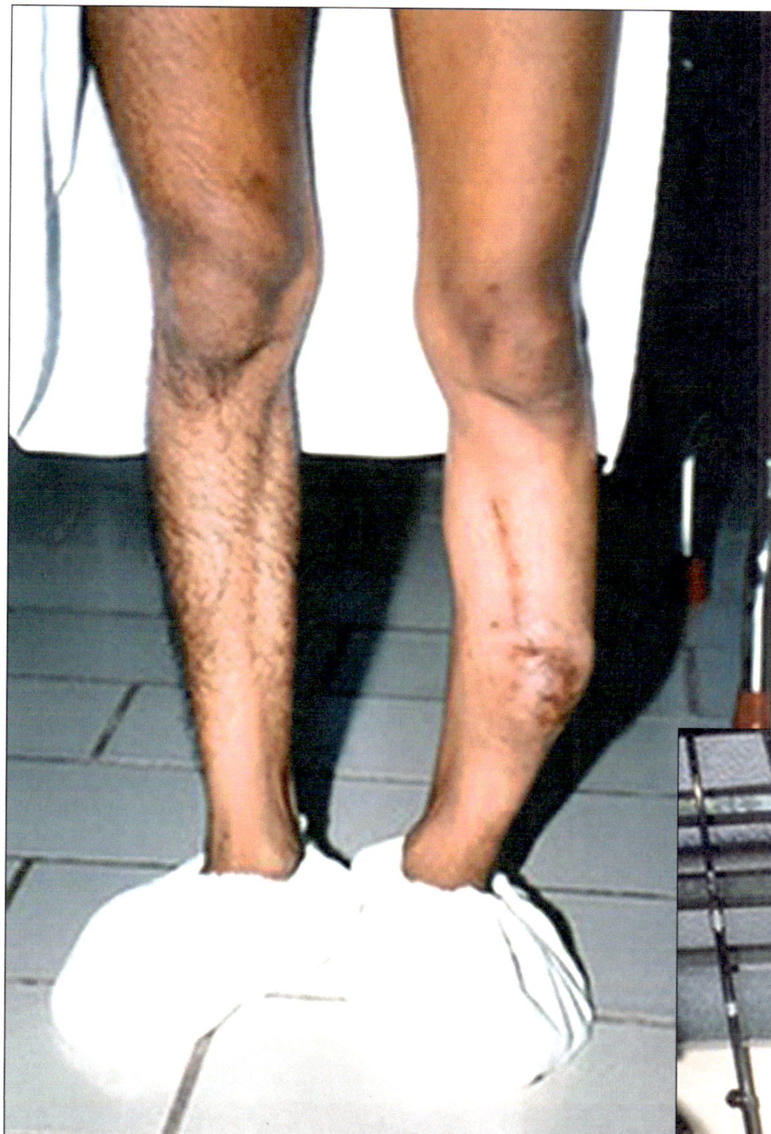

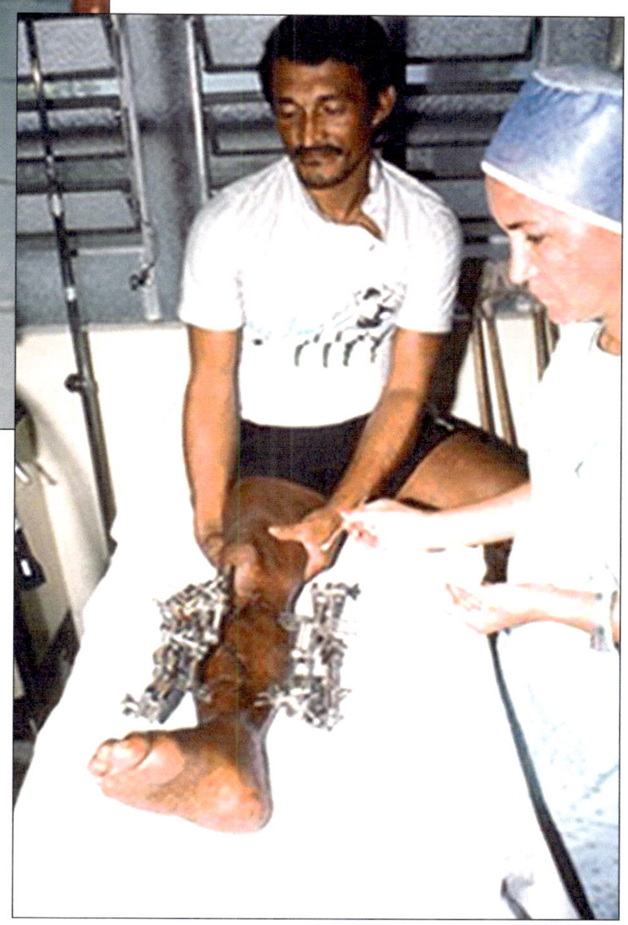

Young girl came to clinic walking on her knees. Had foot surgery 3 months previously, X-ray showed pin protruding onto bottom of her foot. She was given a local anesthetic in the clinic and the pin removed and she walked out.

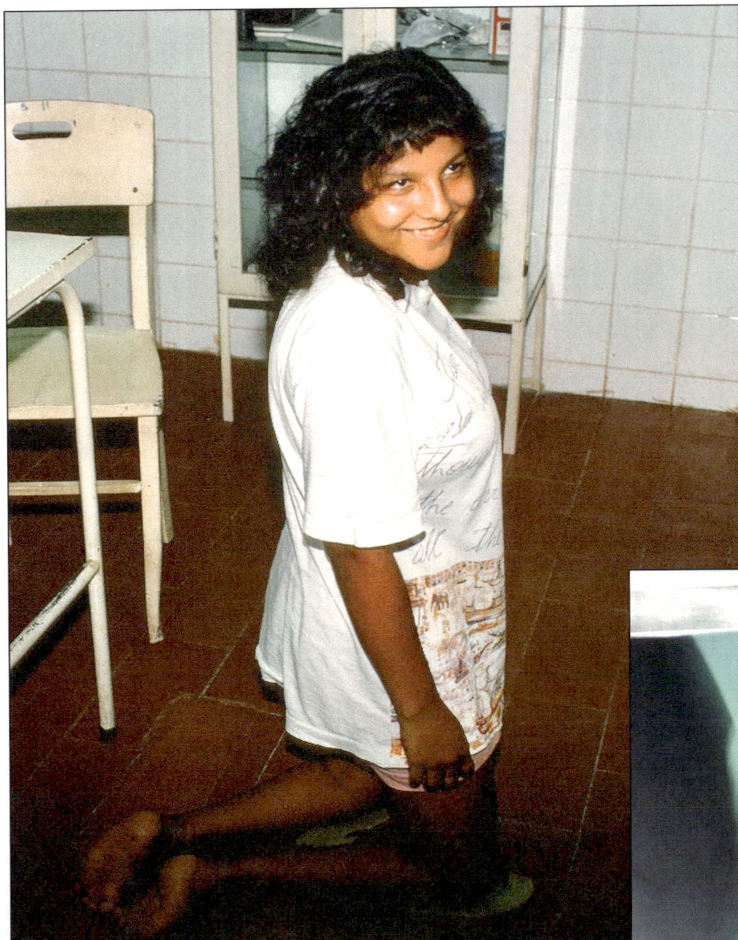

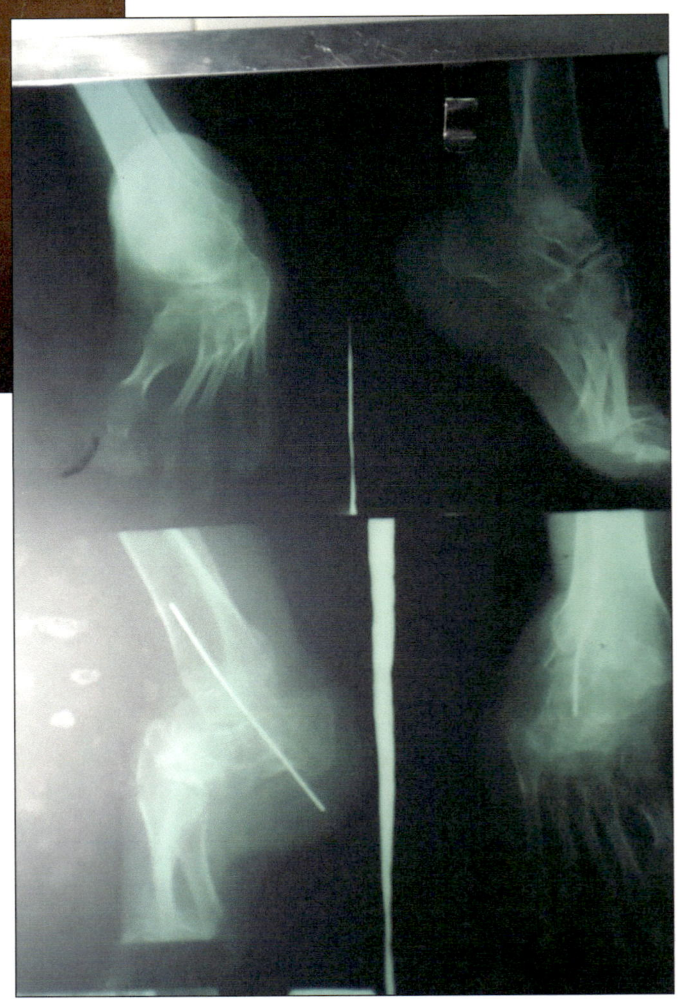

A 16 year old whose father (not in attendance), had told the mother to not allow surgery for fear he would die. After surgery when the mother was brought to see the boy in recovery, she began sobbing, not only because he had survived, but because his foot deformity had been corrected.

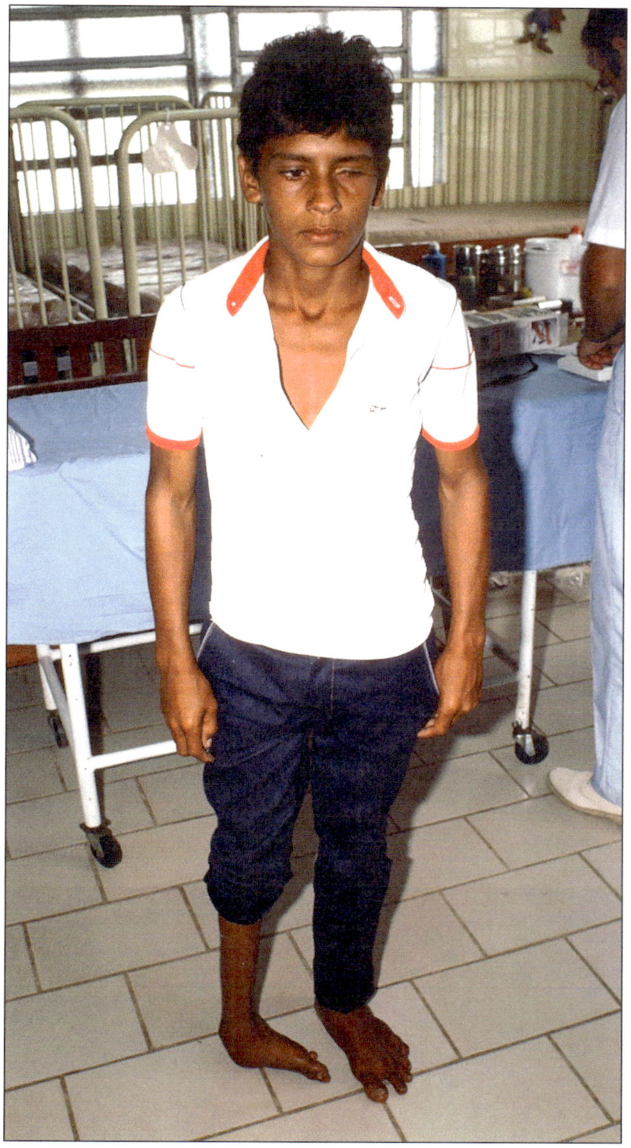

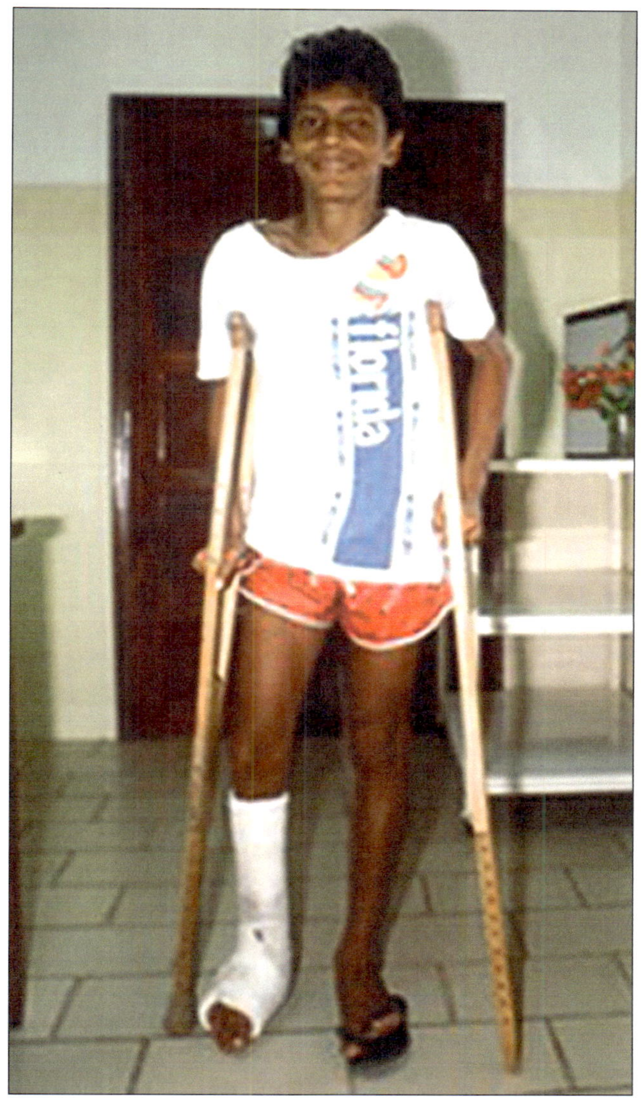

Post-op

On weekends we would on occasion travel up the Tapijos River to a small community called Alter do Chau where there was a pleasant white sand beach, ideal for picnicking and swimming. The Tapijos waters were warm so swimming was enjoyable. On one of these journeys we encountered a young boy walking on the beach on his tip toes on his left foot. I examined him and determined he had a tight Achilles Tendon. After speaking with his mother we brought him back to Santarem and the following day did an Achilles lengthening. Below is his picture walking on the beach and at his post-op visit for cast change with his foot in a neutral position.

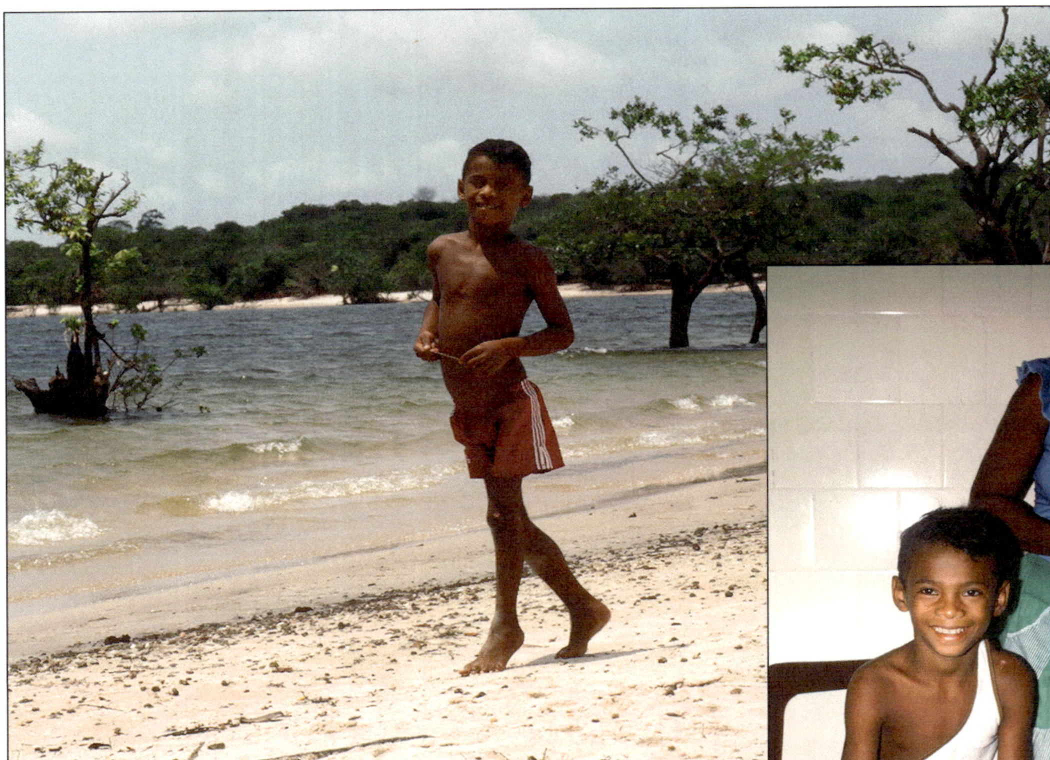

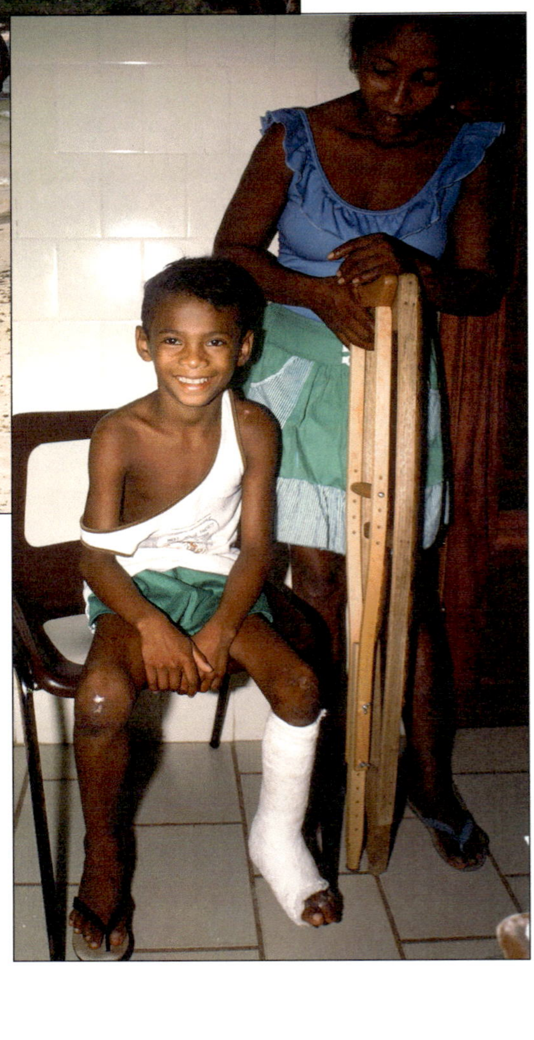

12 year old boy who had fallen some 3 months prior to his visit, with a broken portion of his femur protruding from the skin. His father (who did not accompany him) had forbidden the mother from giving permission for surgery and he thus was turned away as there was no other option for him.

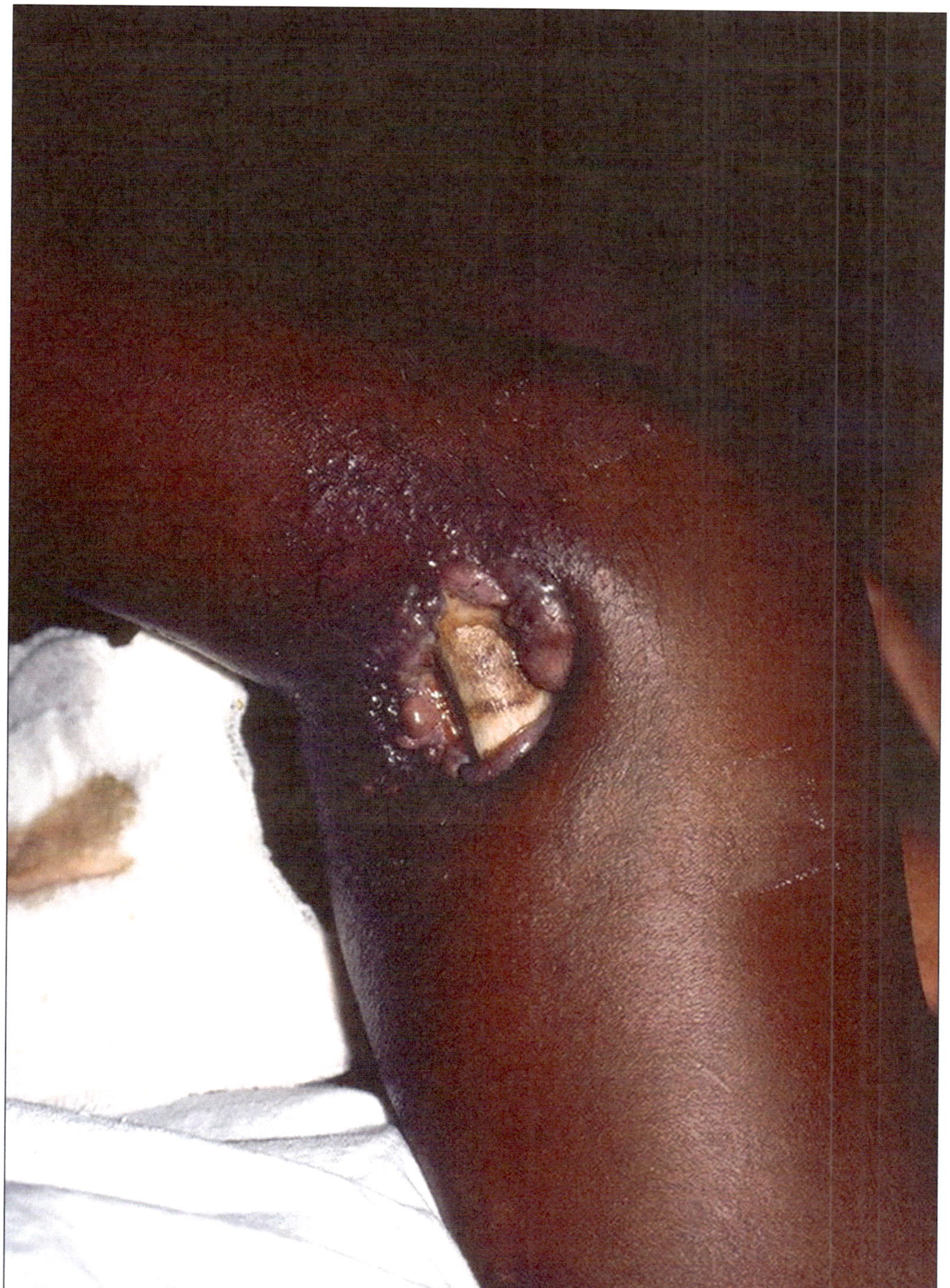

The final 2 days of our trips were devoted to reexamining all of the operative patients, to check their wounds, change dressings and casts and leave written instructions for the remaining post-operative care.

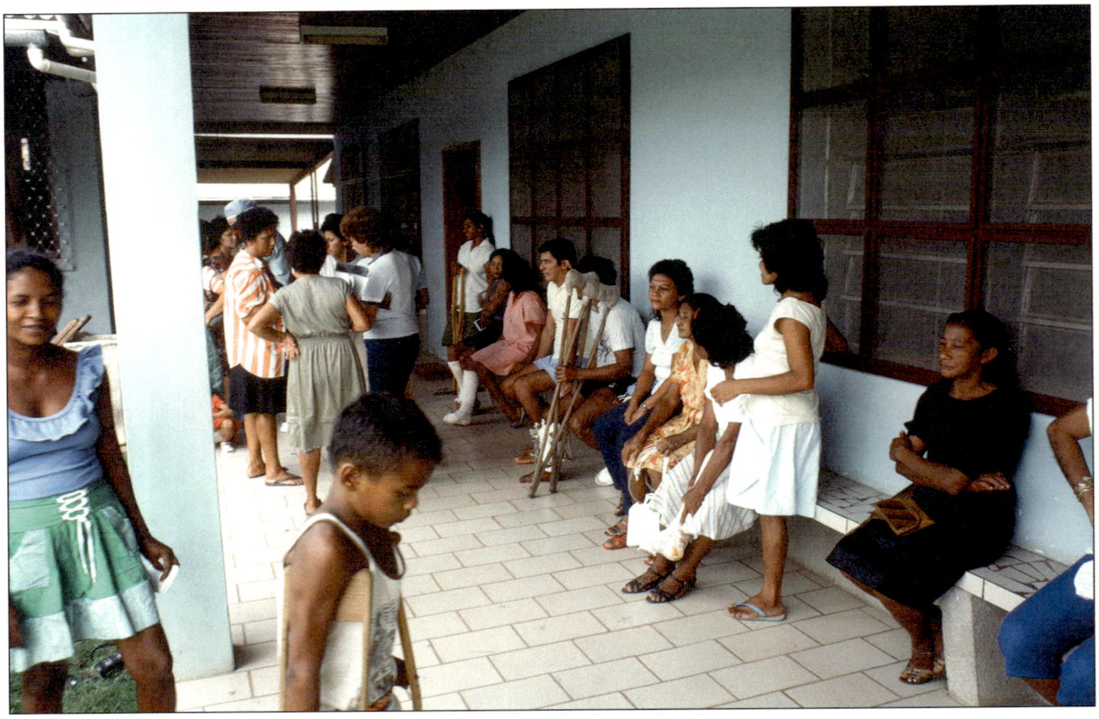

Patients waiting for post-op check and cast change

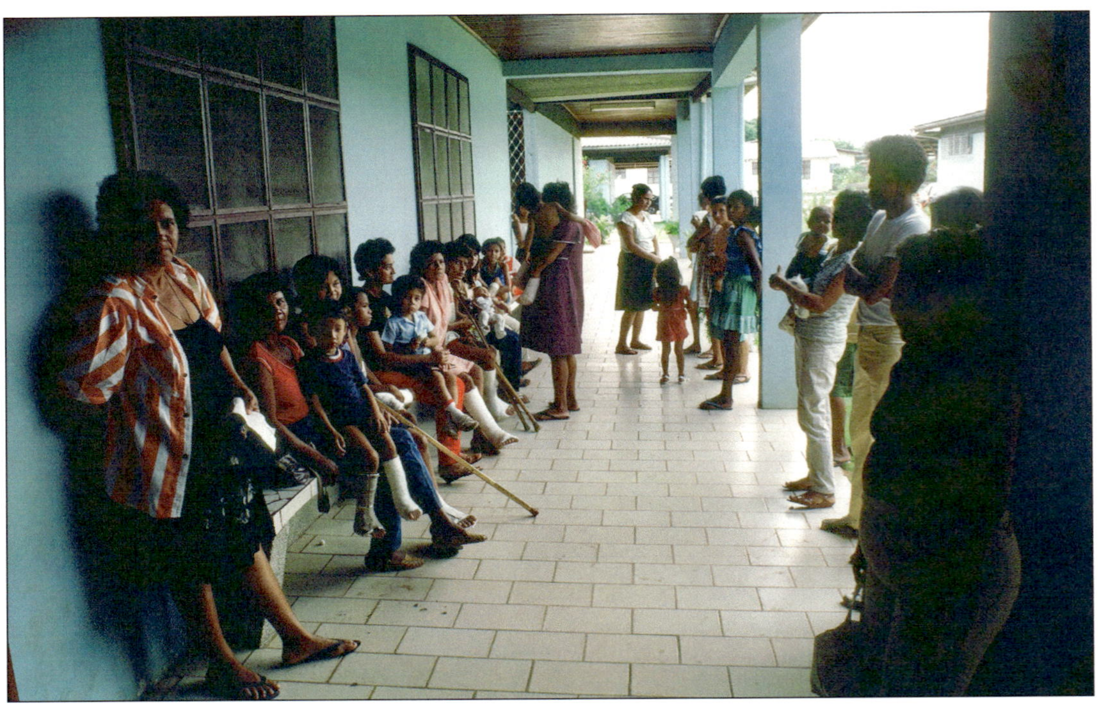

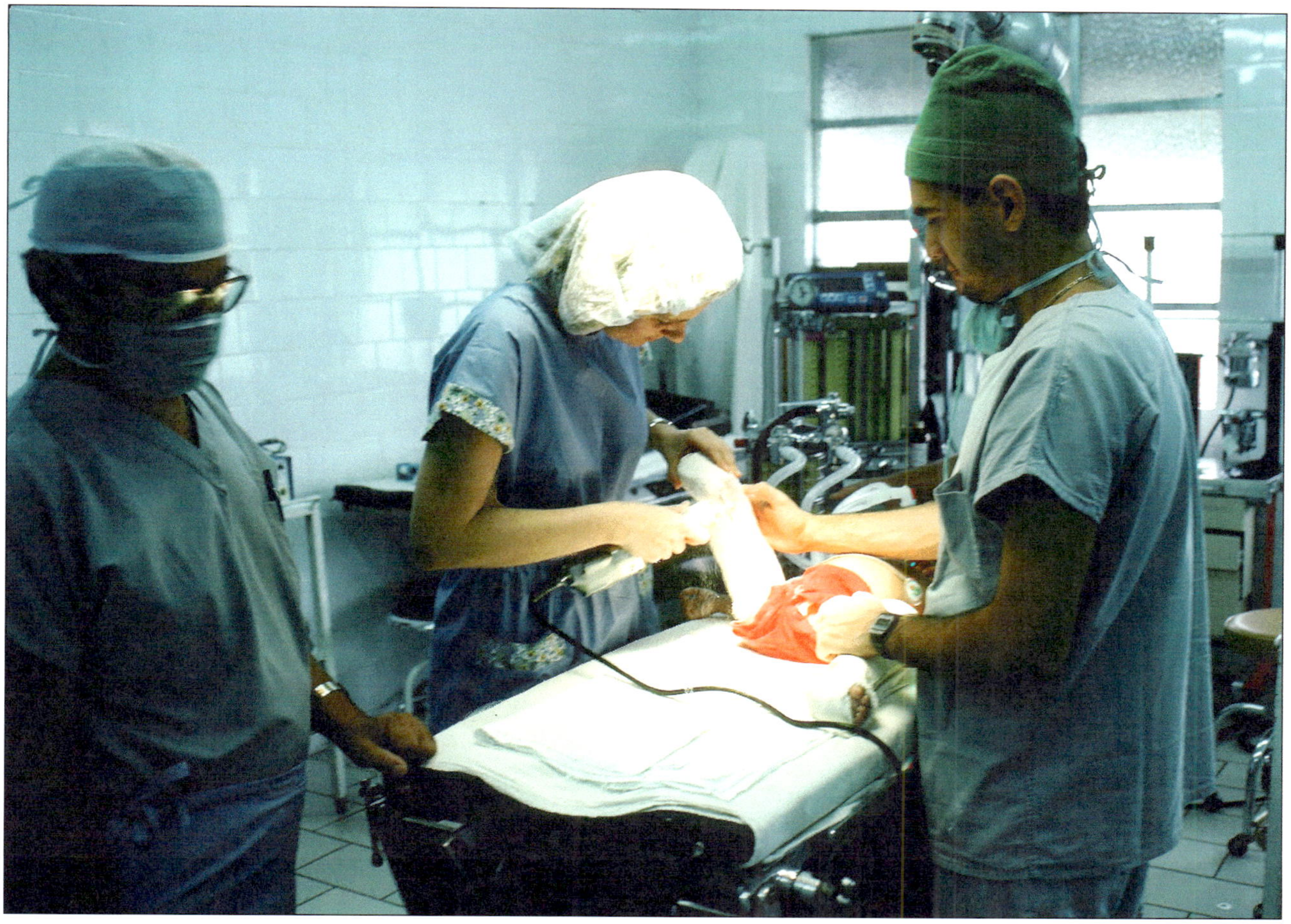

Rita changing a cast

In 1983, the hospital ship was retired and the organization moved to a new land campus that had an out patient facility with a good sized operating room, dorms for the volunteers and an eating facility. A significant improvement from the crowded and often times uncomfortable environment of the ship. Upon departure our team members were exhausted but exhilarated at having the experience of making a lasting impact on the lives of our patients, especially the children. Rita and I made 4 additional trips to Santarem over the next 14 years.

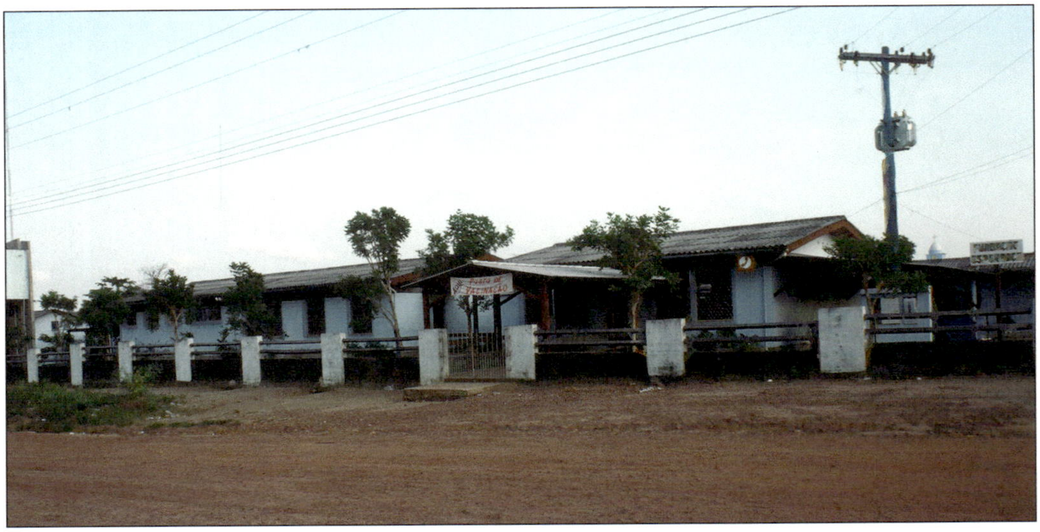

Outpatient facility and operating room

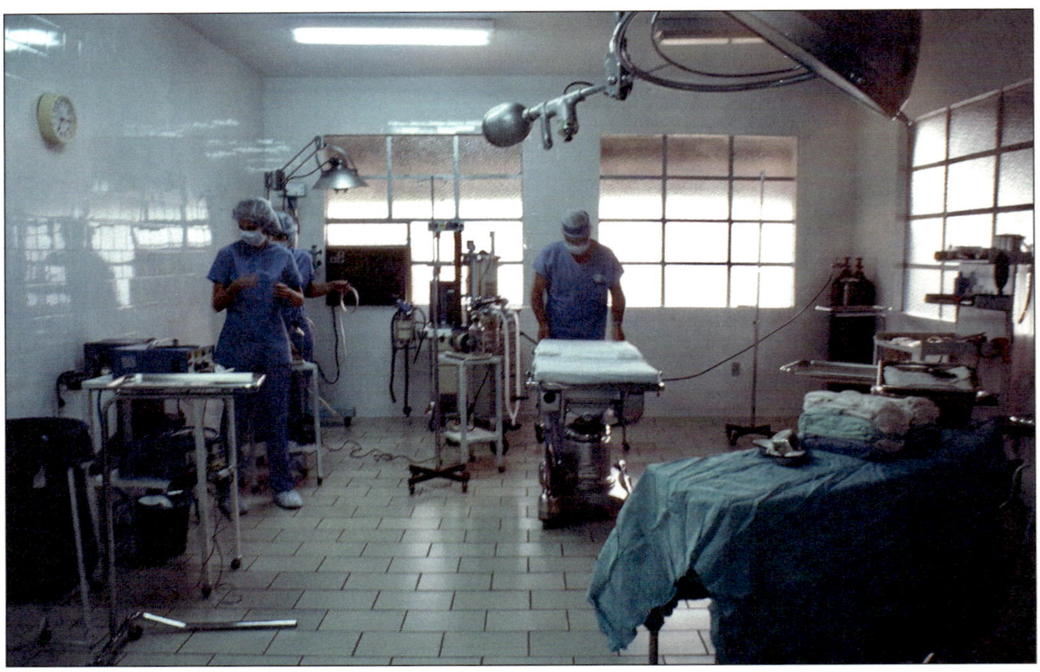

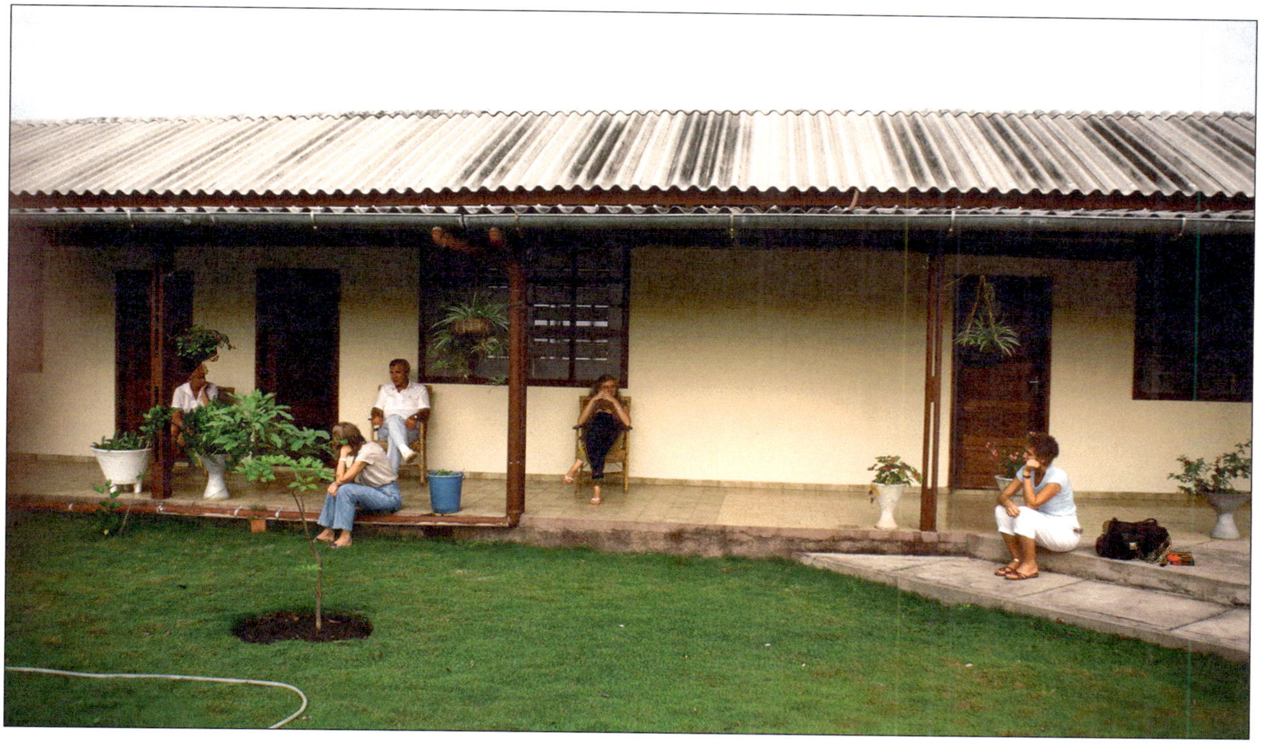

Living quarters for surgical teams

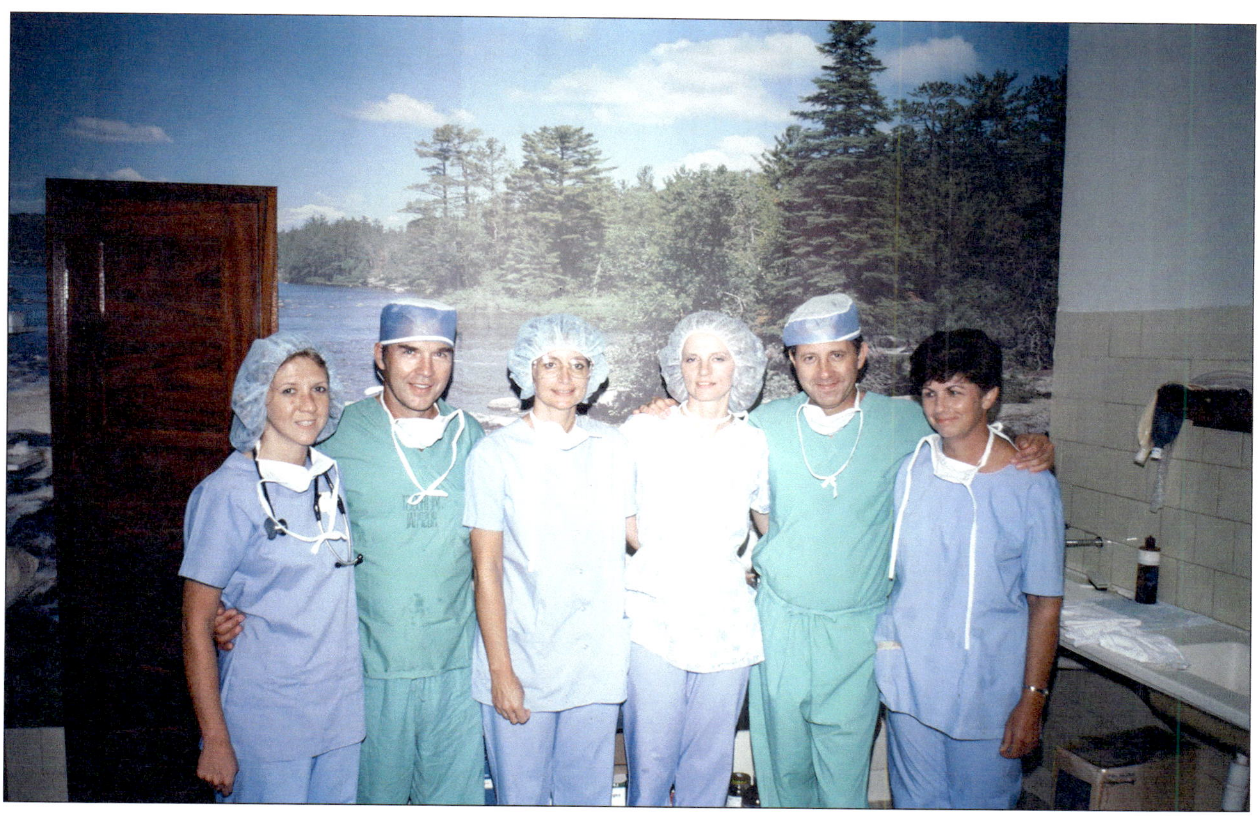

1985 surgical team

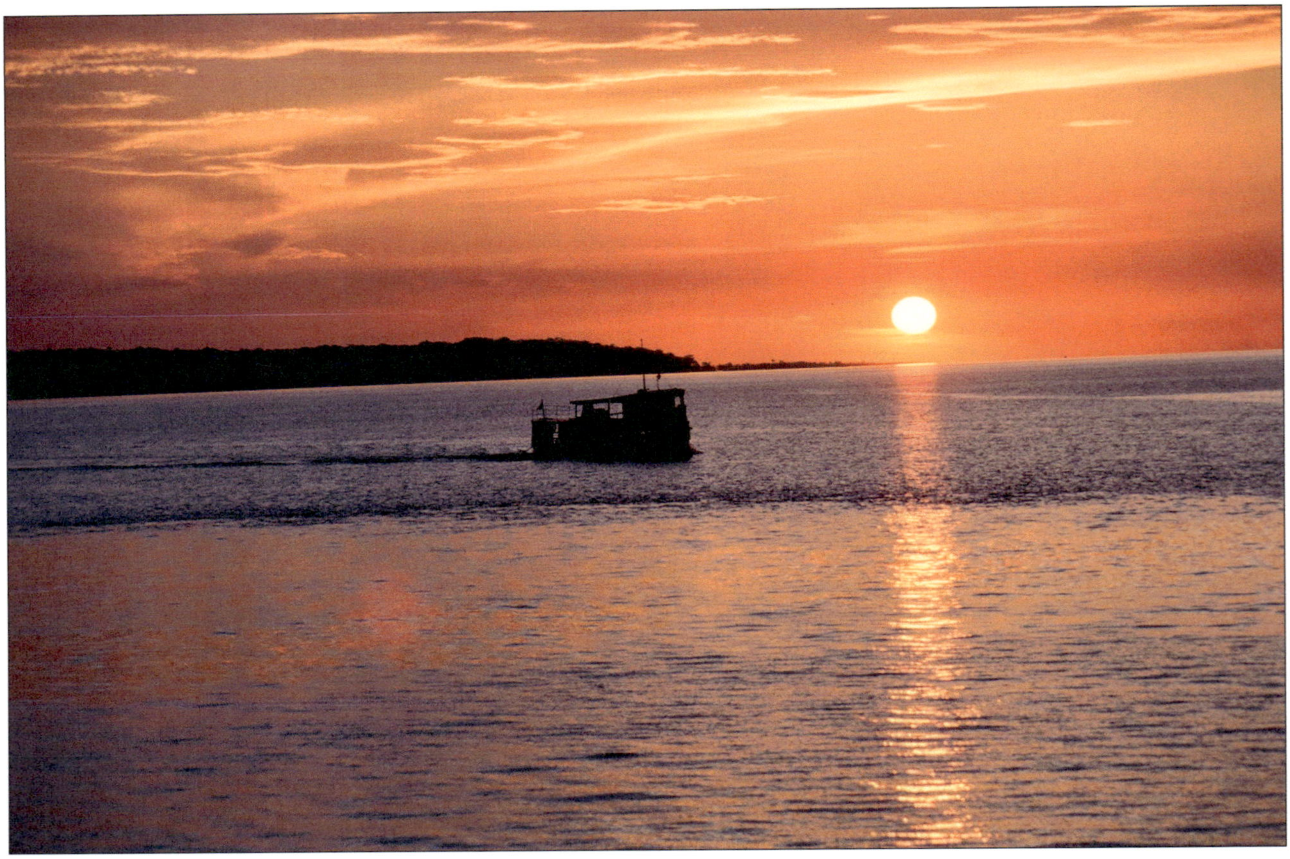

Sun setting on the Amazon

Mexico

In 1978 I obtained my private pilot license and shortly thereafter purchased 1/2 interest in a 1962 Cessna 210. In 1987 Rita and I joined the organization LIGA, which was a group of flying physicians, primarily from Southern California, who would fly to Northern Mexico the first weekend of each month (excluding June, July and August due to the heat) and conduct medical clinics in several rural communities. We were joined by 3 other flying doctors from Mesa, Charlie Gardner, an orthopedist, Ed Fenstermacher, a plastic surgeon and Nick Morrison a general surgeon. We would depart Mesa on Friday and fly to Guaymas, Mexico, our port of entry and then on to Alamos, a small community approximately 70 miles south of the city of Oregon to meet up with the California group. Alamos is lovely community with many US expats. The town is remarkable for its cleanliness and beautiful flowers. Friday evening we would all gather to go over the next day's village assignments and plan to reunite in Guaymas late Saturday afternoon. The Mesa group went to El Fuerte in the northern state of Sinaloa, departing at 7am arriving around 8:00. We were greeted by locals and usually transported by ambulance or truck to the clinic.

Alamos is lovely community with many US expats. The town is remarkable for its cleanliness and beautiful flowers.

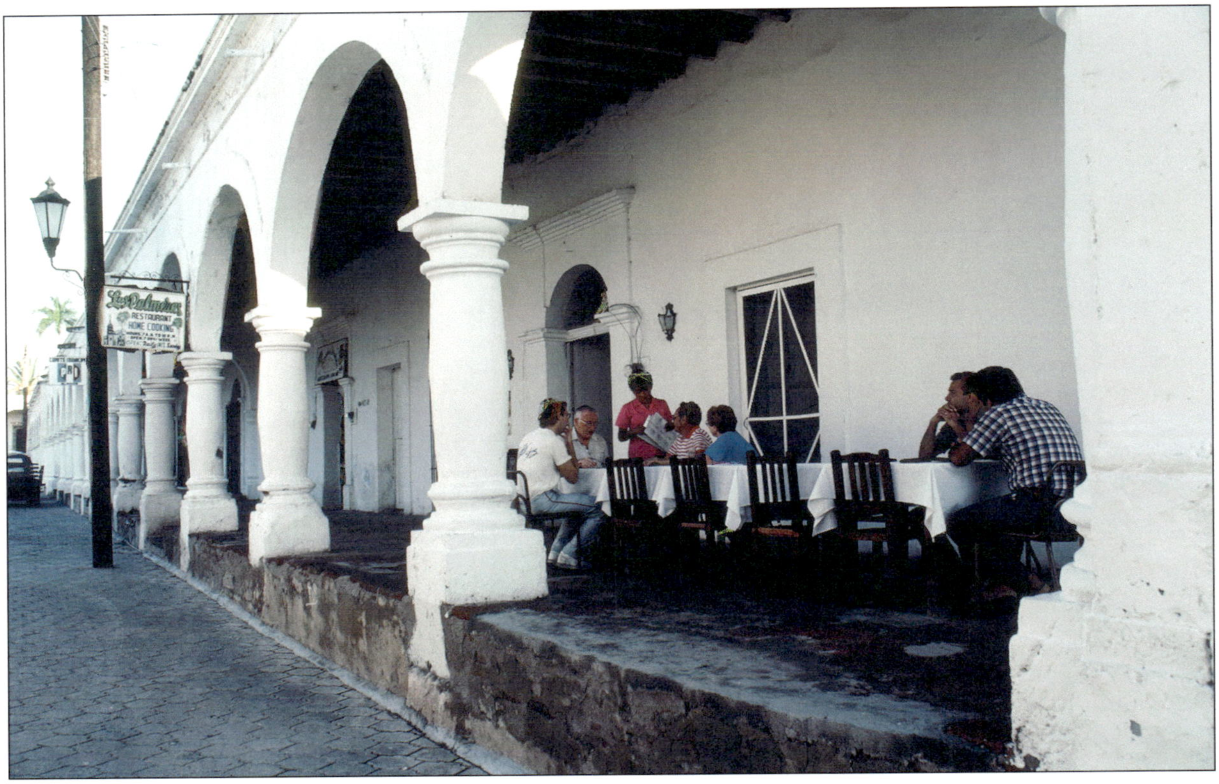

Images of Alamos, Mexico

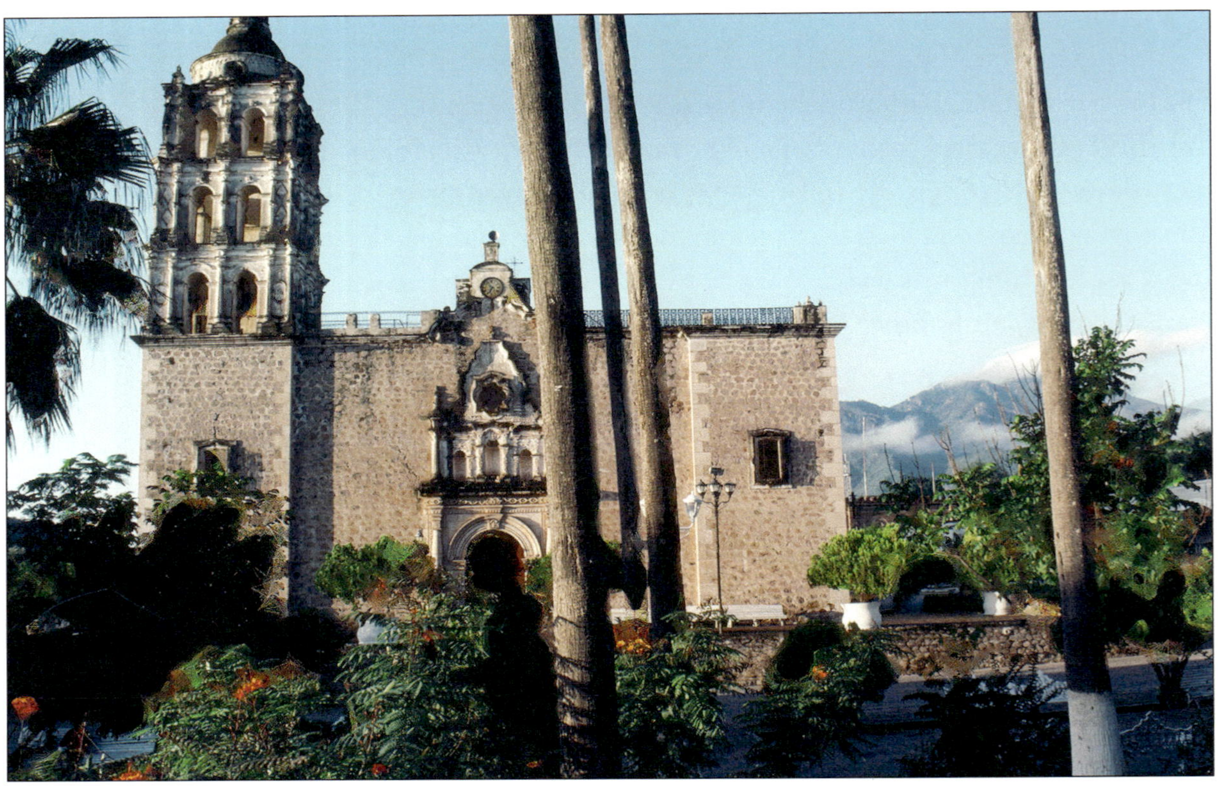

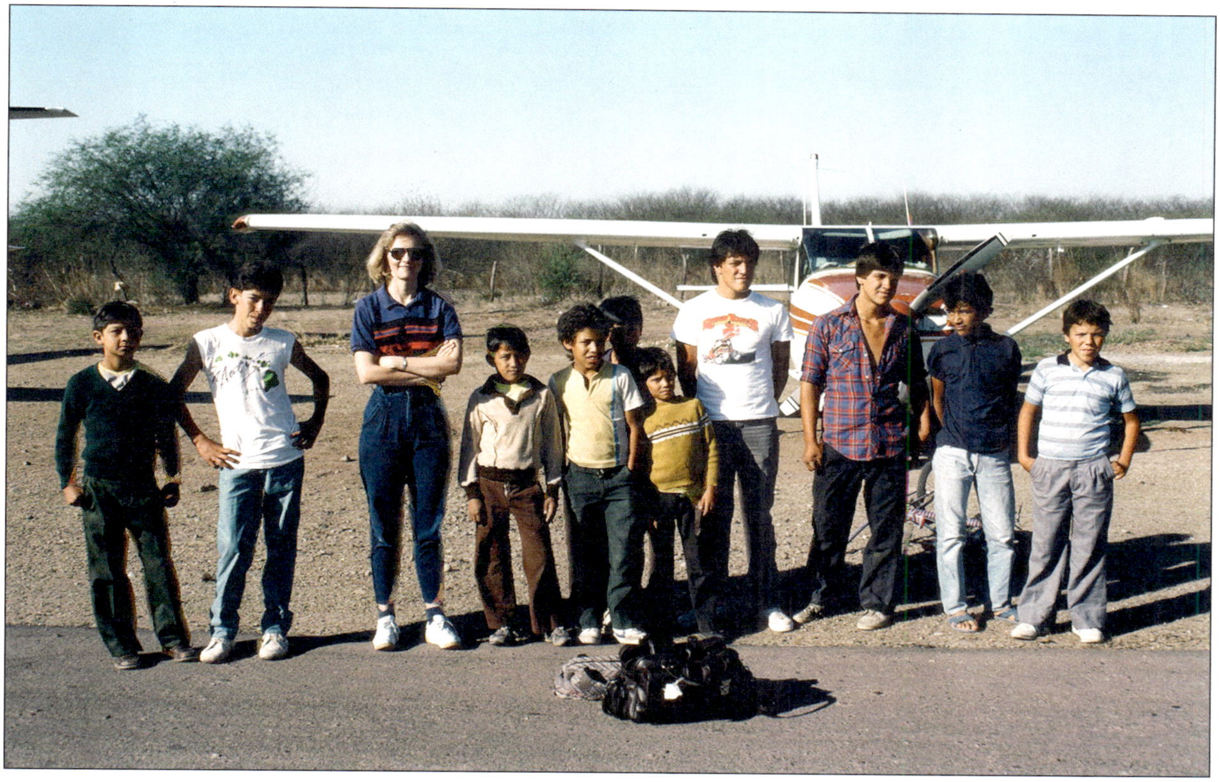

Airport greeters in El Fuerte

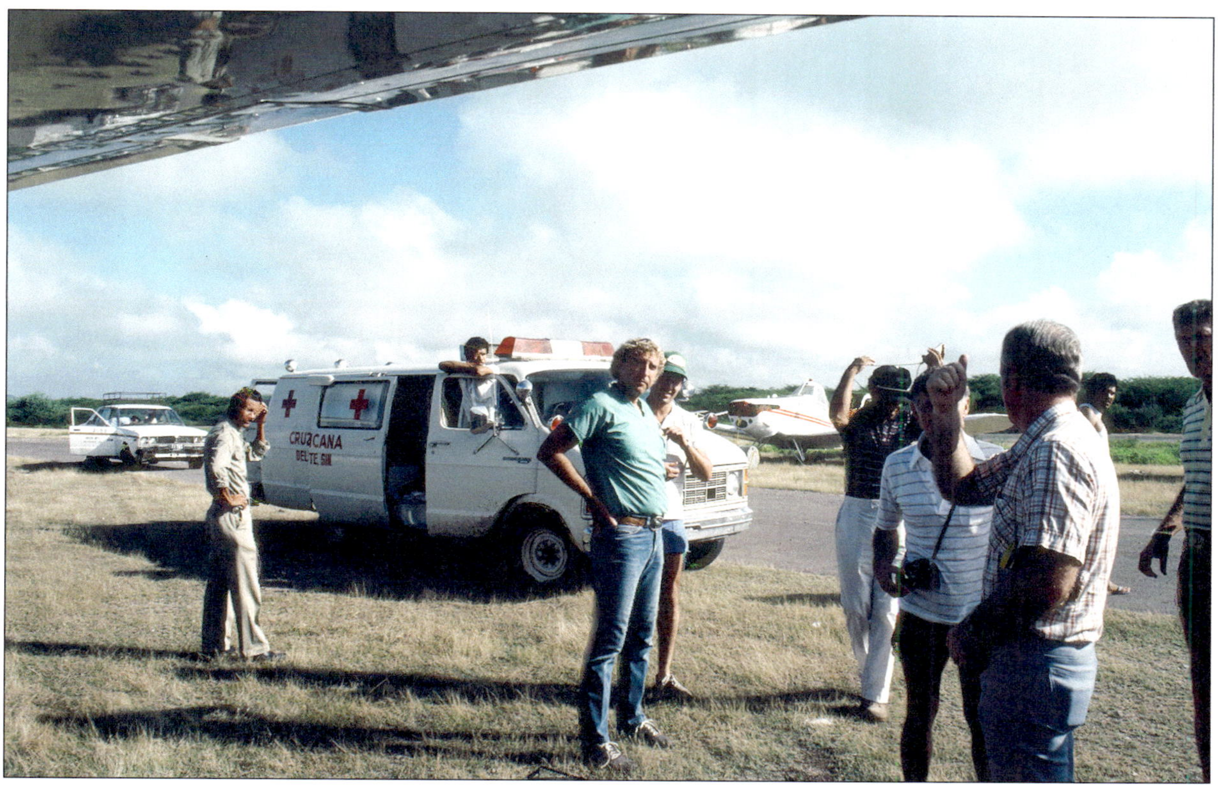

Ambulance transport

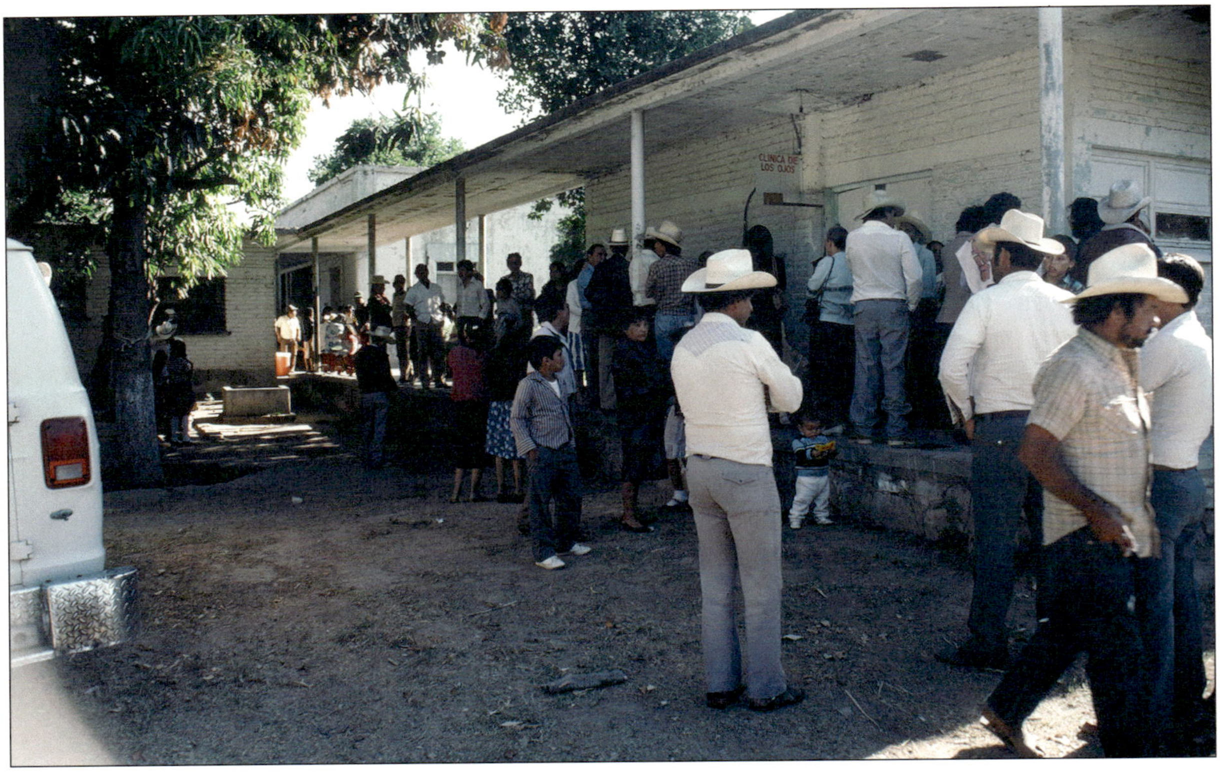

Patients waiting to be seen at clinic in El Fuerte

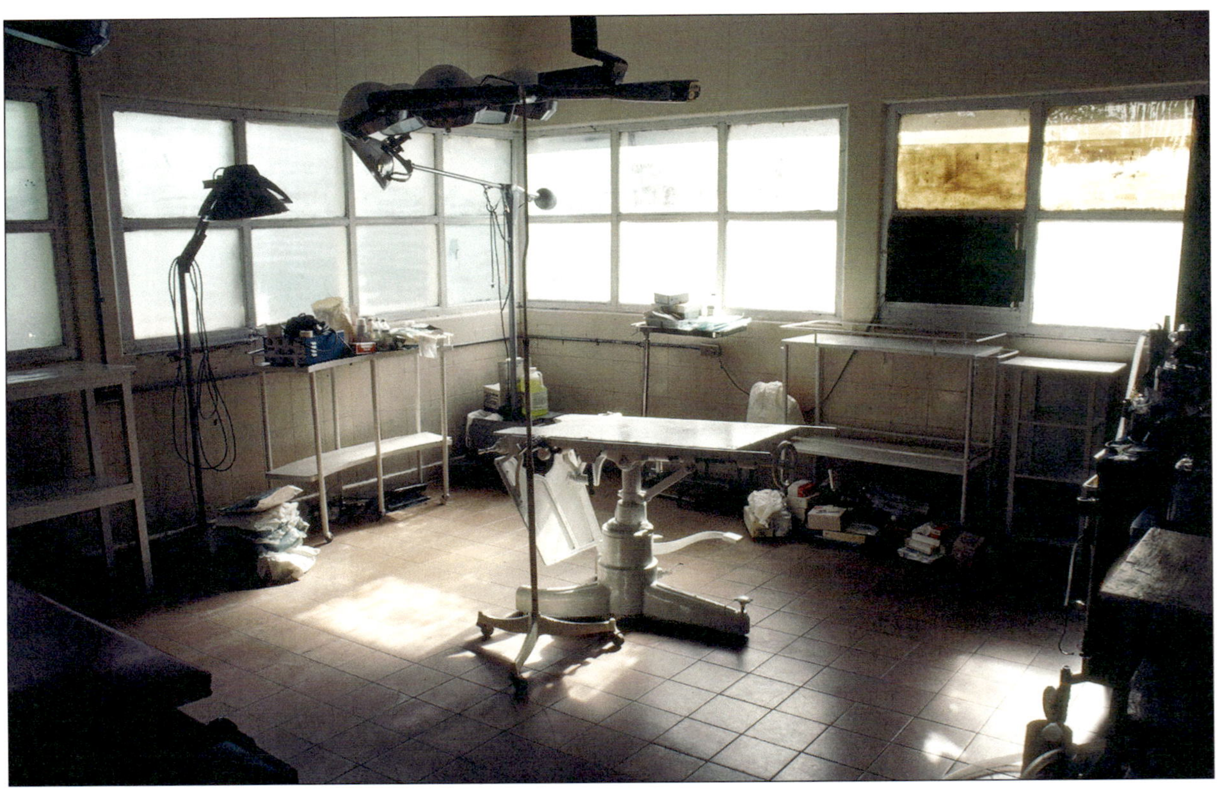

Operating room, El Fuerte for minor surgeries

We would see and treat patients until around 4 in the afternoon, then fly to Guaymas and reunite with the other teams and enjoy a night reliving our encounters that day. Most of the patients I saw had various musculoskeletal complaints that were treated with anti inflammatory medications and exercise. On occasion minor surgeries would be performed but the facility limitations and lack of general anesthesia prevented major surgeries from being performed. The patients were very excited to see an American Doctor believing we could cure any malady. Unfortunately we left many disappointed due to the limitations of the clinic.

One young woman of 18 years came to me seeking a cure for a neurological disorder that left her with marked lower extremity weakness. When I explained that her condition was not amenable to surgical correction she broke down and sobbed. It was always difficult to tell these patients they couldn't be helped.

Unfortunately we left many disappointed due to the limitations of the clinic.

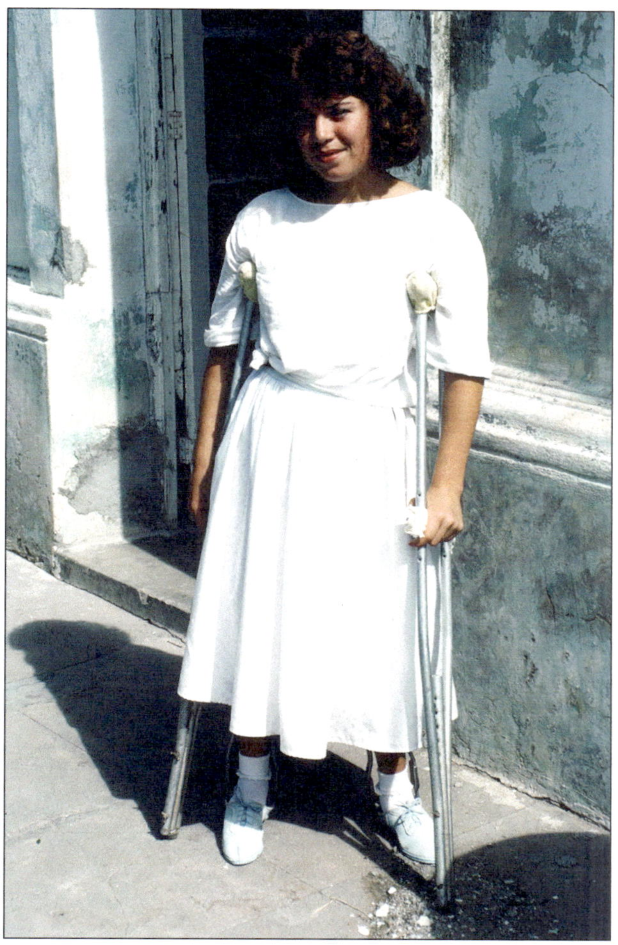

Young girl with neurological weakness in legs

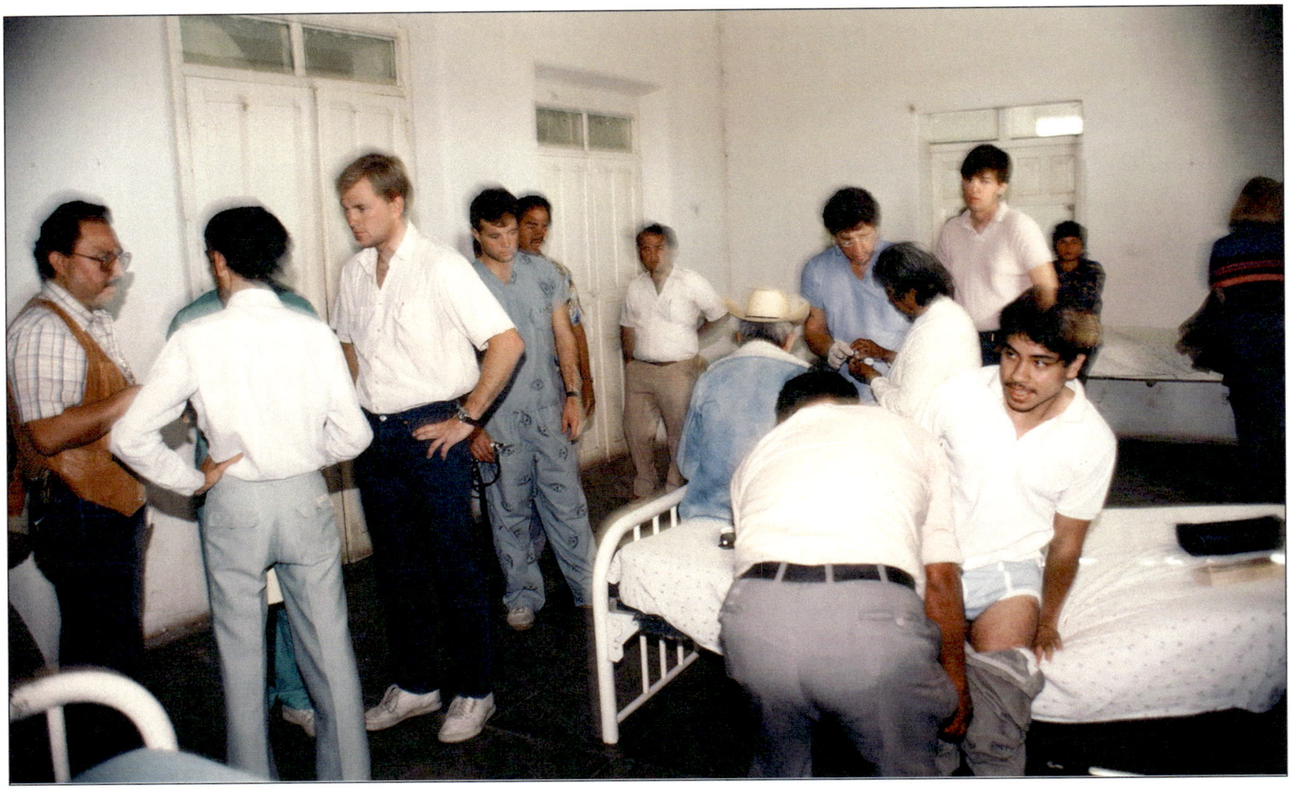

Exam "rooms"

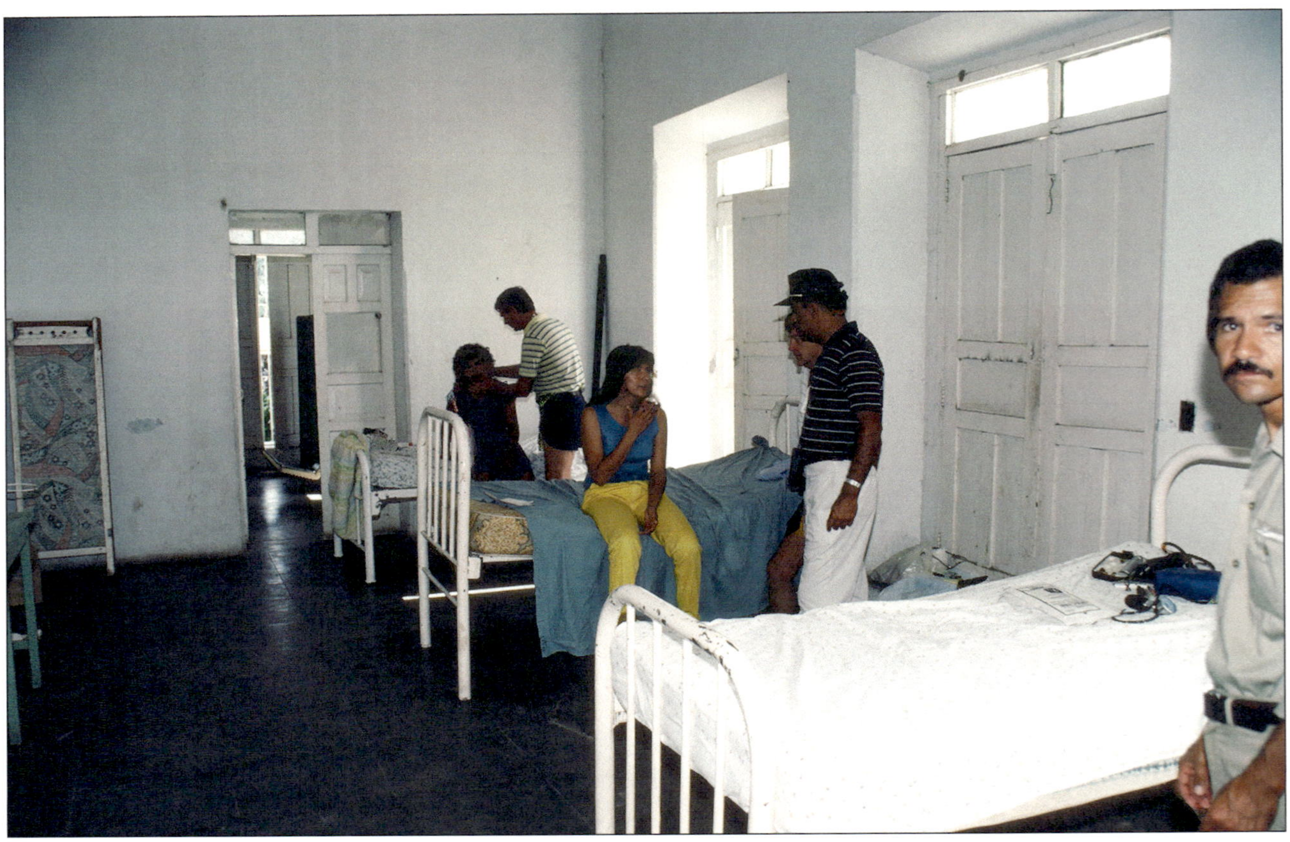

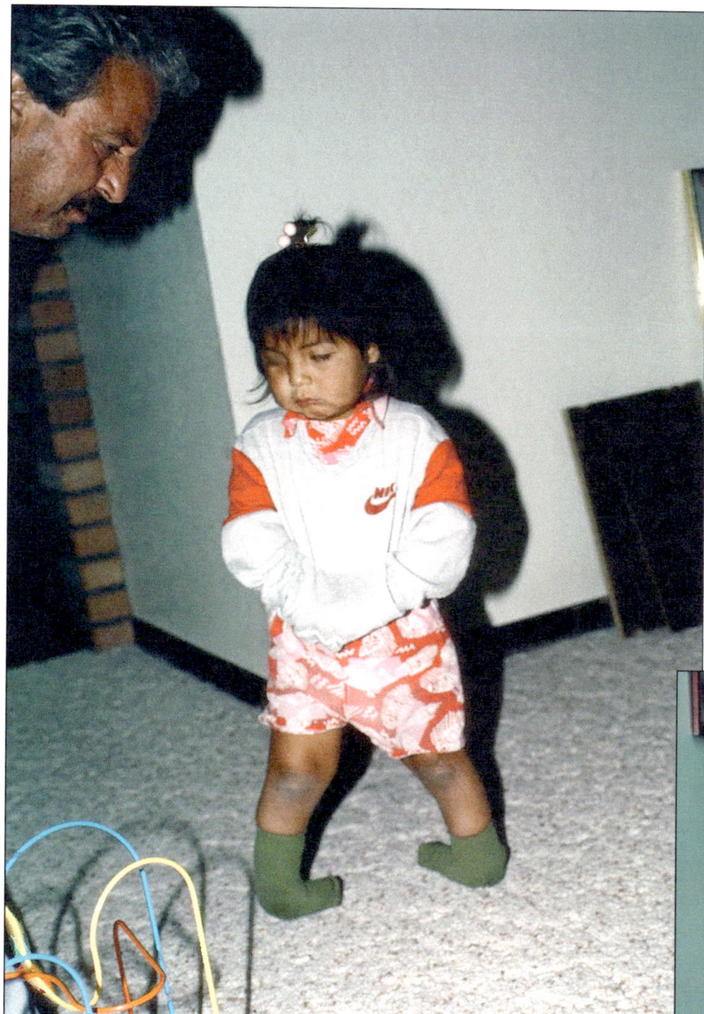

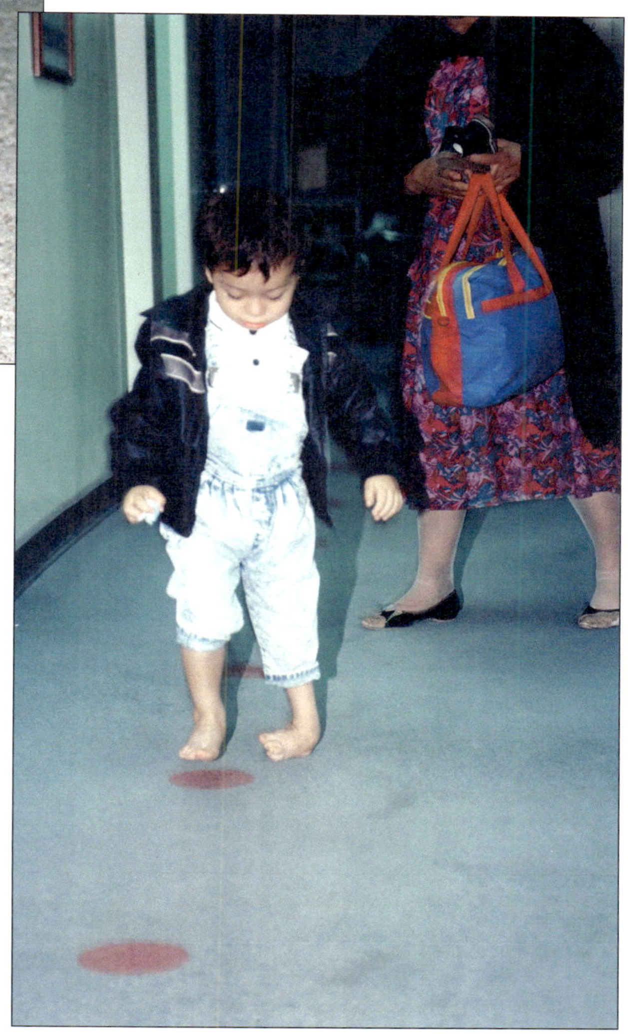

Two young boys aged 3 and 4 with clubfeet.

Since surgery could not be performed in the local facility, I conferred with our local hospital administrator and was given approval to do surgery on the two boys in Mesa. The following month I flew the boys and their fathers to Mesa, and we performed the surgical corrections. Five days later, I flew them back to Mexico. We changed their casts and continued their follow-up care on our return trips over the next two months.

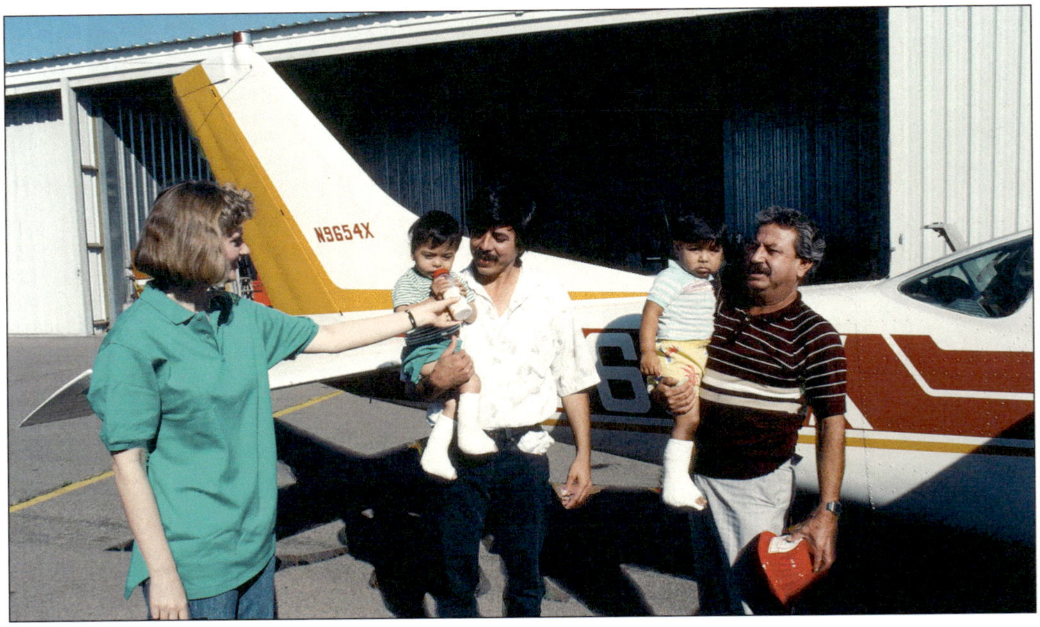

At airport prior to return to El Fuerte

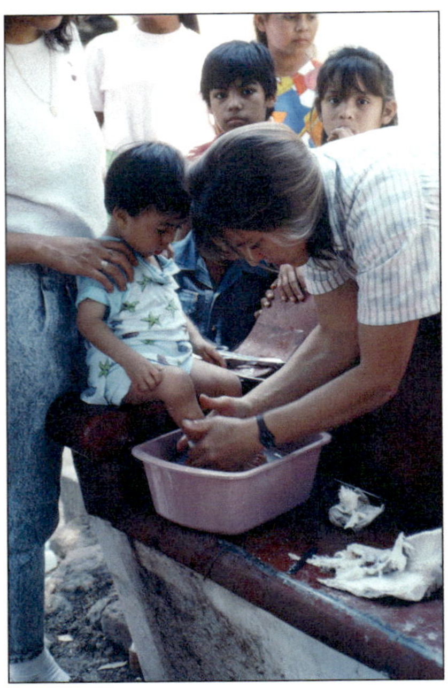

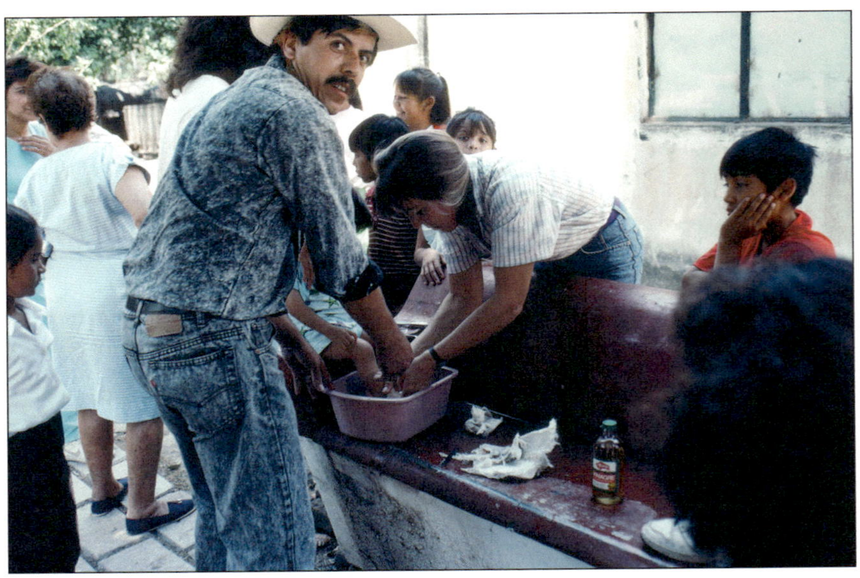

Cast removal after two months

Patients unable to be treated at clinic

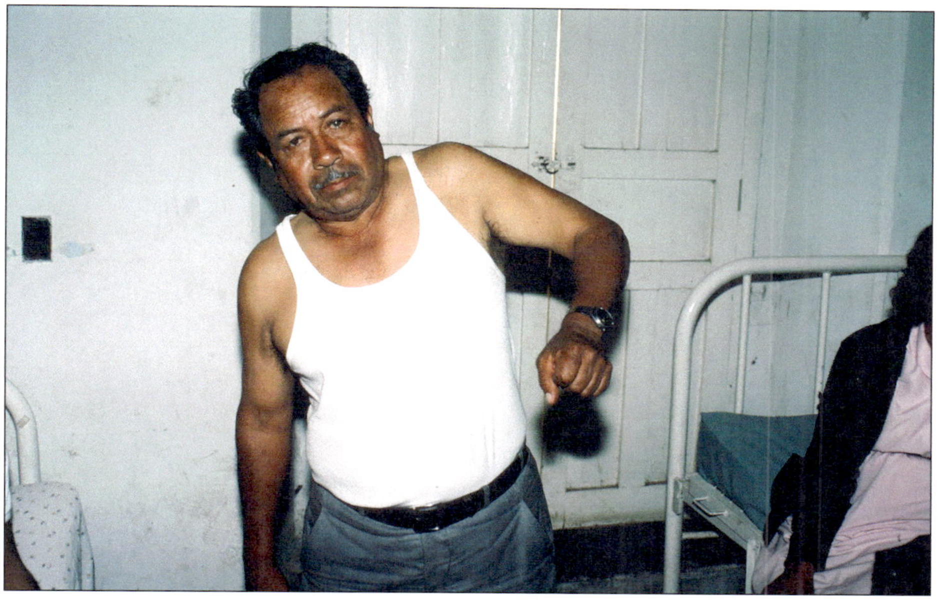

Man with rotator cuff tear unable to raise shoulder

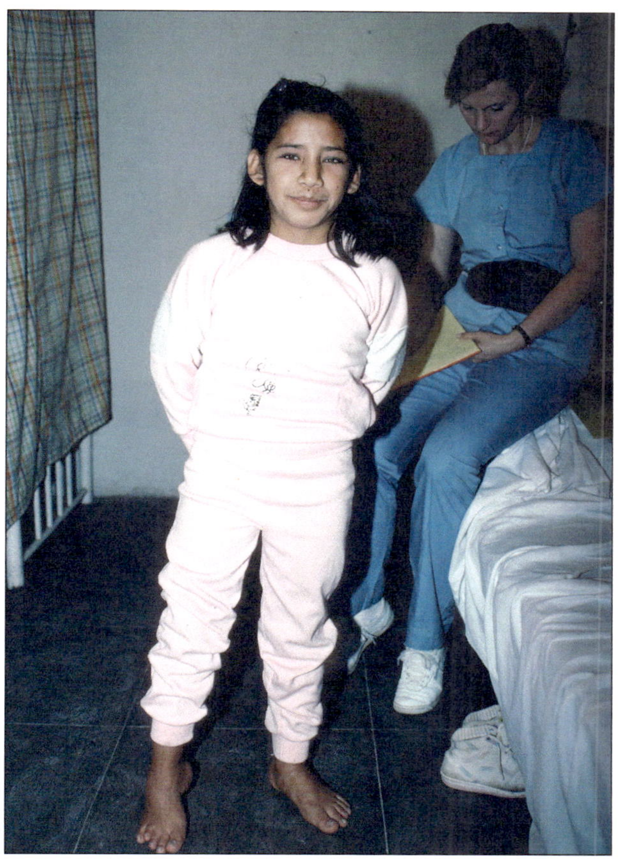

Young girl with foot deformity secondary to polio

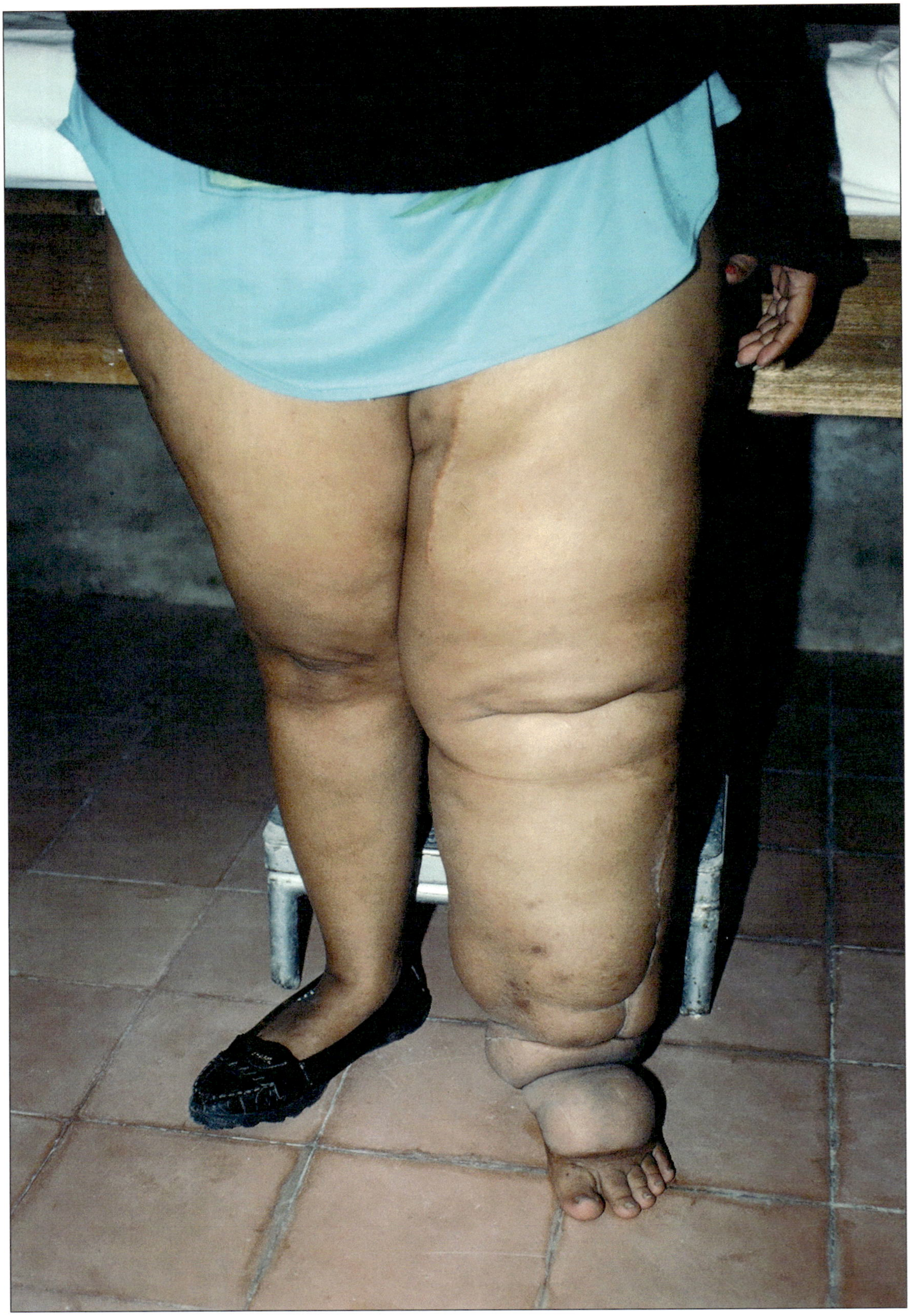

Woman with severe lymphedema of leg

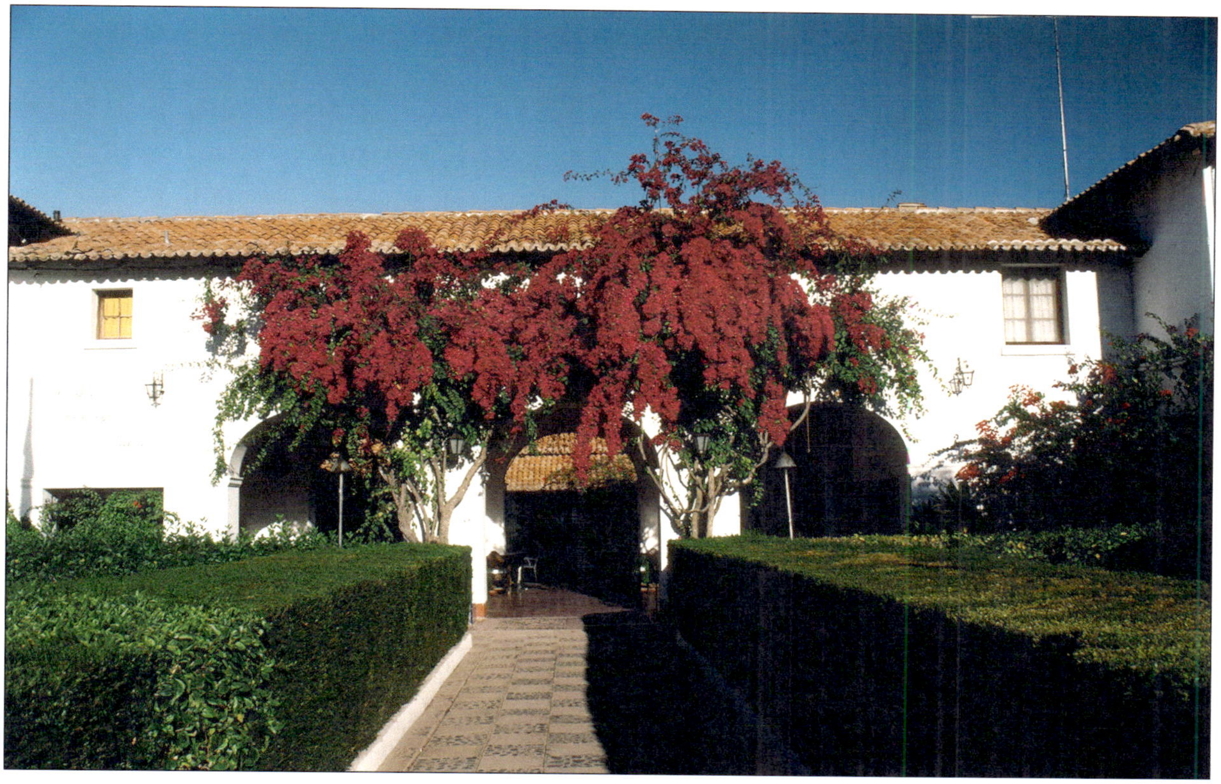

Playa de Cortez, Guaymas, Mexico

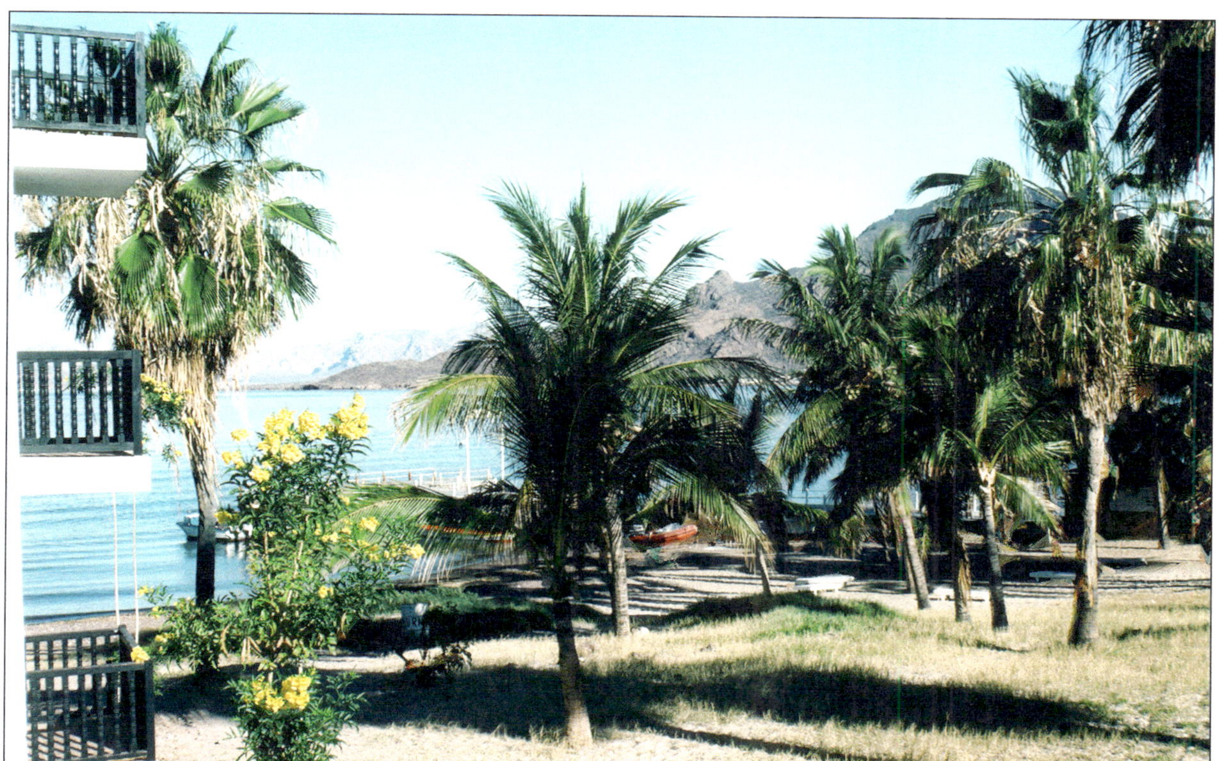

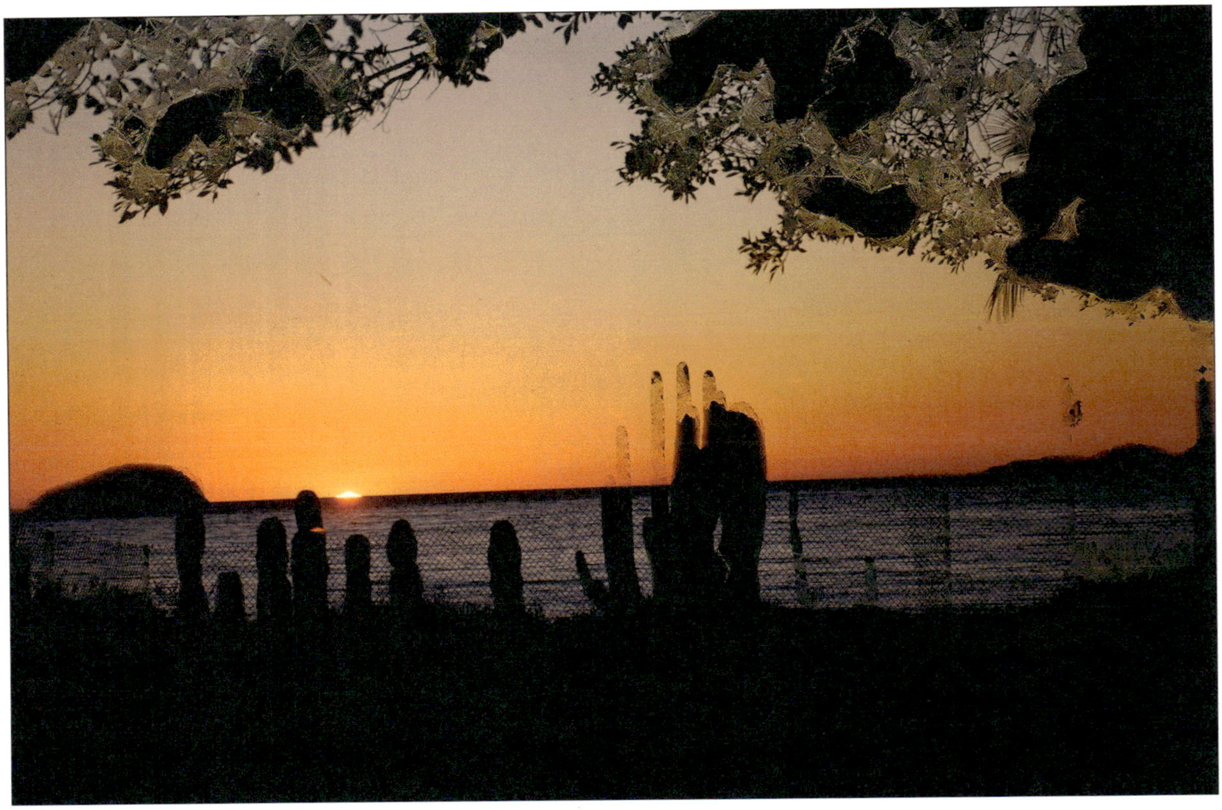

Sunset, Guaymas

Ecuador

During one of our weekend trips to Mexico, we spent the night in El Fuerte. Our group went to dinner on the roof of a local hotel enjoying the view and some appetizers when a group of women nearby struck up a conversation with us. One of them was from Ecuador and ran an orphanage; she invited us to come to Ecuador and do surgery at their local hospital. Doctors Morrison, Fenstermacher, and I were interested and the following summer took four surgical teams, including anesthesiologists, nurses, and OR technicians to Ambato, Ecuador for a week of intense surgical care. For these trips, it required us to bring all of our own supplies, including dressings, anesthetics, casting material, pain meds, and, of course, toys for the children. This entailed extensive pre-trip preparation and packing up to 40 trunks for transport and getting these items through customs, which, at times, was quite frustrating. Our routine was similar to that of Esperanza, evaluating patients on arrival and making up a surgical schedule for the week, saving the day before departure for dressing and cast changes and leaving written instructions with the local physicians for follow-up care. Patients, however, continued to stream in throughout our stay seeking treatment. We found that protecting our supplies was a major concern, and, ultimately, we had them locked in a room and posted a guard at the door for further protection.

For these trips, it required us to bring all of our own supplies, including dressings, anesthetics, casting material and, of course, toys for the children.

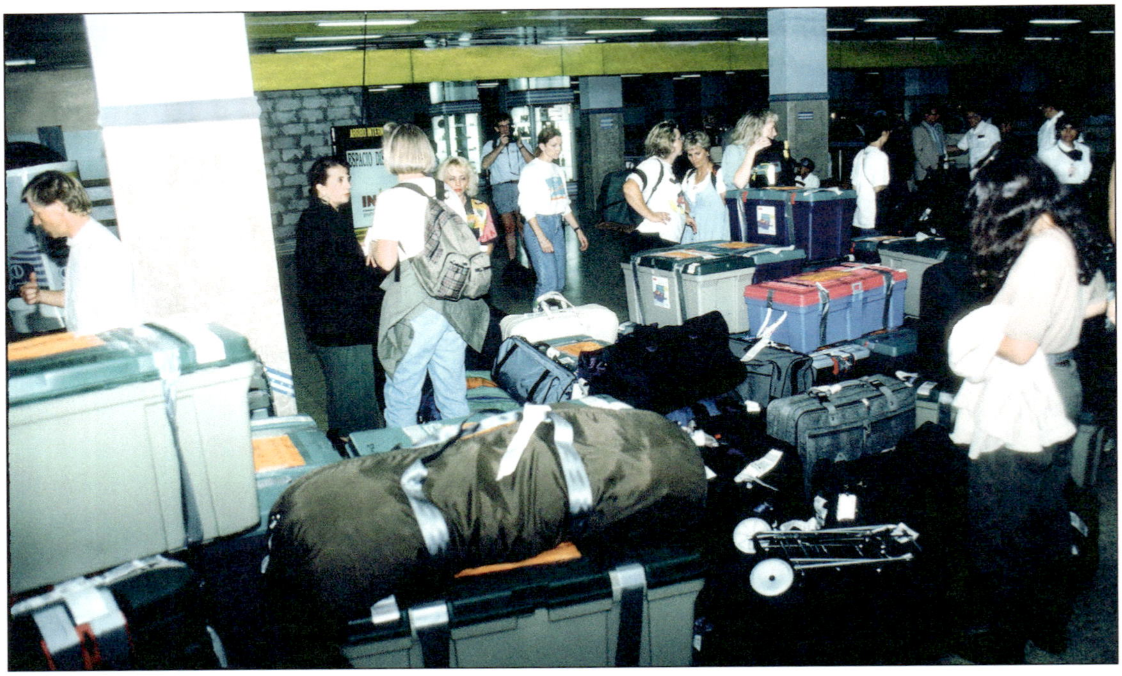

Supply trunks at Quito airport

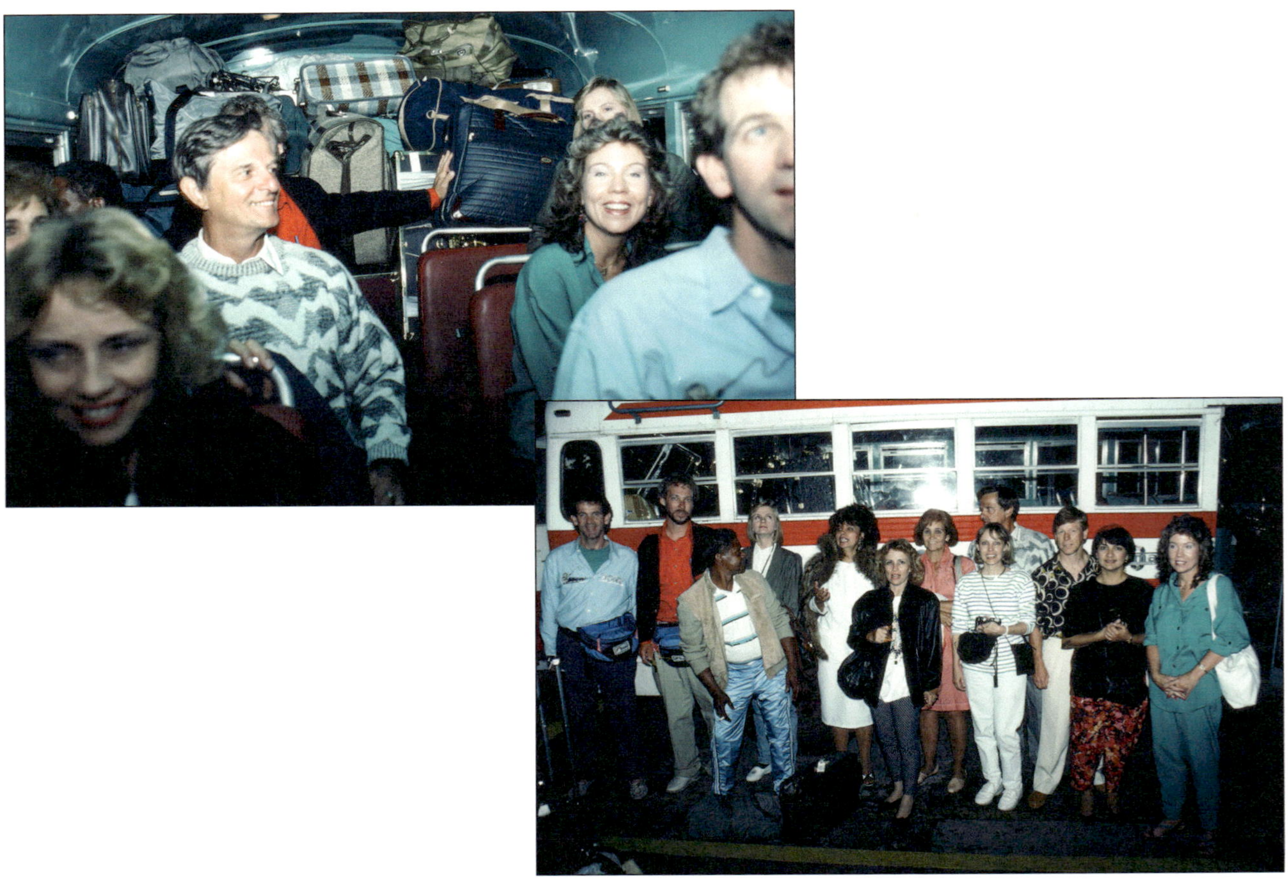

Bus transport from airport

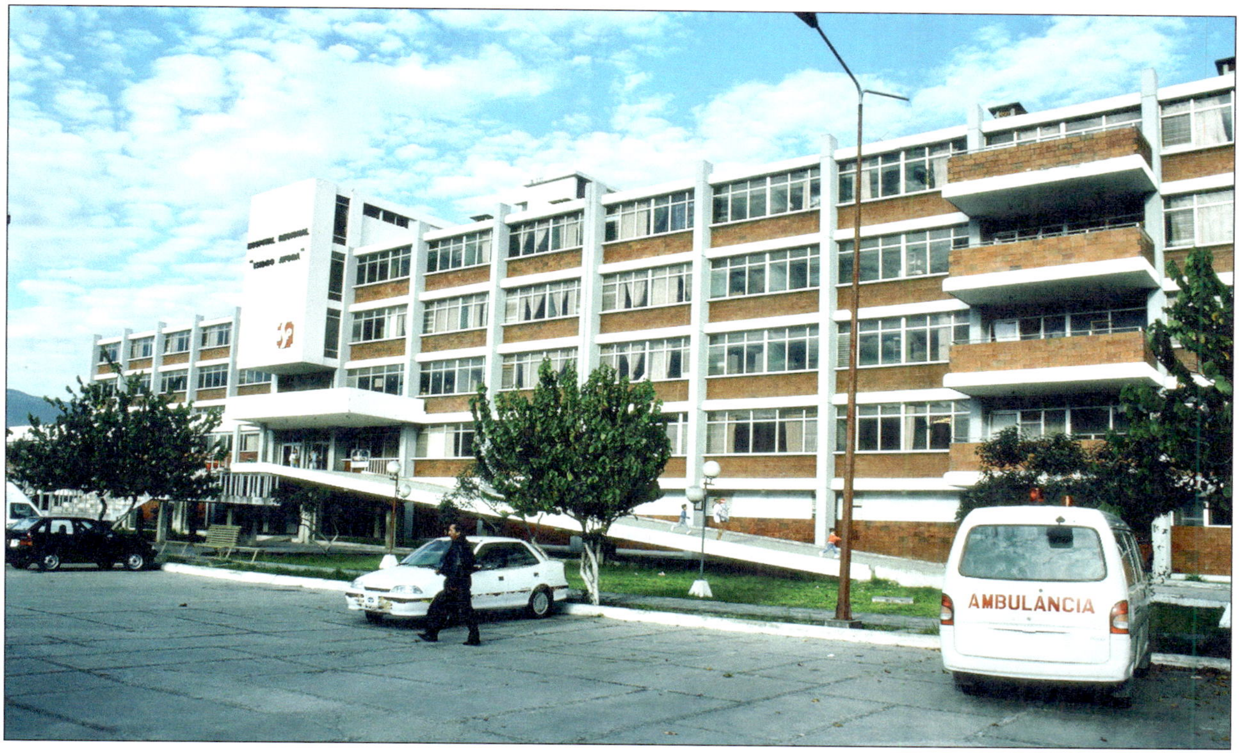

Ambato Hospital

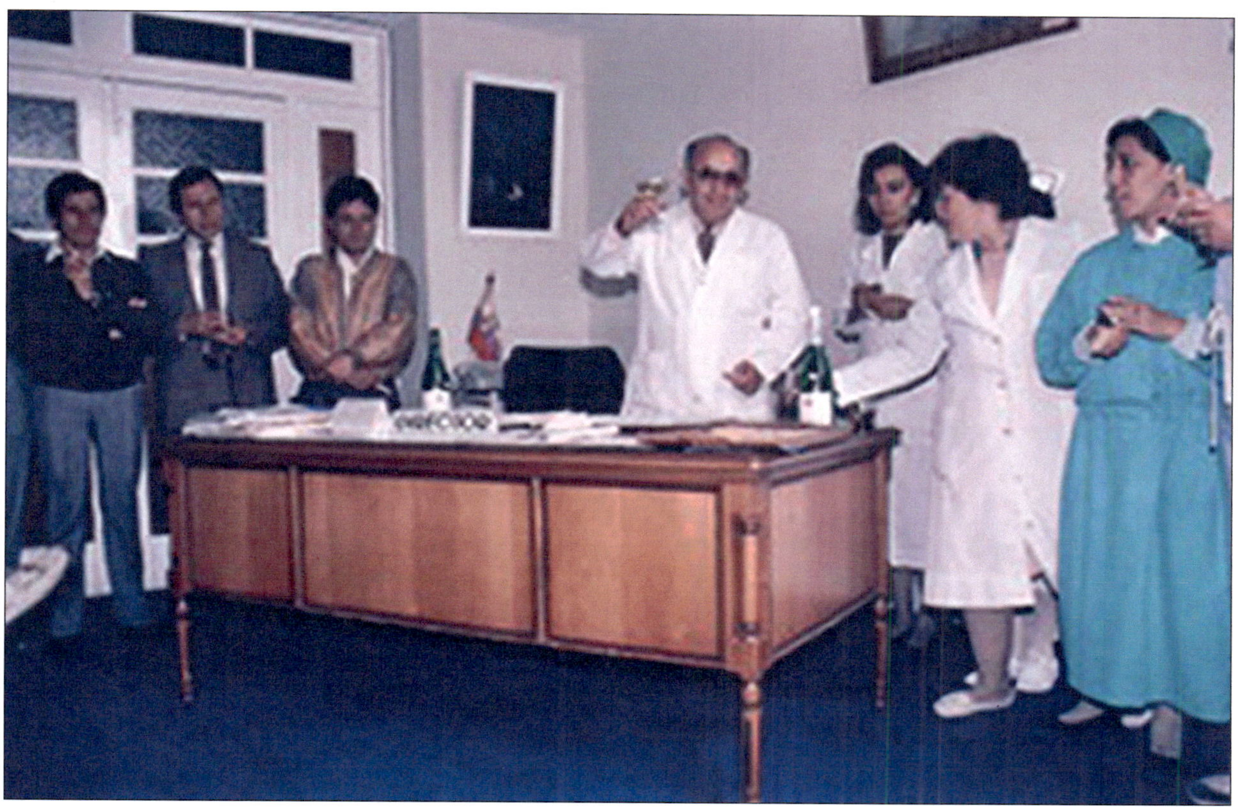

Being welcomed by hospital director

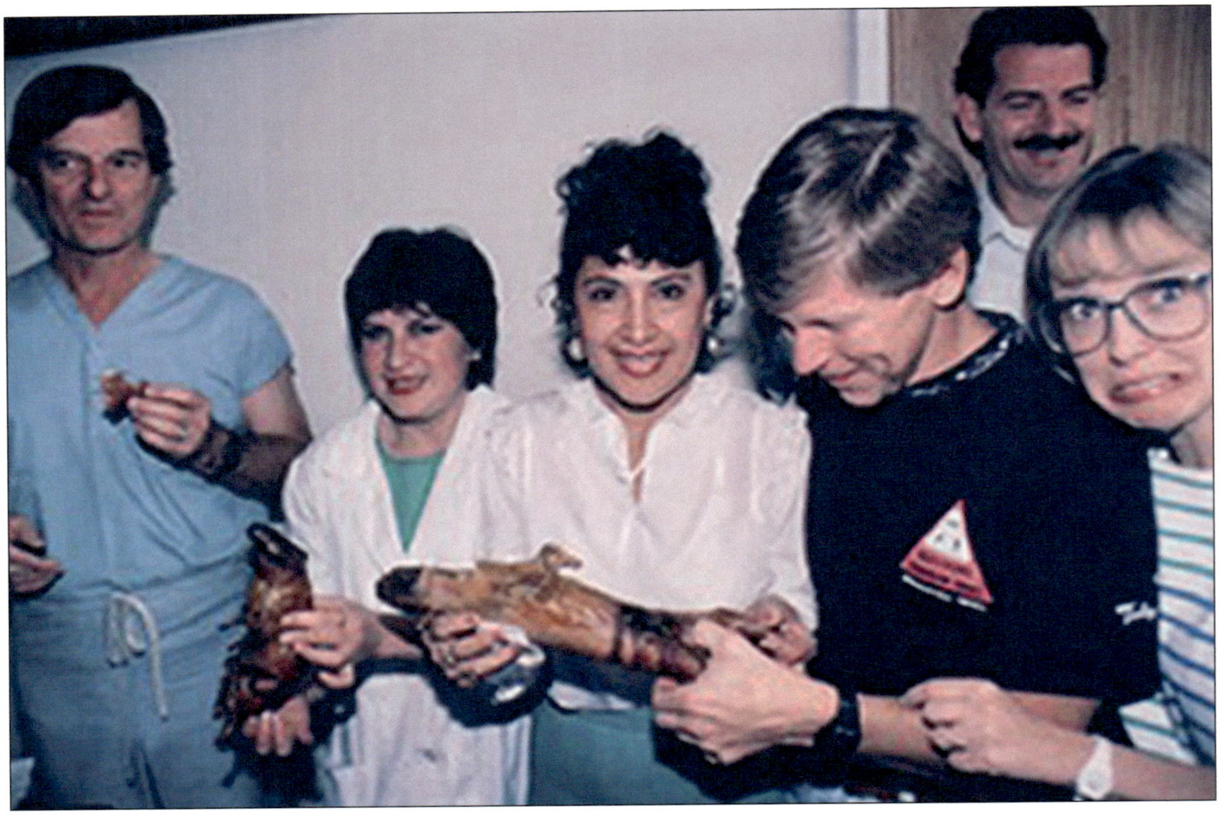

Eating Ecuadorian delicacy, fried guinea pig

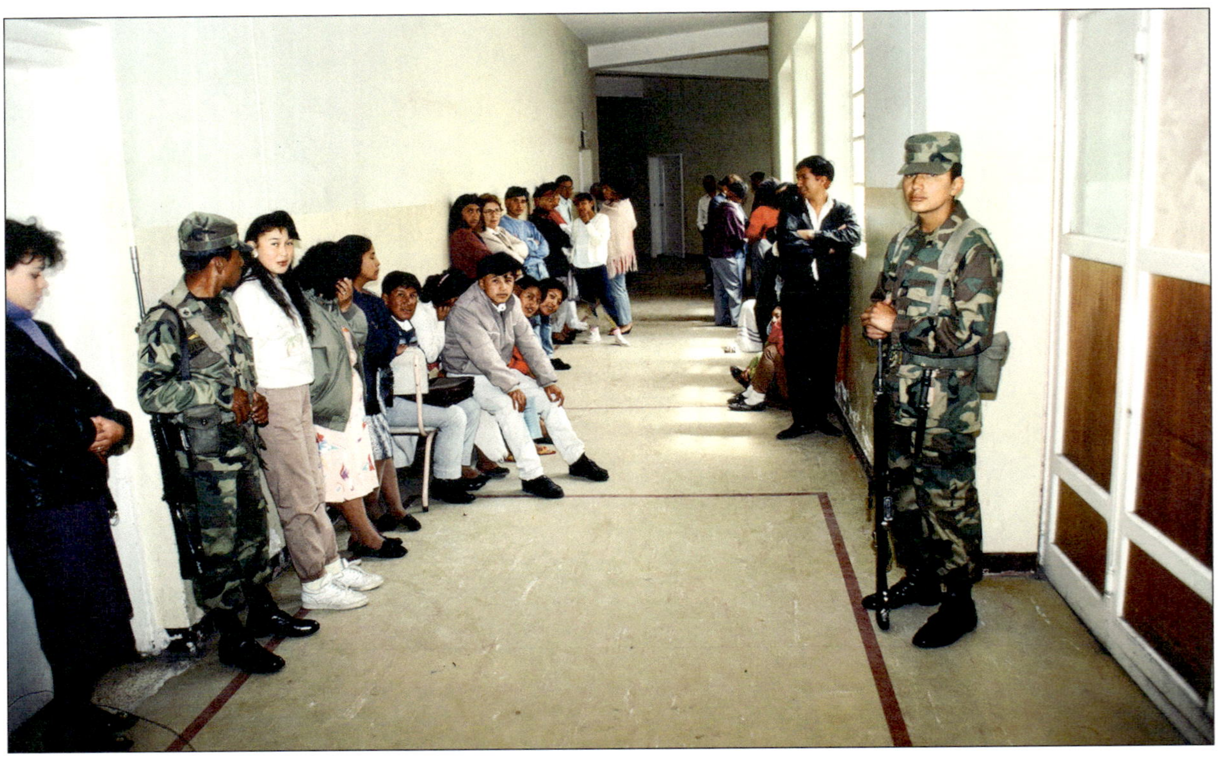

Patients waiting to be seen in the hospital. Guard in front of supply room

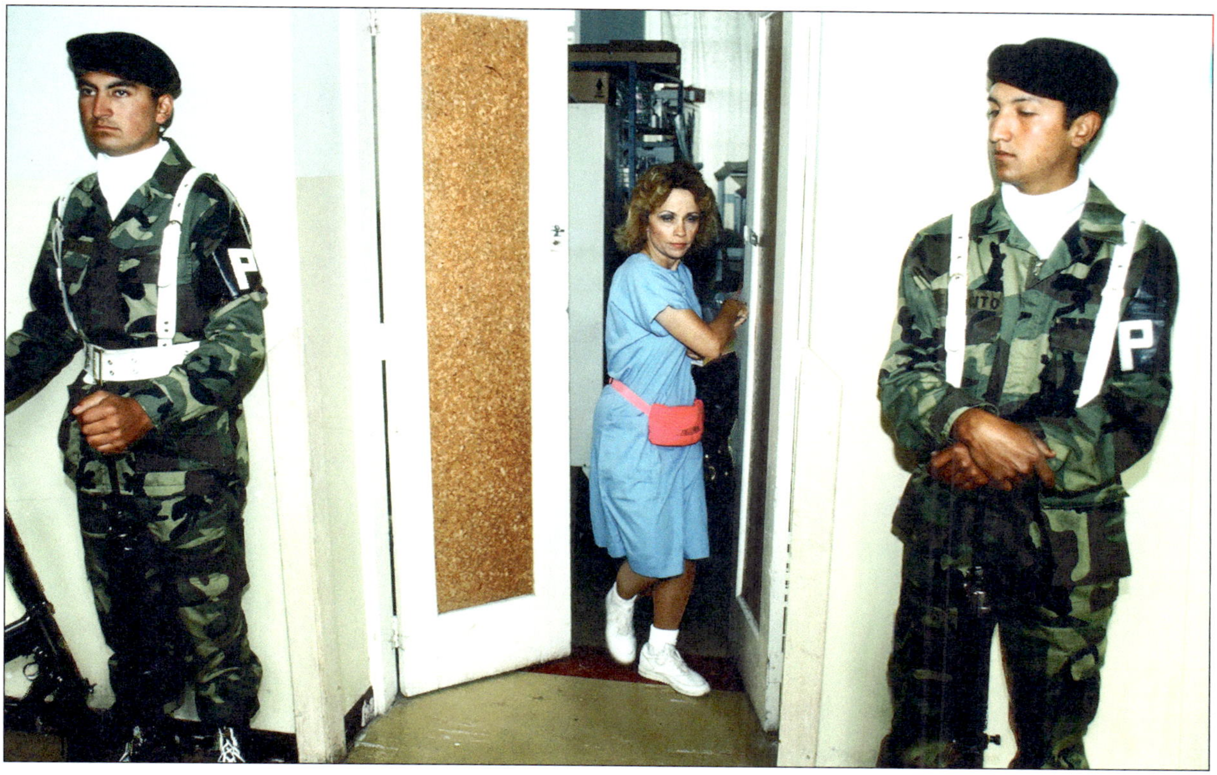

Terri Morrison leaving guarded supply room

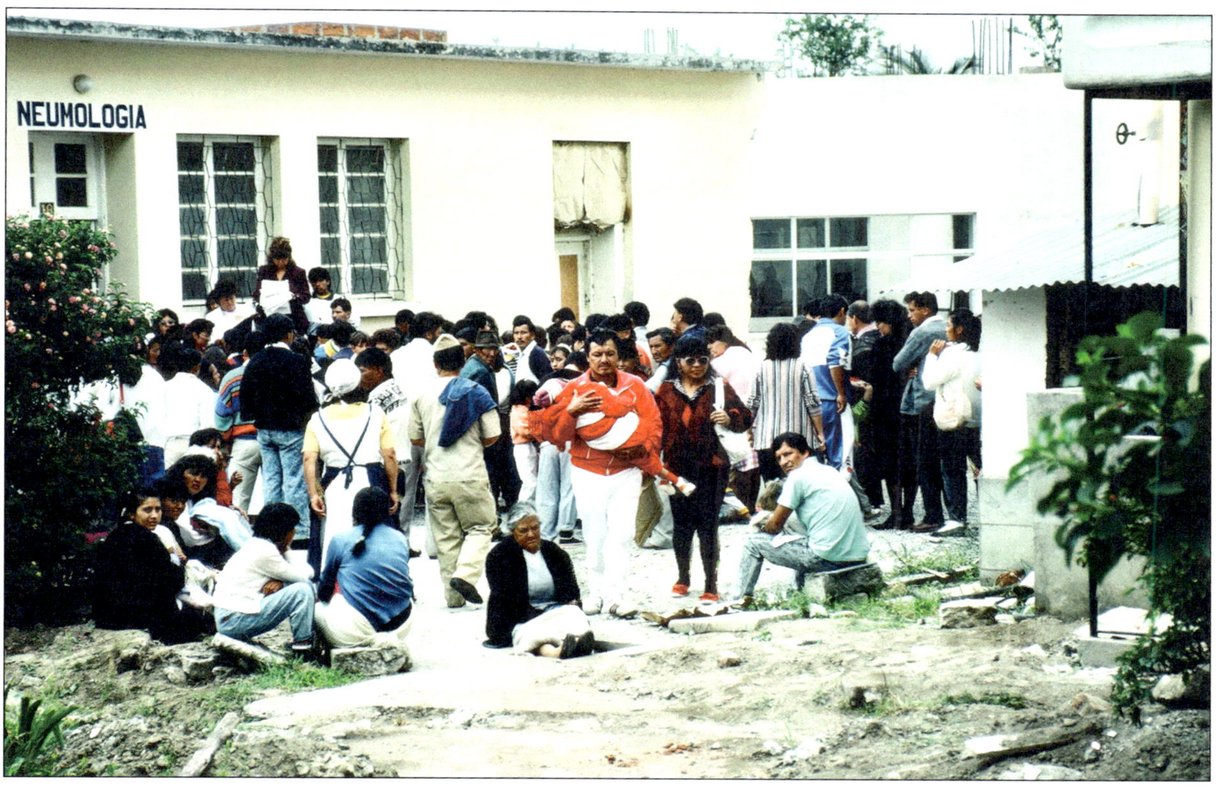

Patients waiting outside the hospital to be seen

Burn patients

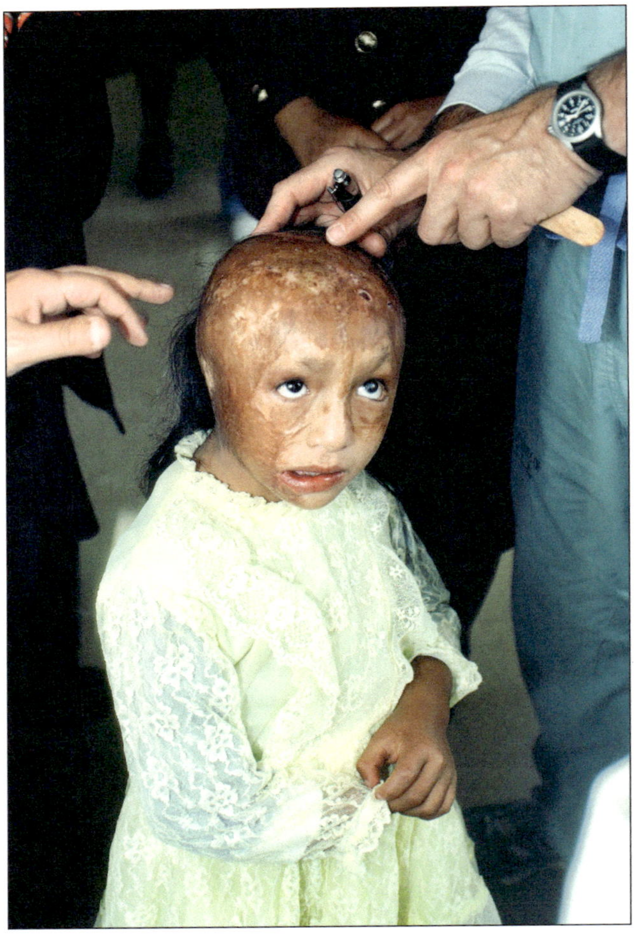

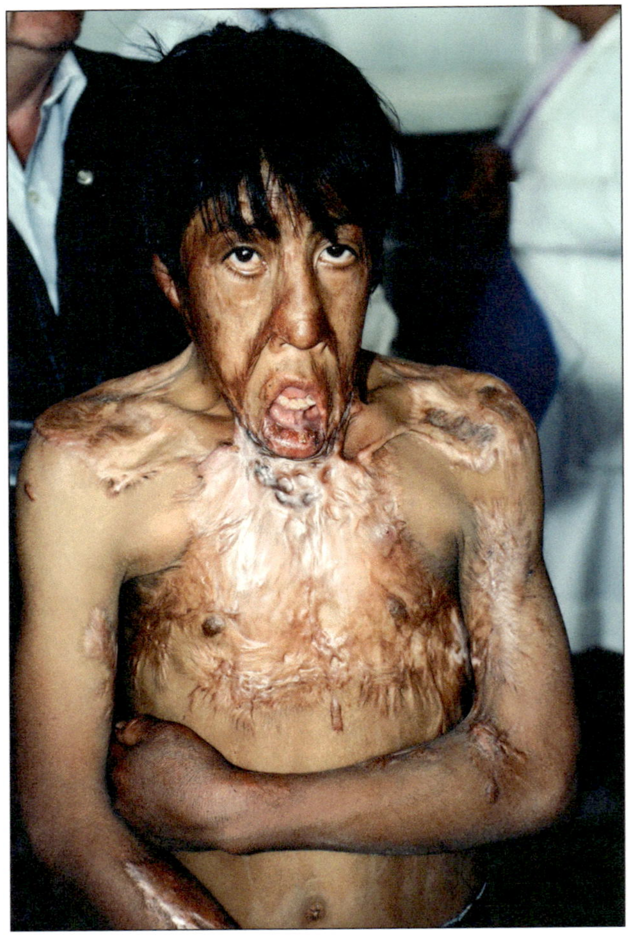

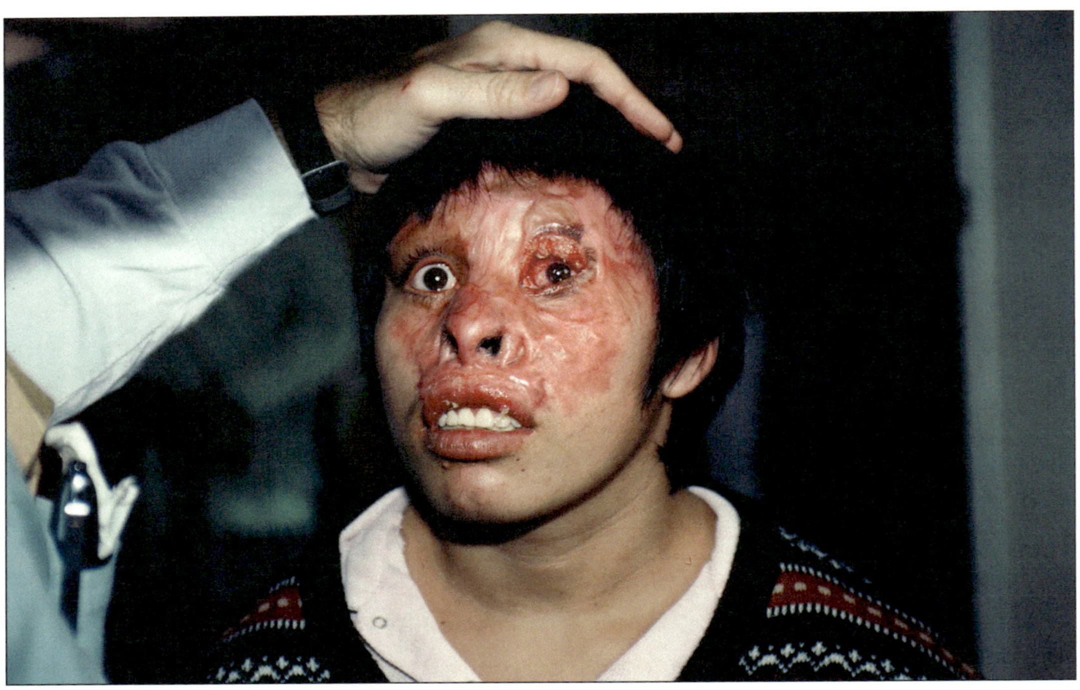

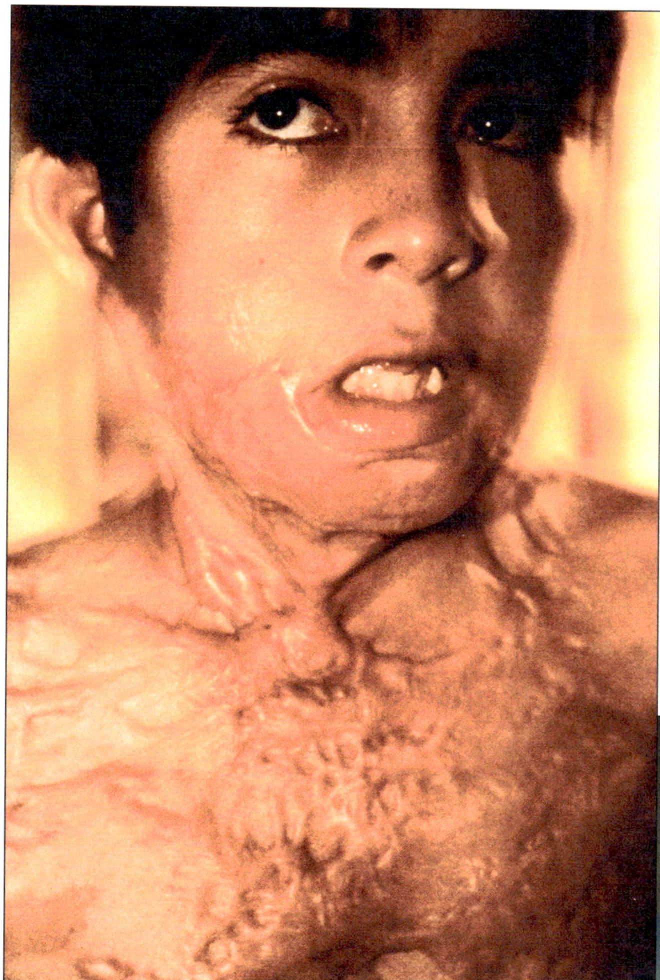

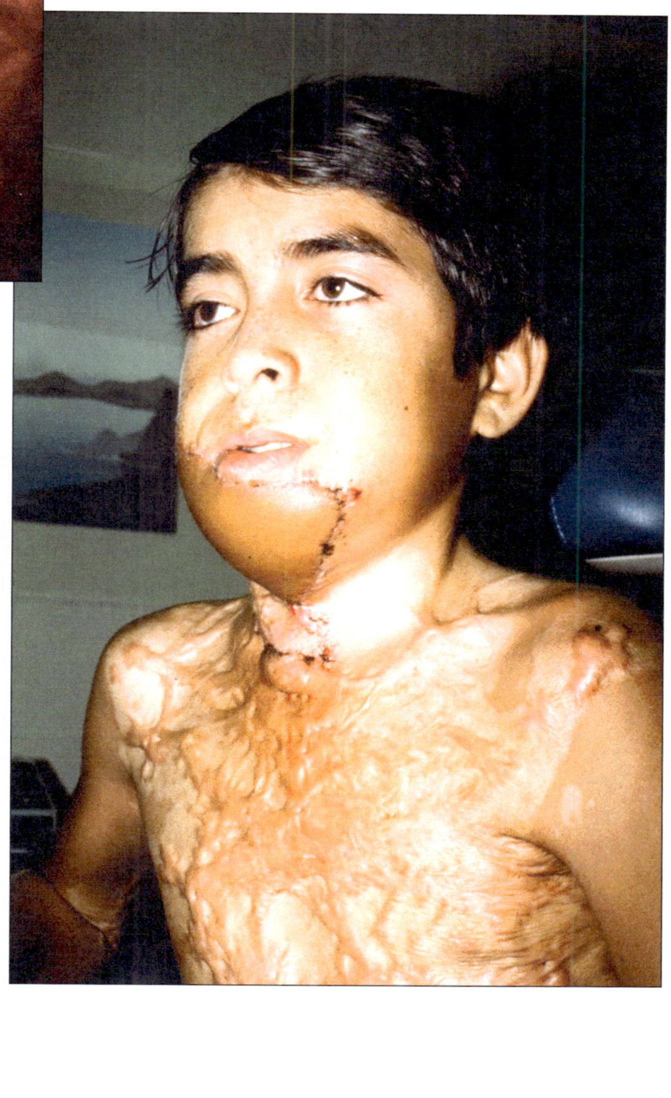

Post surgery

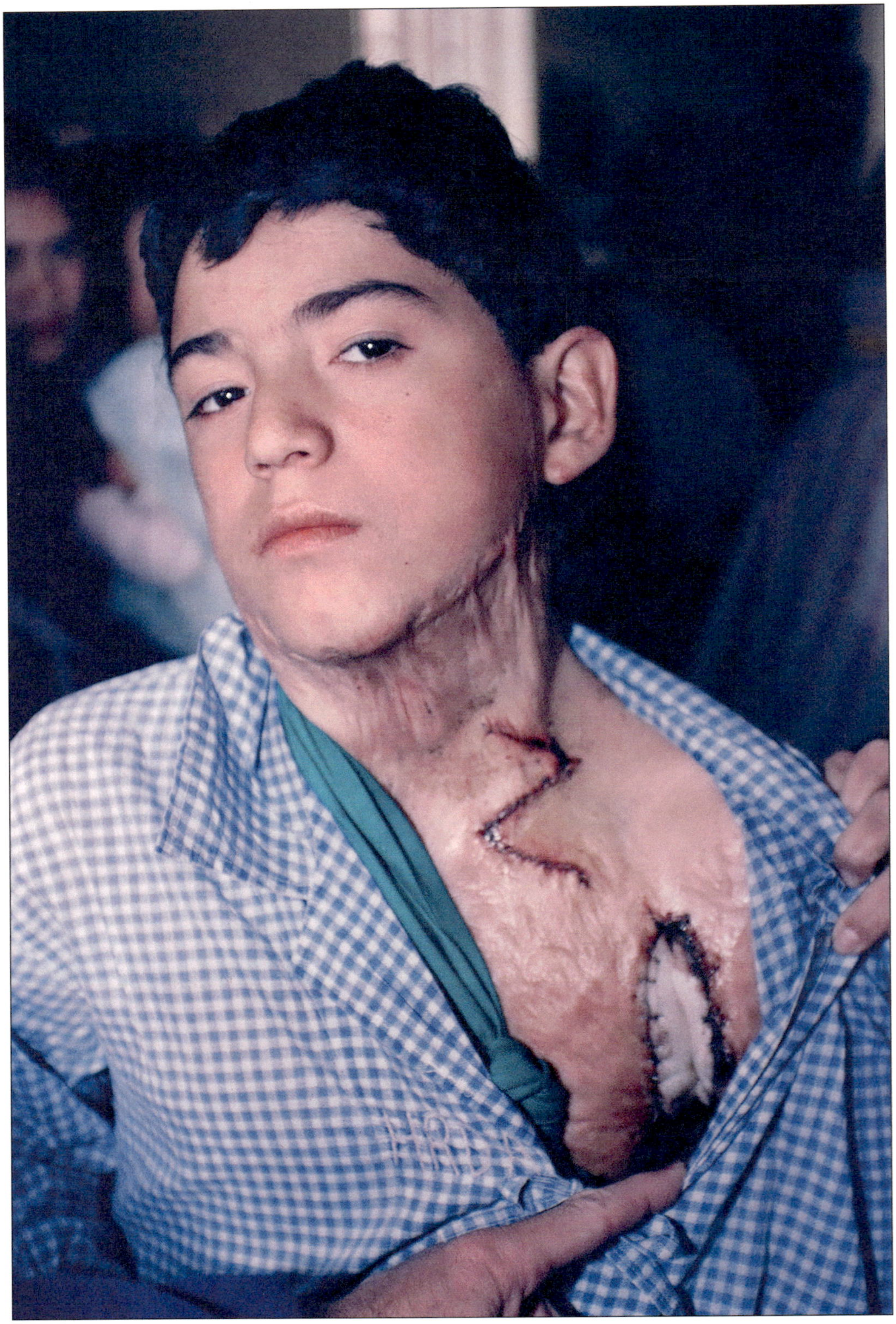

After first-stage surgery

More clubfeet repairs

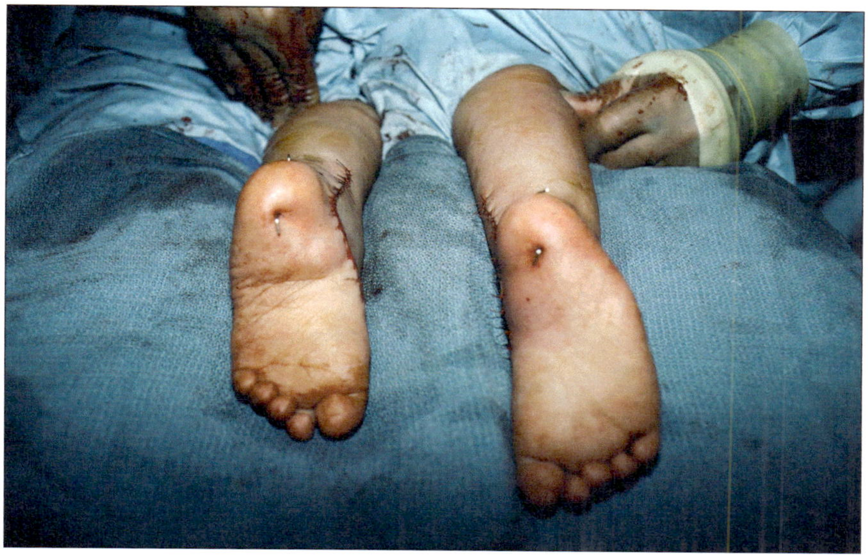

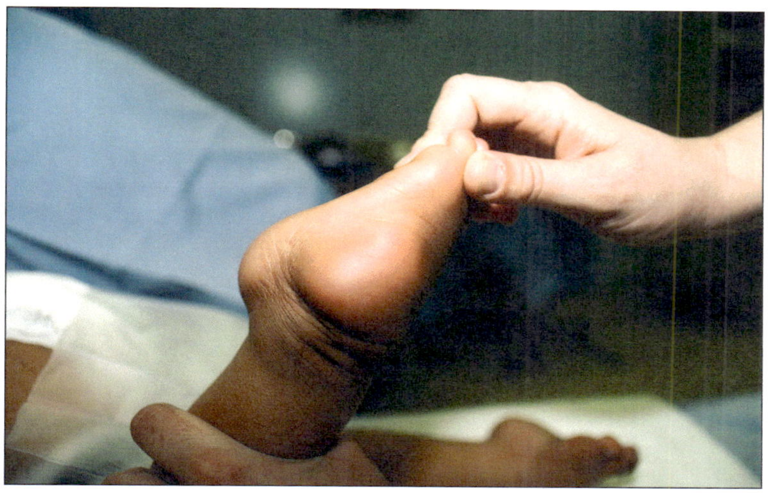

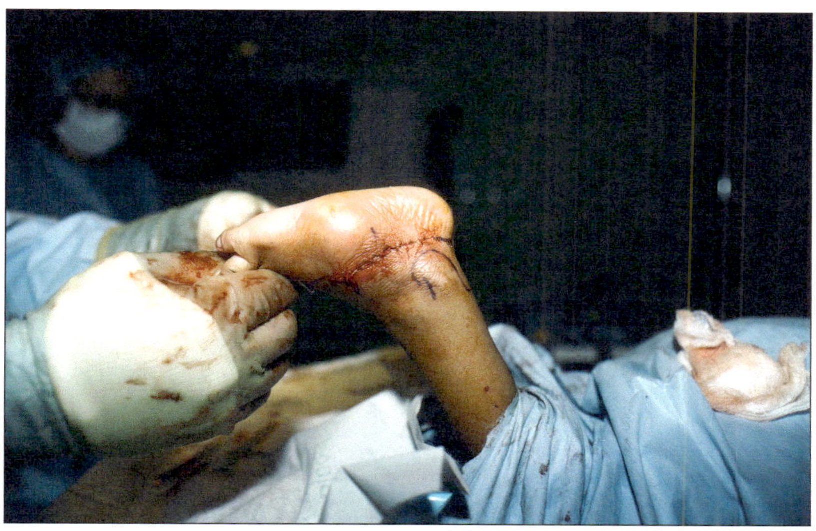

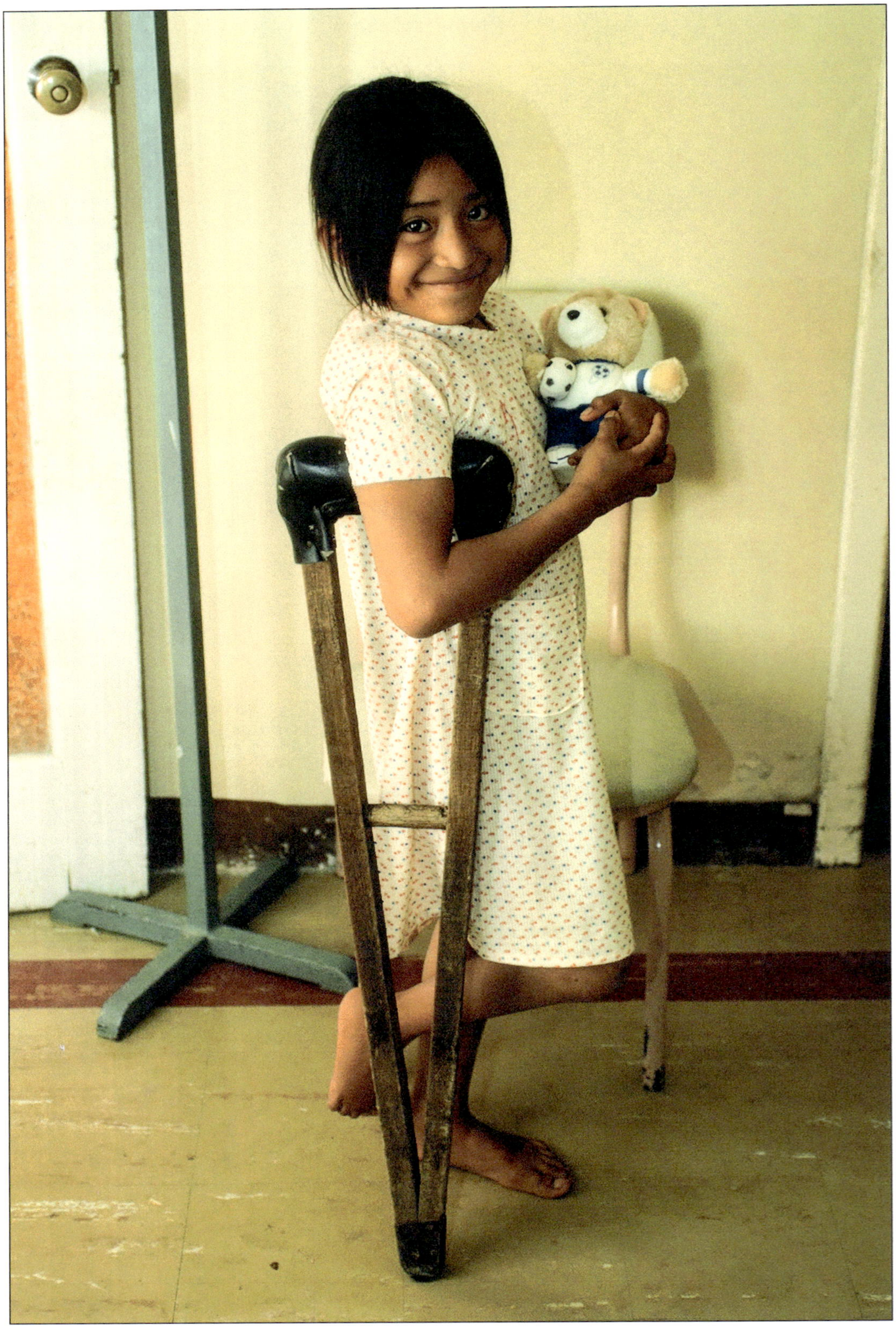

11-year-old with severe knee flexion contracture (and stuffed animal)

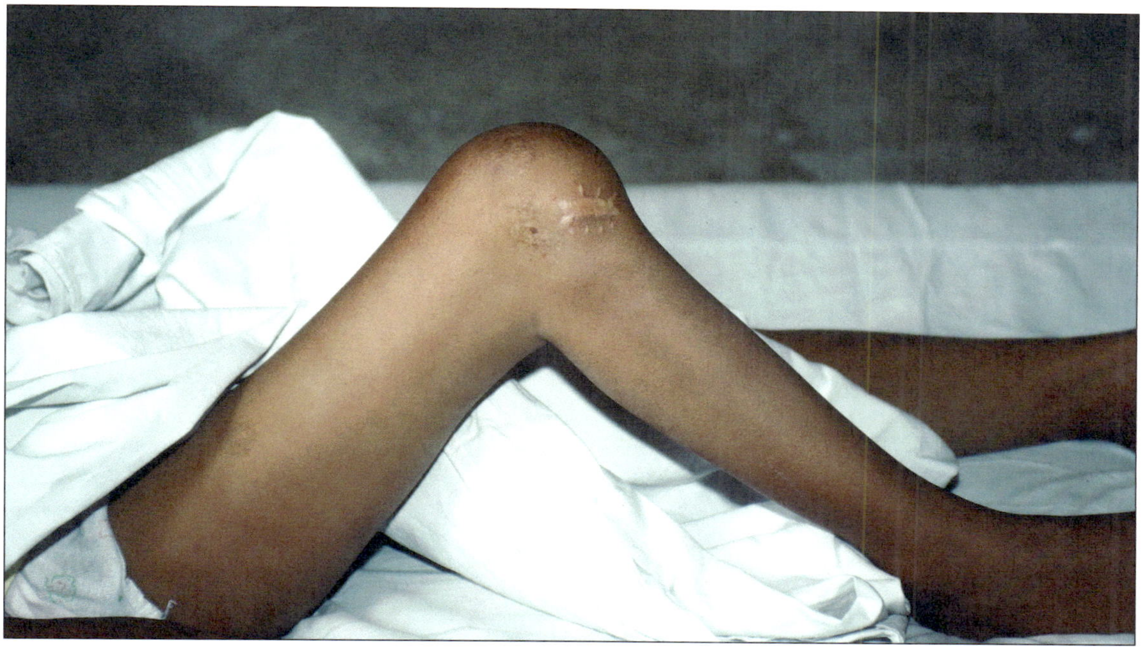

On operating table

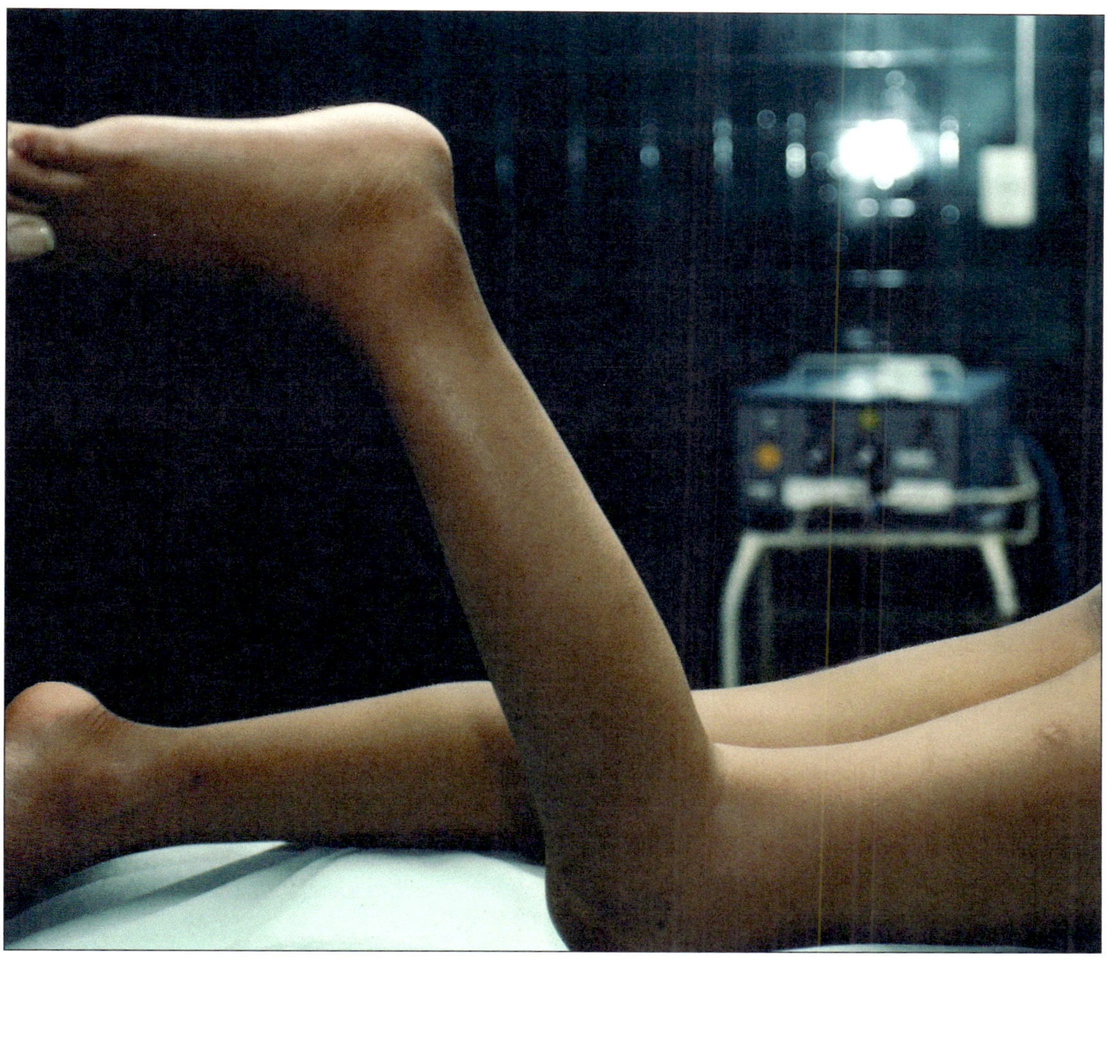

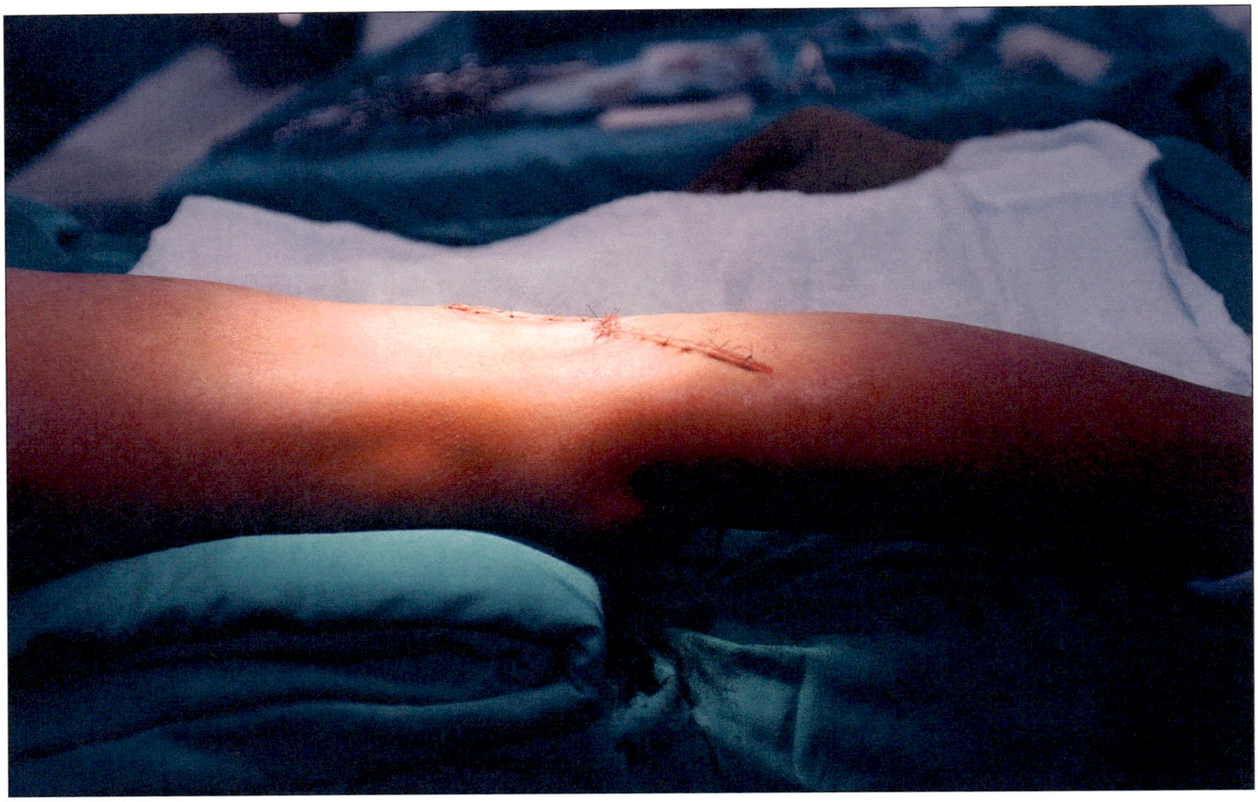

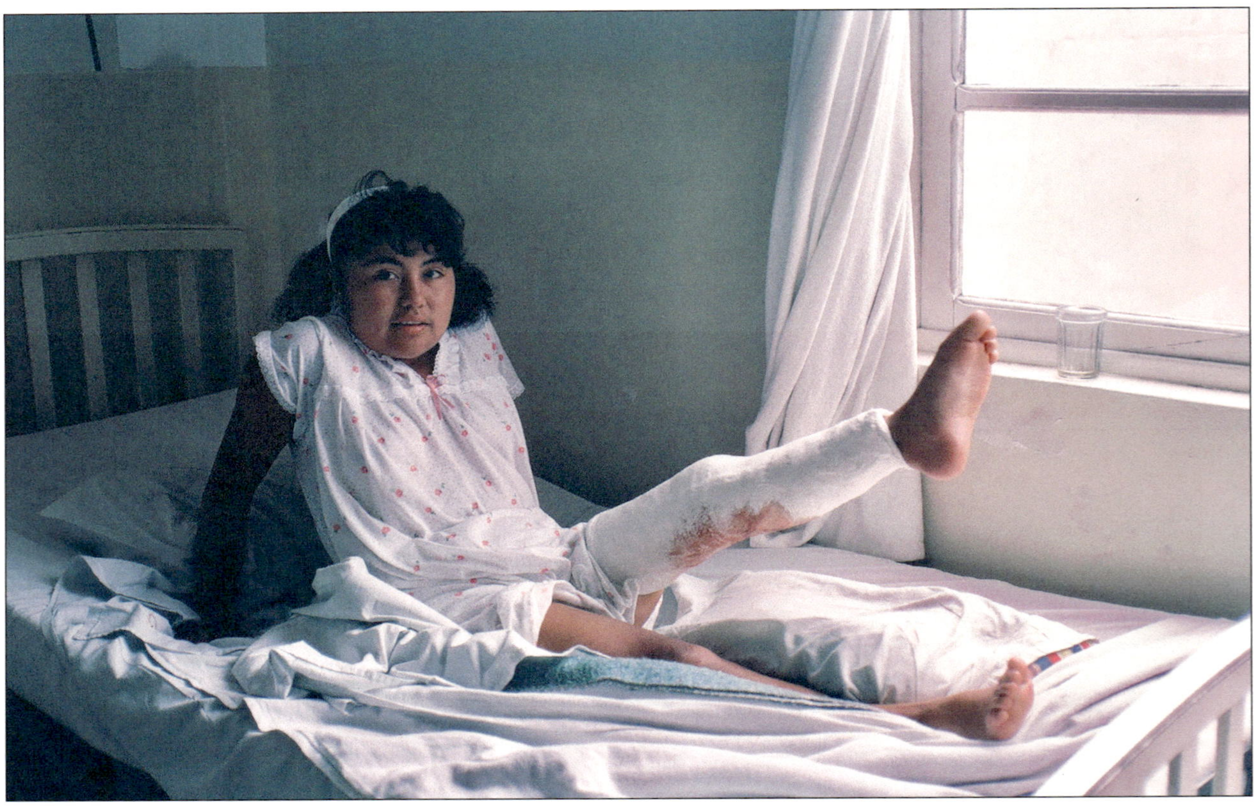

Post surgery

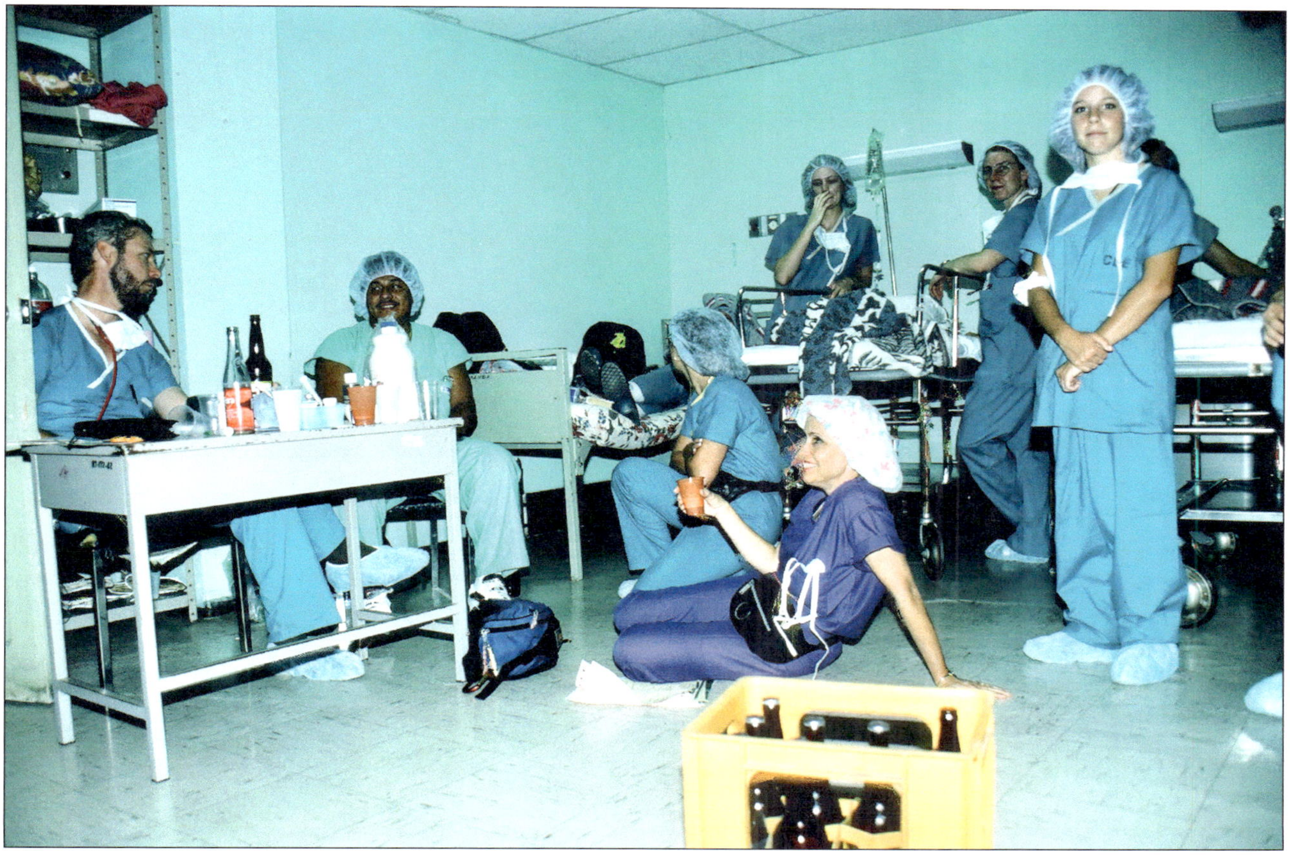

Lunch break

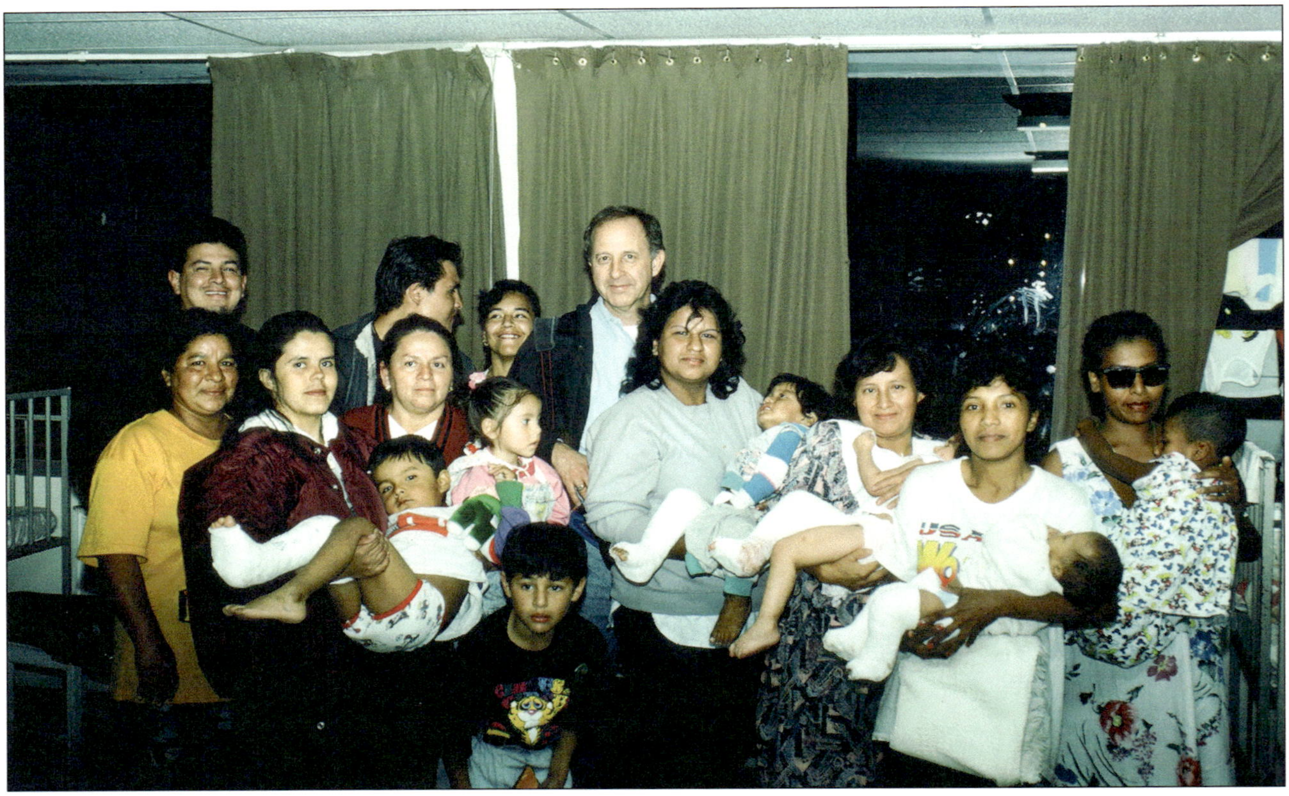

With patients post-op

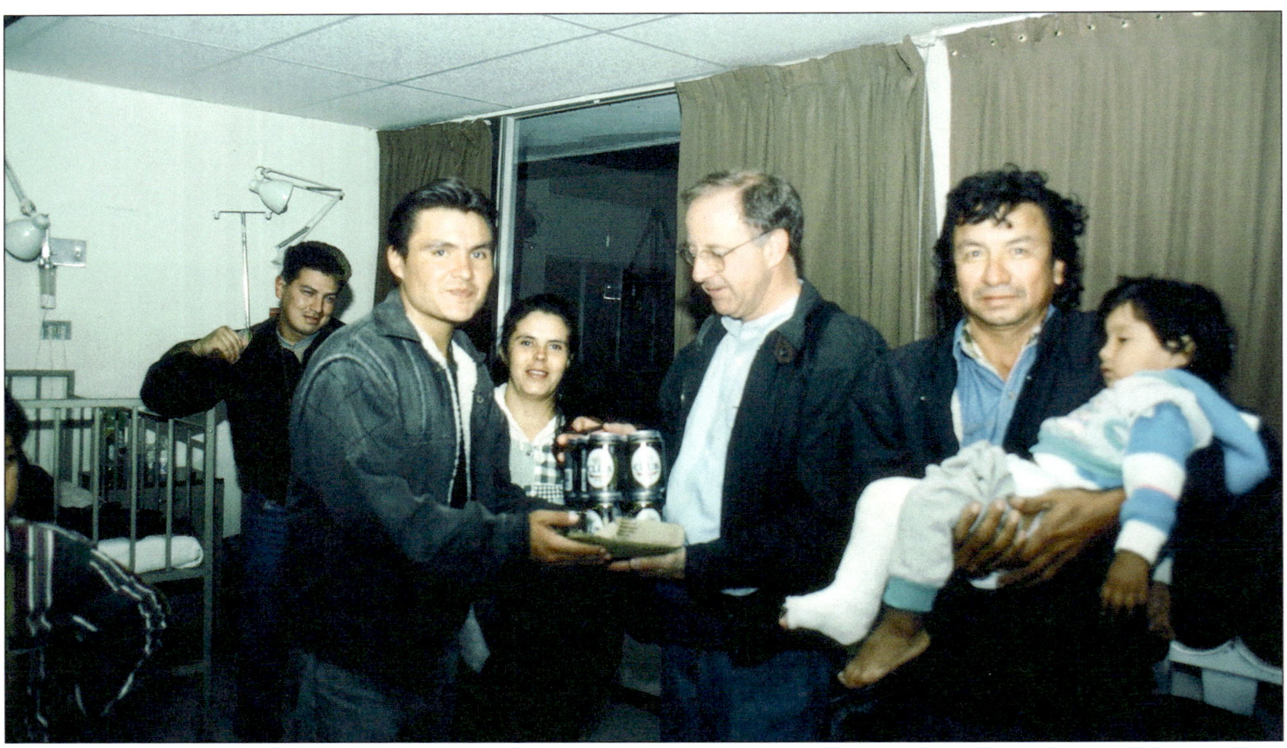

Showing gratitude with six pack of beer

Two years later we returned to Ecuador to the community of Loja. We flew to Guayaquil and were transported by military aircraft to Loja. At the military airport, dozens of patients showed up, so we ended up conducting a clinic, which delayed our departure for about an hour. We were housed in private homes during our stay, and our hosts relegated us to a very small room with a double bed with a huge sag in the middle, such that it was an effort for either one of us to climb out of bed, and, due to the small size of our room, our suitcases took up most of what was left after the mattress. The family was very accommodating, however, and we tolerated the minor inconveniences.

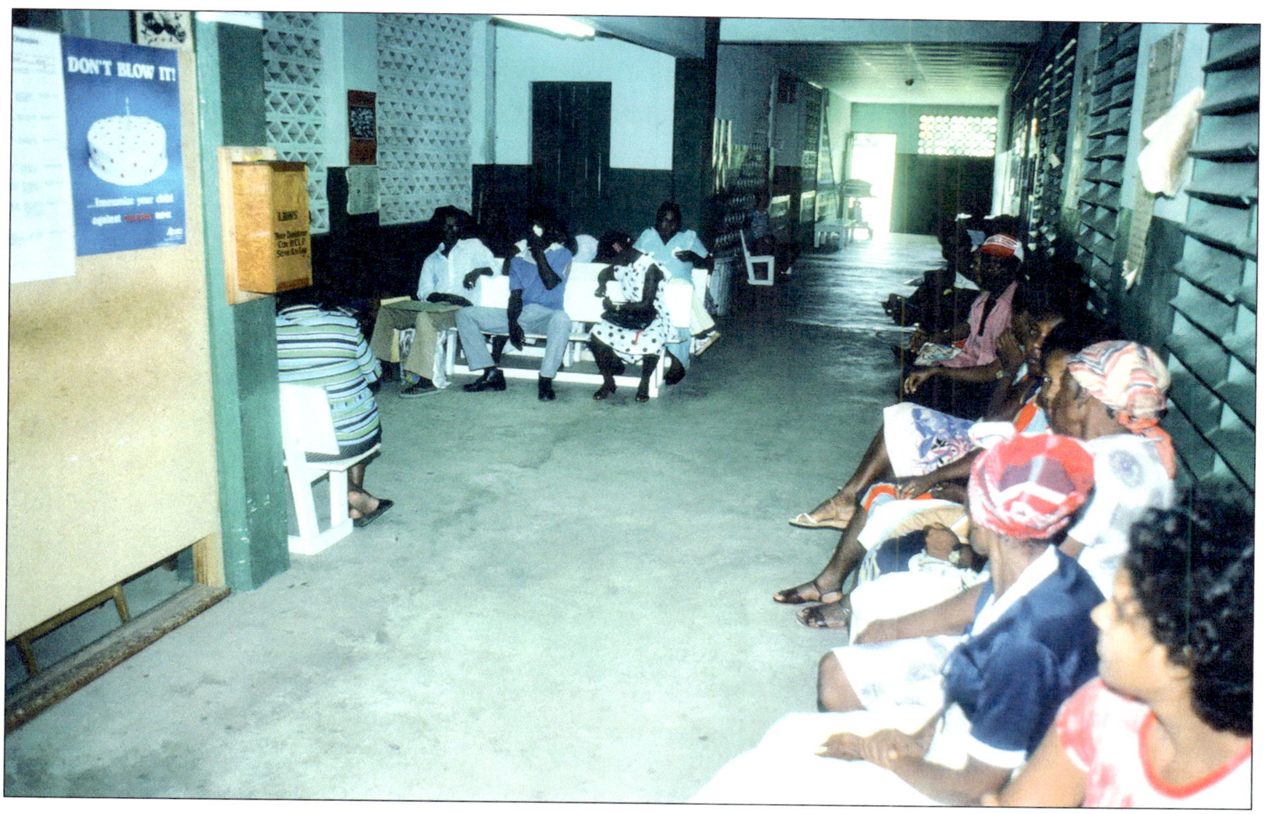

Patients waiting to be seen at military airport

Dr. Morrison has continued to make annual trips to Ecuador and has founded an organization for these efforts titled Fundacion de Paz y Salud, Foundation for Peace and Health.

Pakistan

We traveled under the auspices of several different organizations, one of which was Orthopedics Overseas. There were three countries we visited under this umbrella, and the first was Pakistan in 1986, during the Russian invasion of Afghanistan. We traveled to the northern city of Peshawar, situated some 30 miles from the Khyber Pass and Afghanistan and a rather parochial city and hotbed of Islamic Fundamentalism. We worked at the Afghan Surgical Hospital, treating injured Afghan soldiers who had been transported from the battlefield, often aboard mules, since ambulances and motorized vehicles were easy targets for the Russian airships. The hospital contained two floors constructed in a square with a central courtyard separating four wings. It was staffed by Pakistani and Afghan surgeons. Supplies were scarce, and patients abundant. There were two operating rooms, and they were busy most every day, oftentimes two surgeries being performed simultaneously in the same operating room. Needless to say, there were many wound infections secondary to the operating room environment, wound contamination, and the delay in treatment due to transportation difficulties.

Supplies were scarce, and patients abundant.

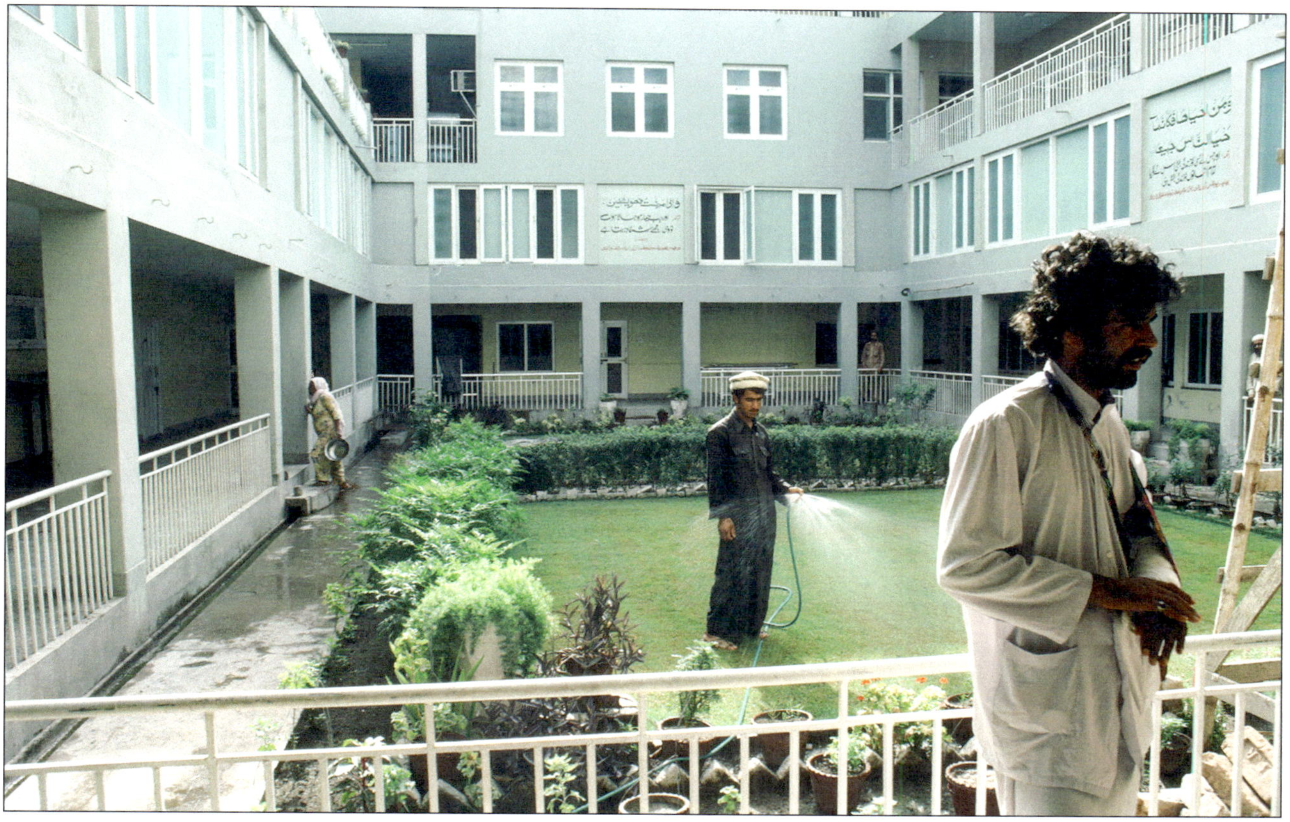

Hospital courtyard

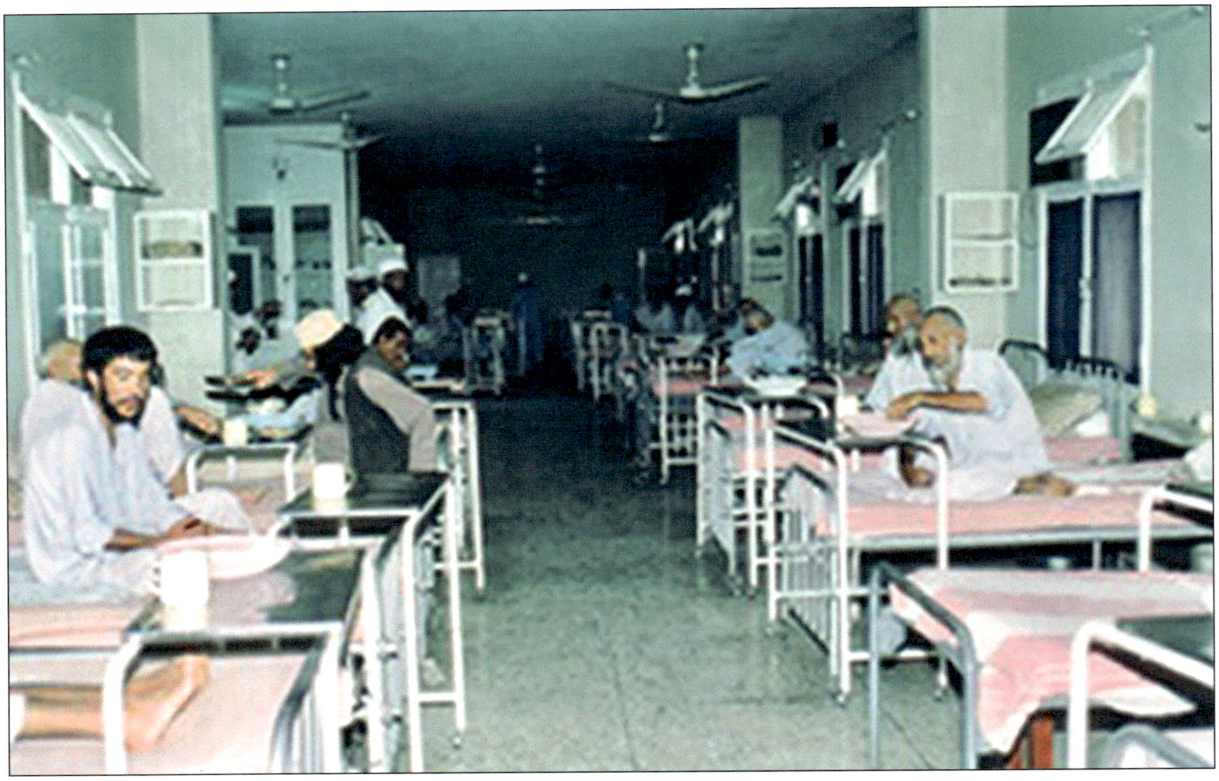

Hospital ward

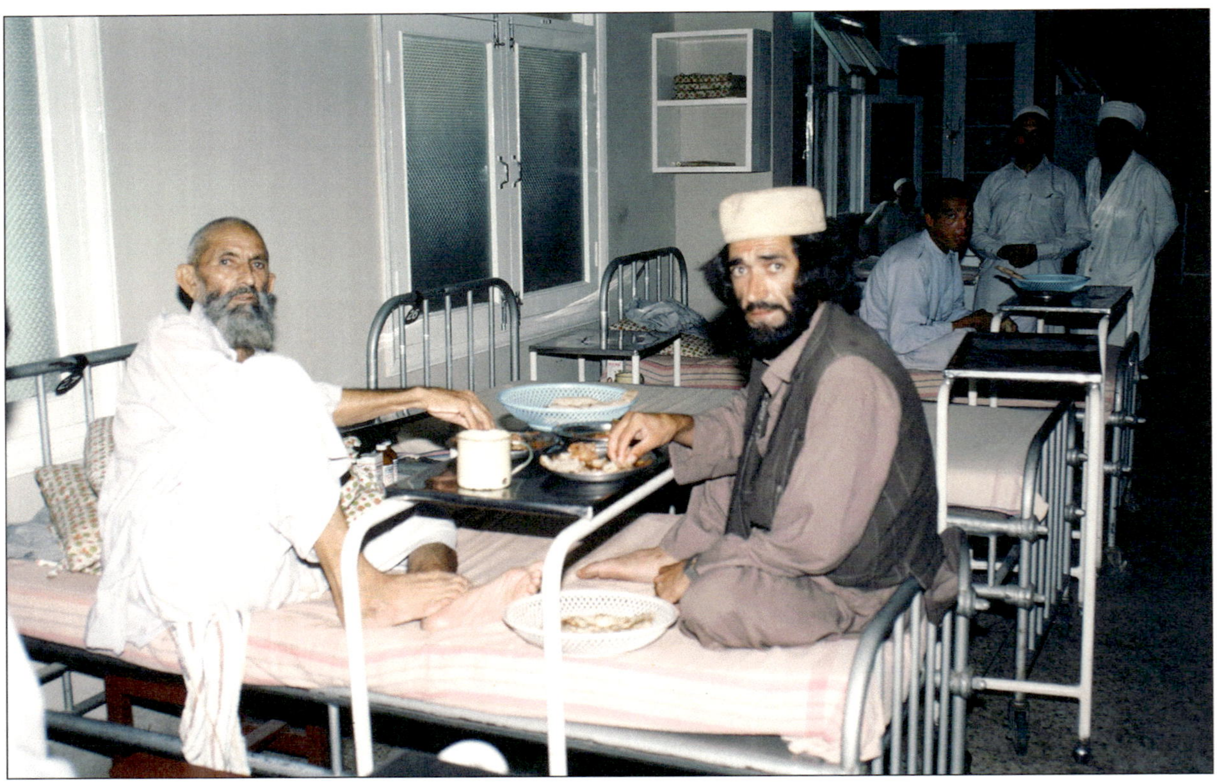

Family members or friends at bedside to assist with patient care

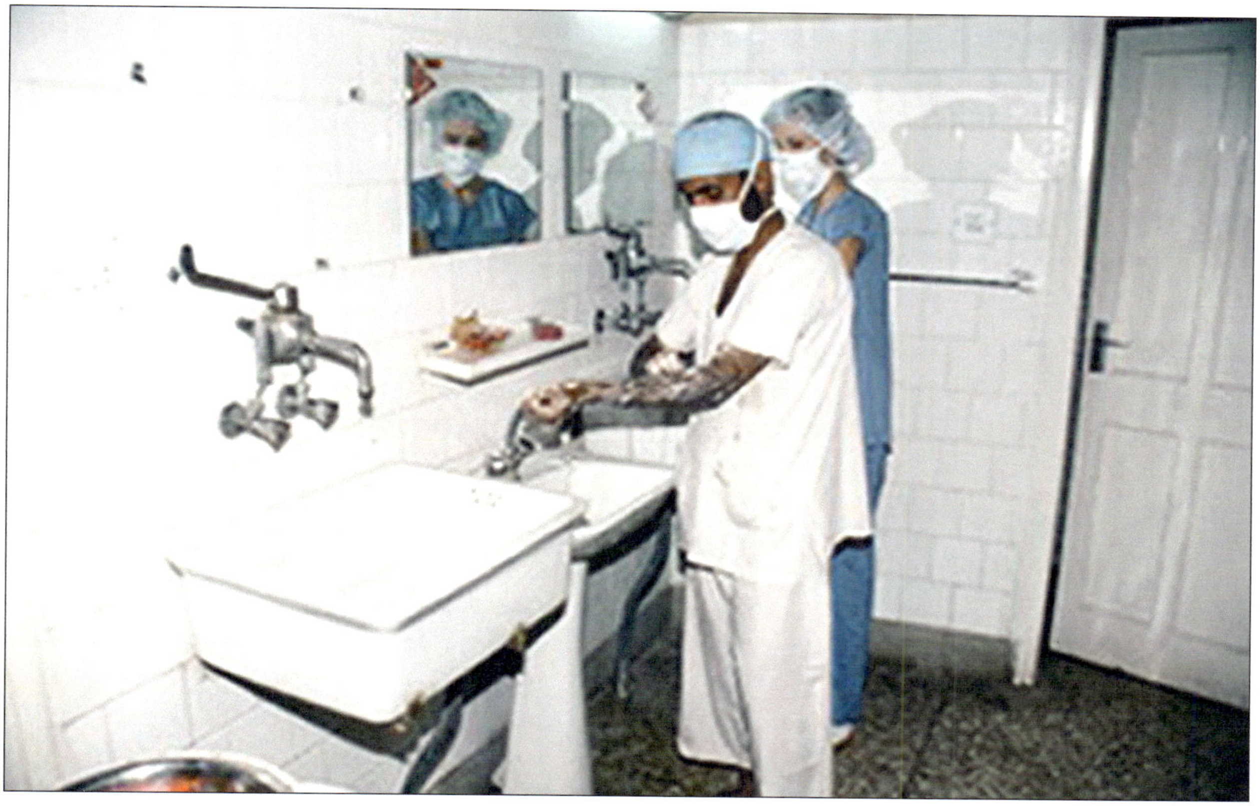

Scrubbing for surgery

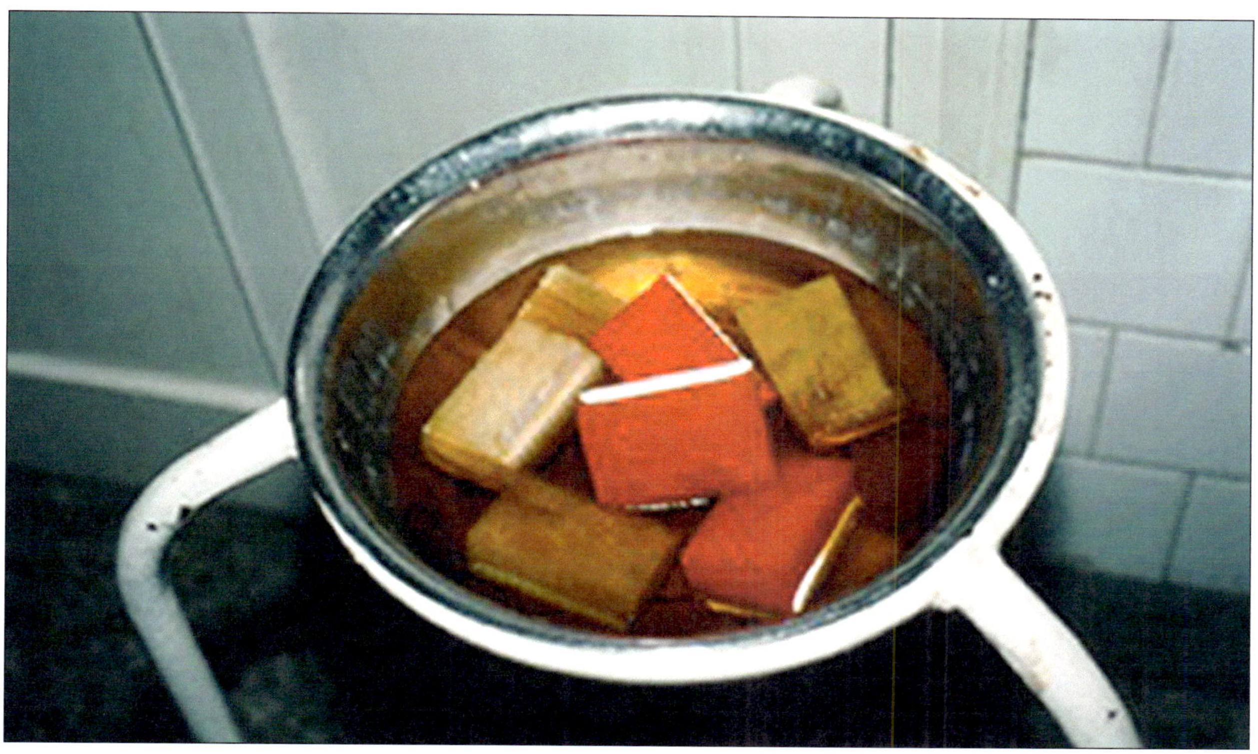

Reusing "disposable" scrub brushes

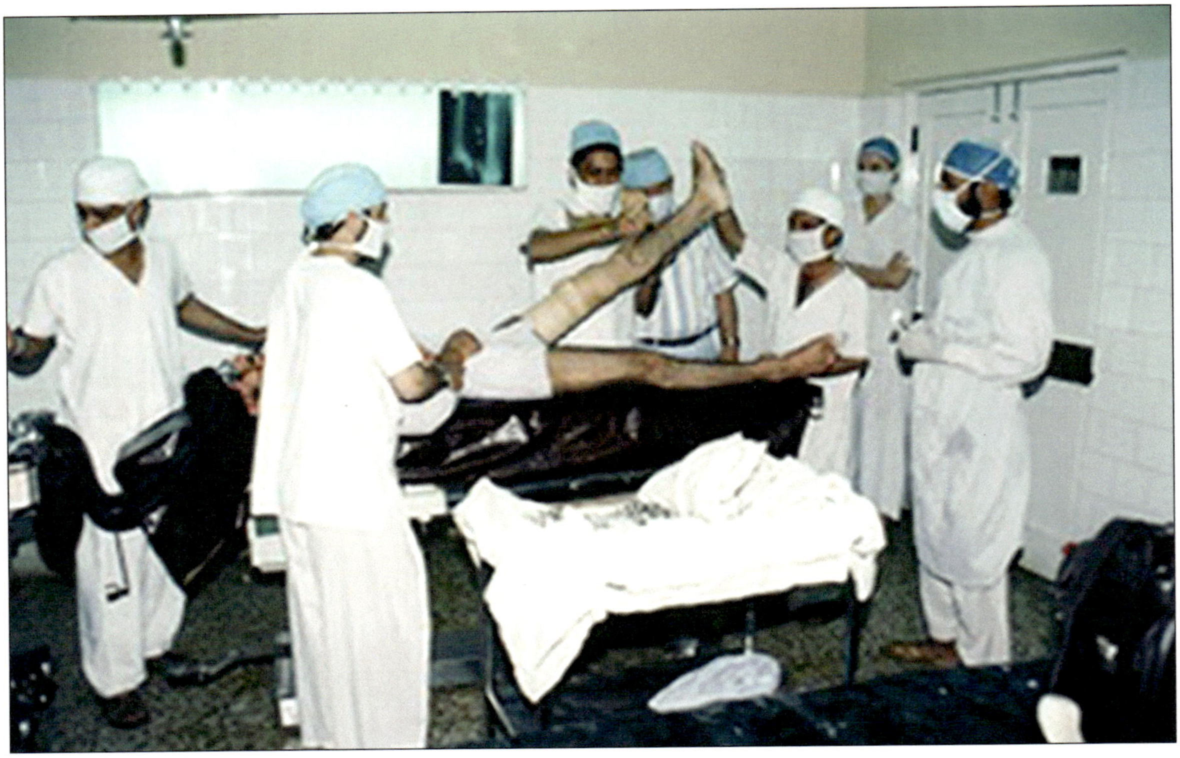

Operating Room

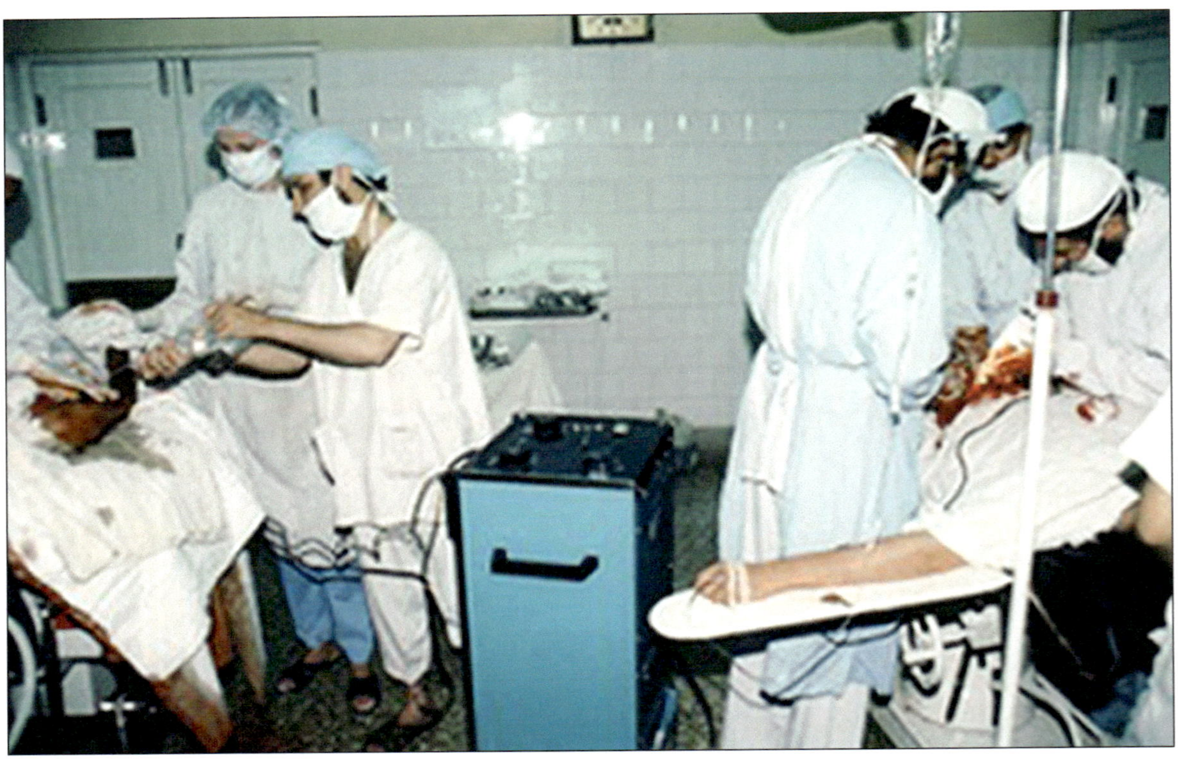

Simultaneous surgeries

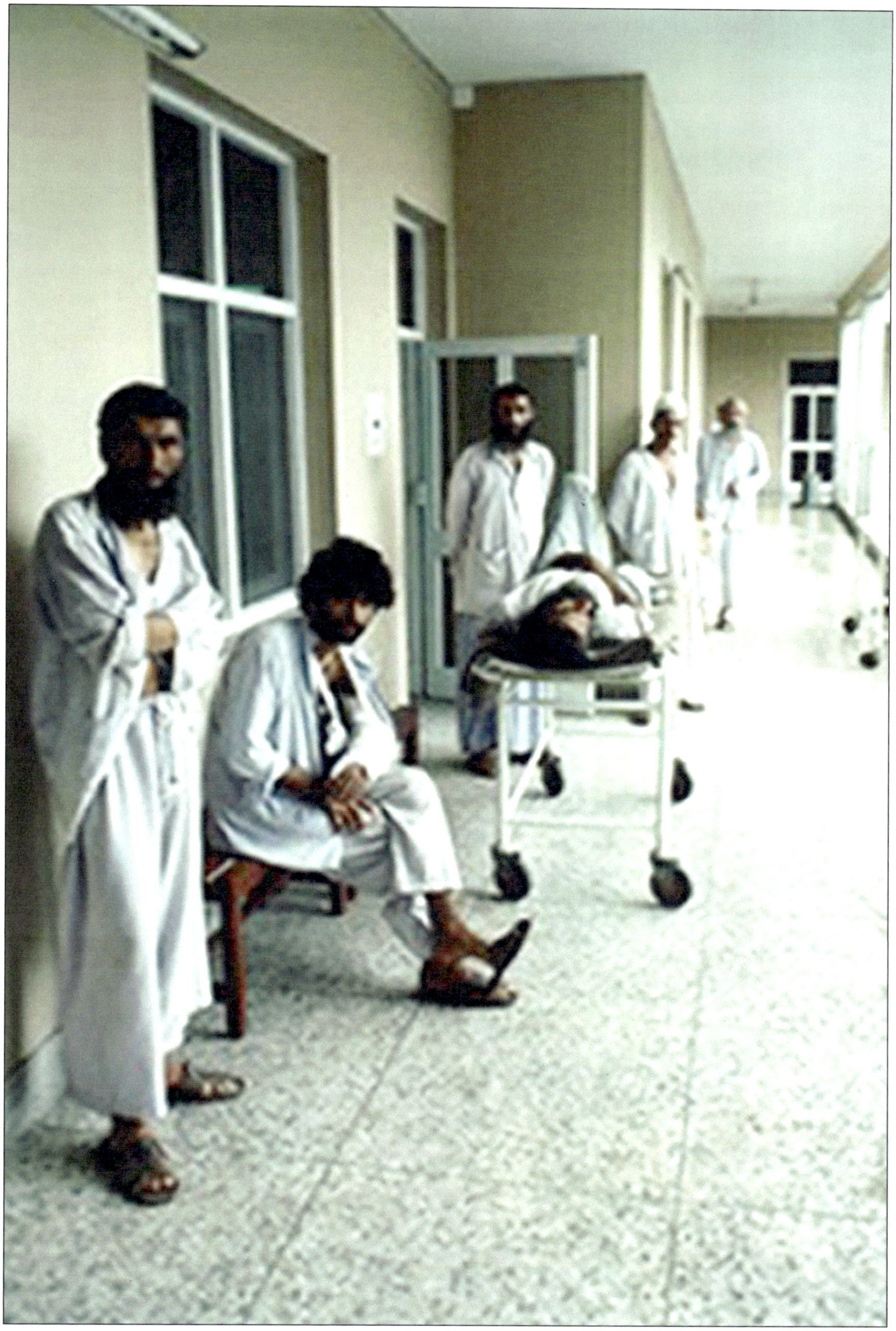

Patients in “pre-op holding area” waiting to be taken into surgery

I was impressed by the loyalty and dedication of the wounded regarding their desire to be cured so they could return to their country and fight the Russians. I suspect many of these were members of the Taliban, which we eventually faced in our own Afghanistan war. Outside the hospital there was a wall with photos of the soldiers who had entered martyrdom. There were also several children in the hospital with various fractures, amputations, and burns that were said to have been caused by the Russians dropping toys into the villages, only to have them explode once they were handled.

I was impressed by the loyalty and dedication of the wounded regarding their desire to be cured so they could return to their country and fight the Russians.

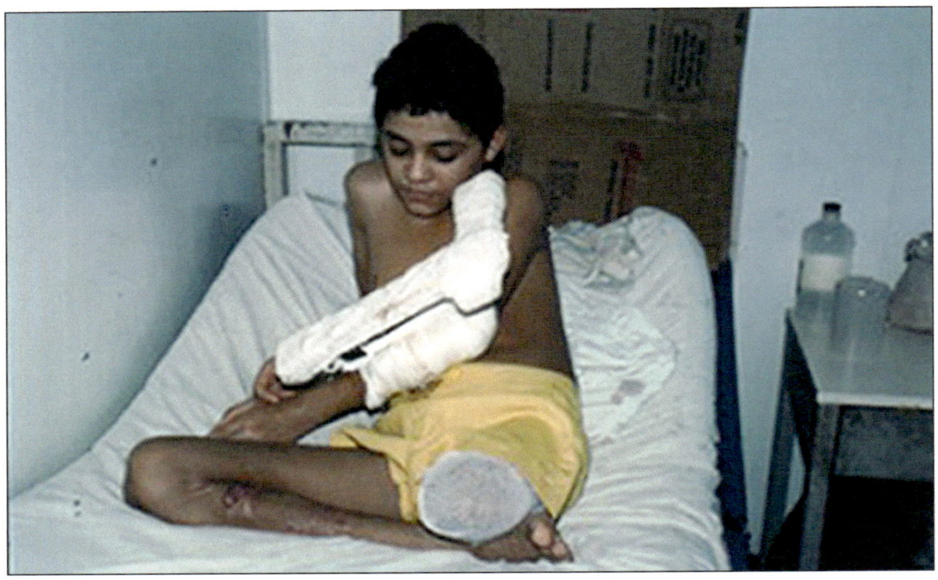

Boy with fractured arm and amputated left leg

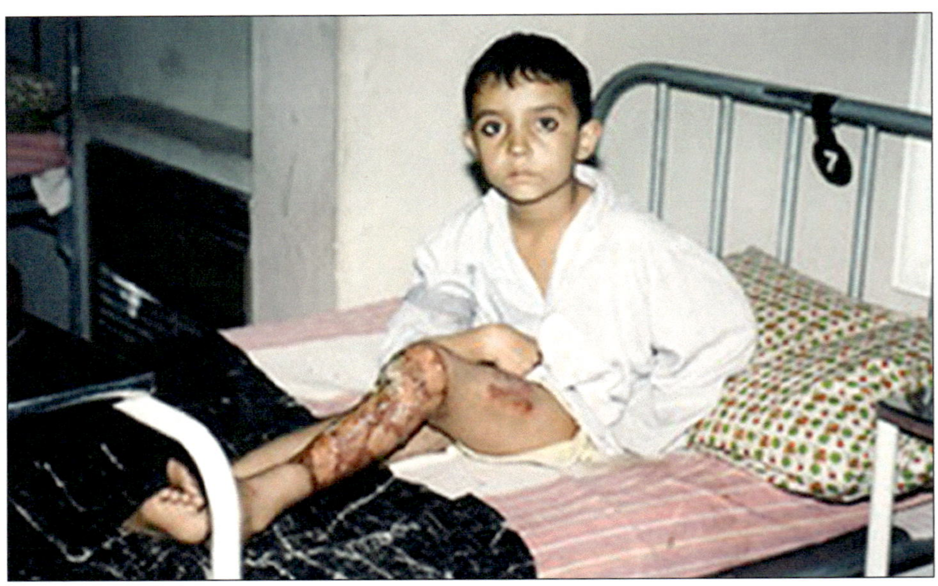

Severe burns left leg

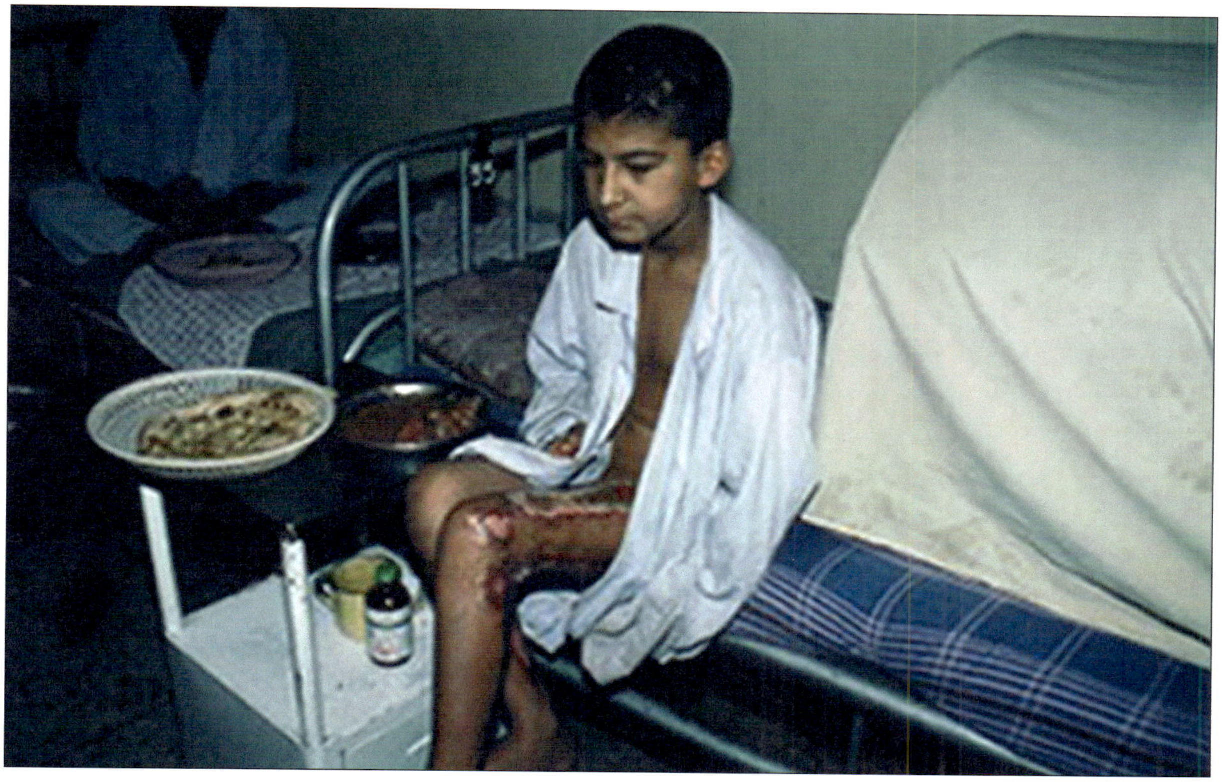

Left leg burns

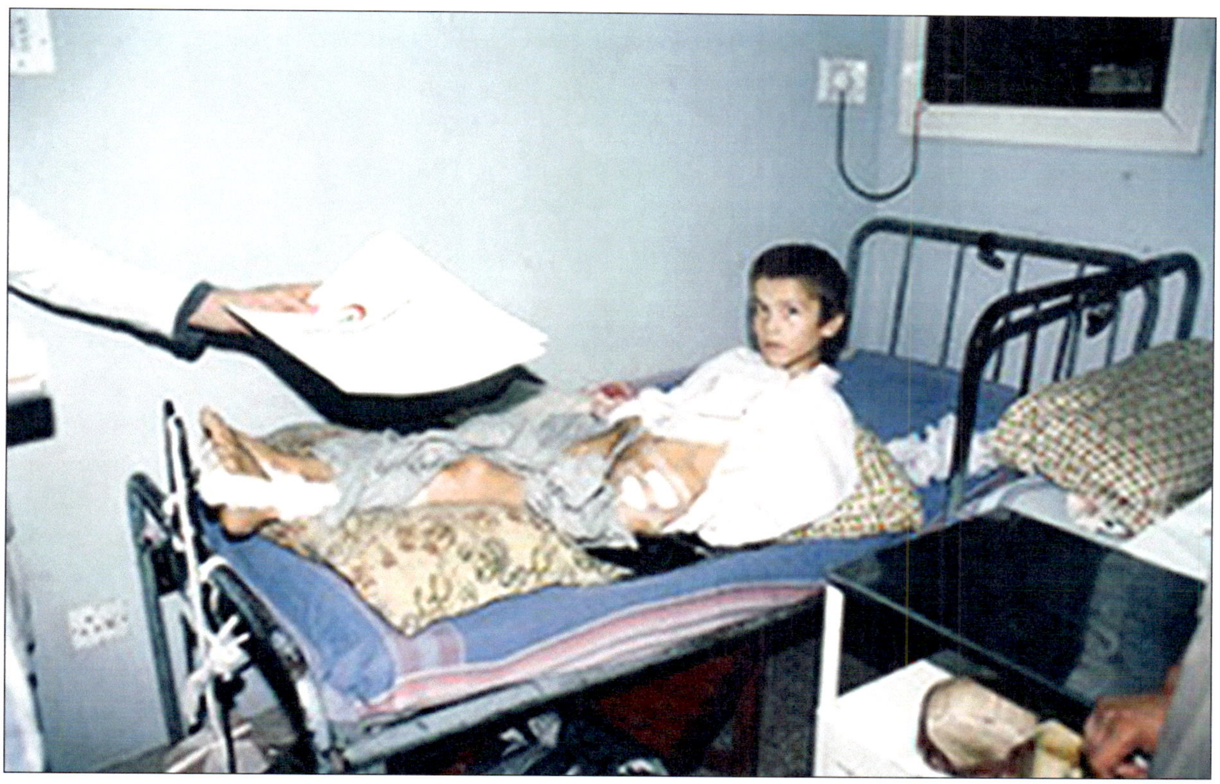

Fractured left femur in traction

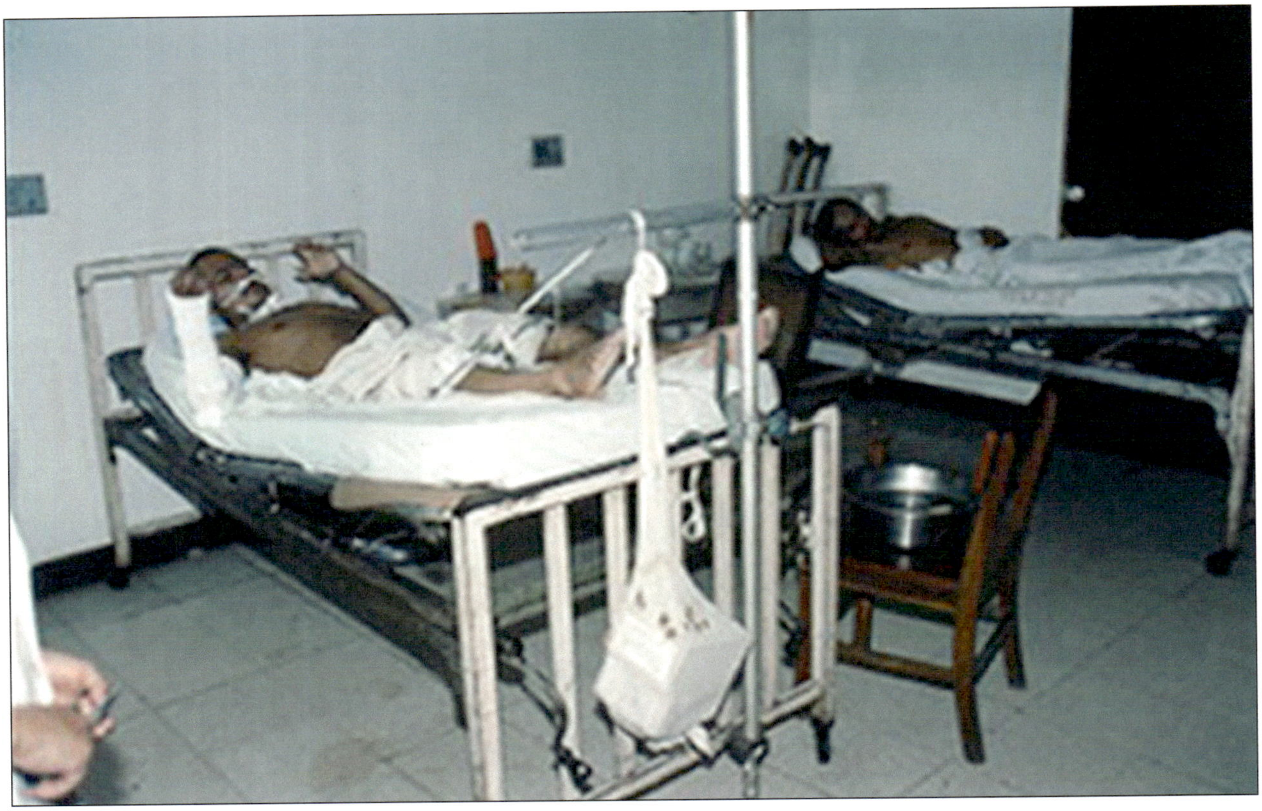

Improvised weights for traction

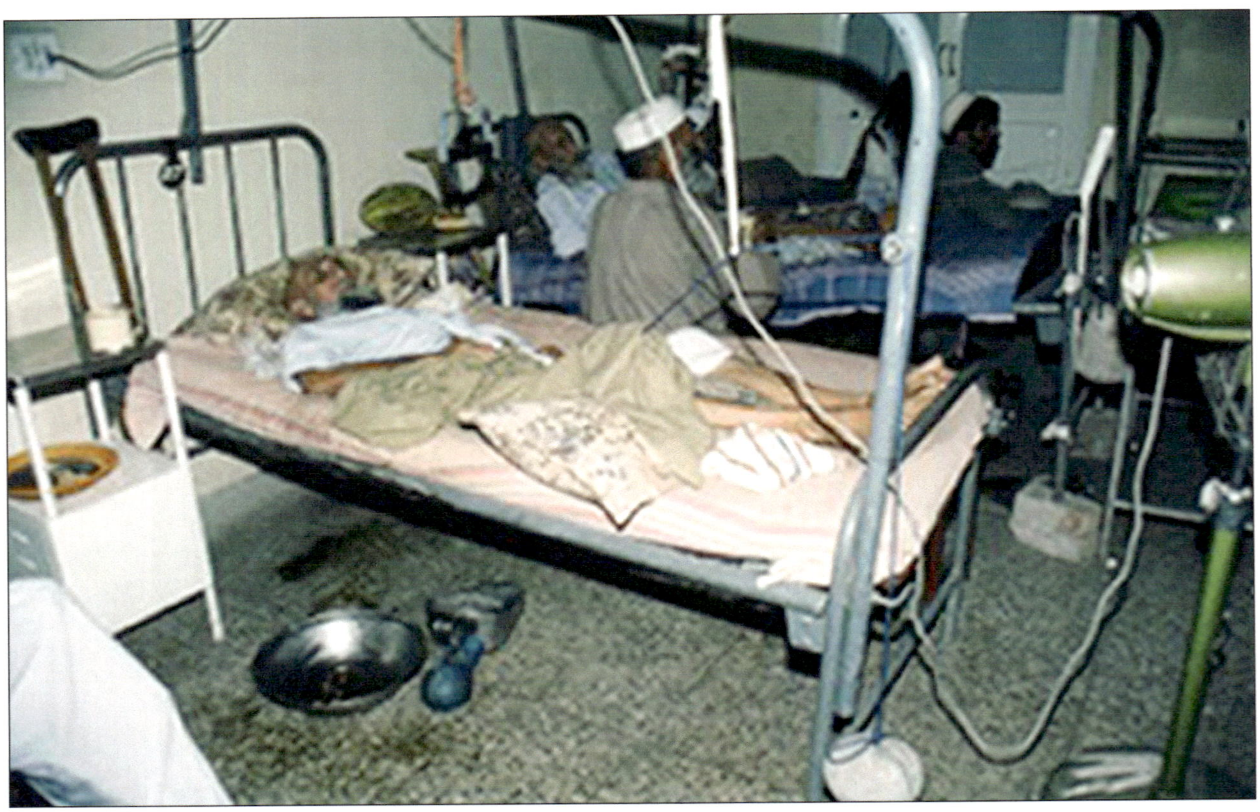

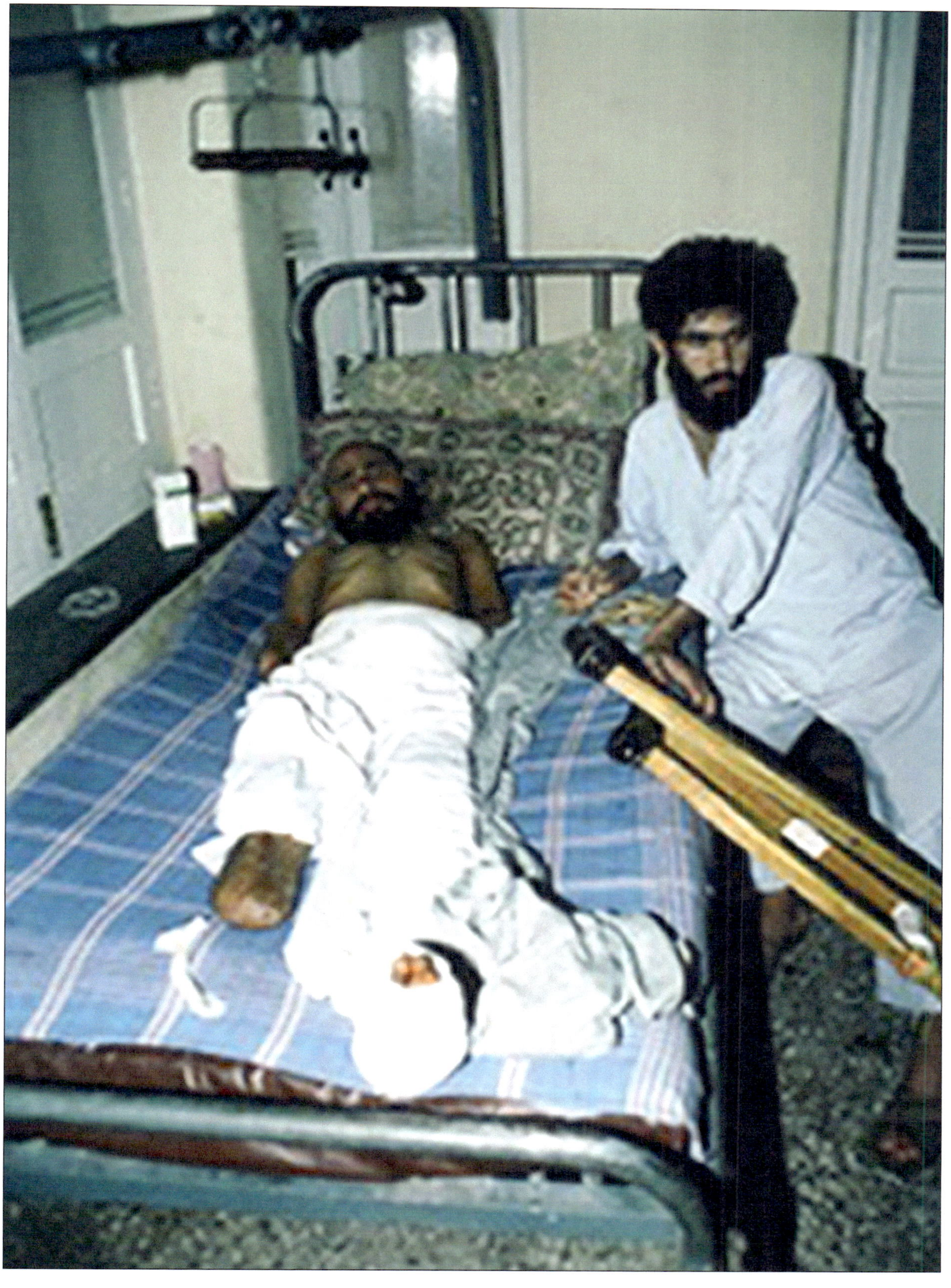

Amputated right leg and severe loss of skin on left hand attached to abdomen for skin flap coverage

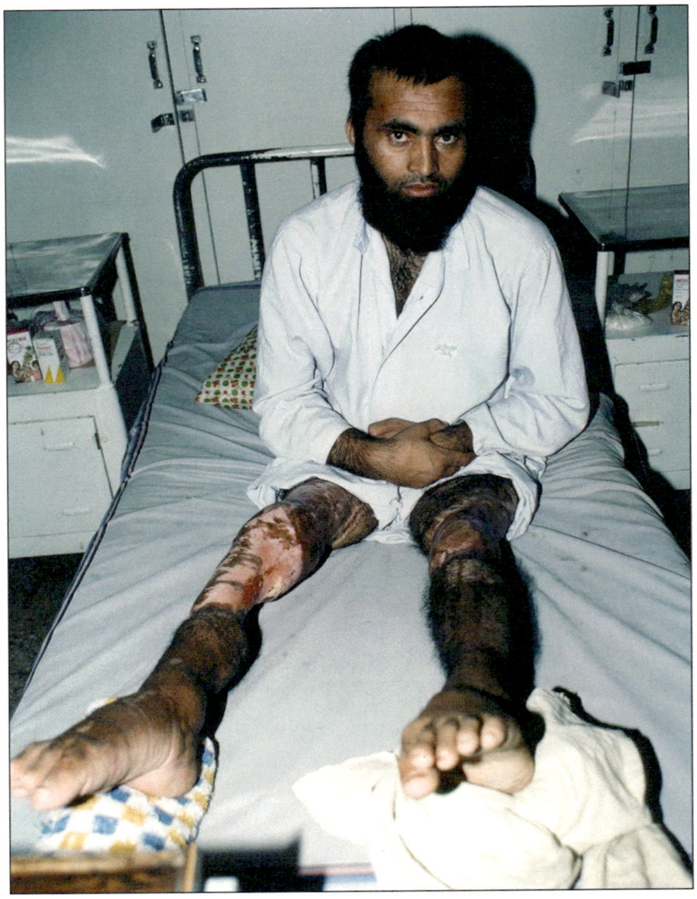

Man run over by an armored personnel carrier

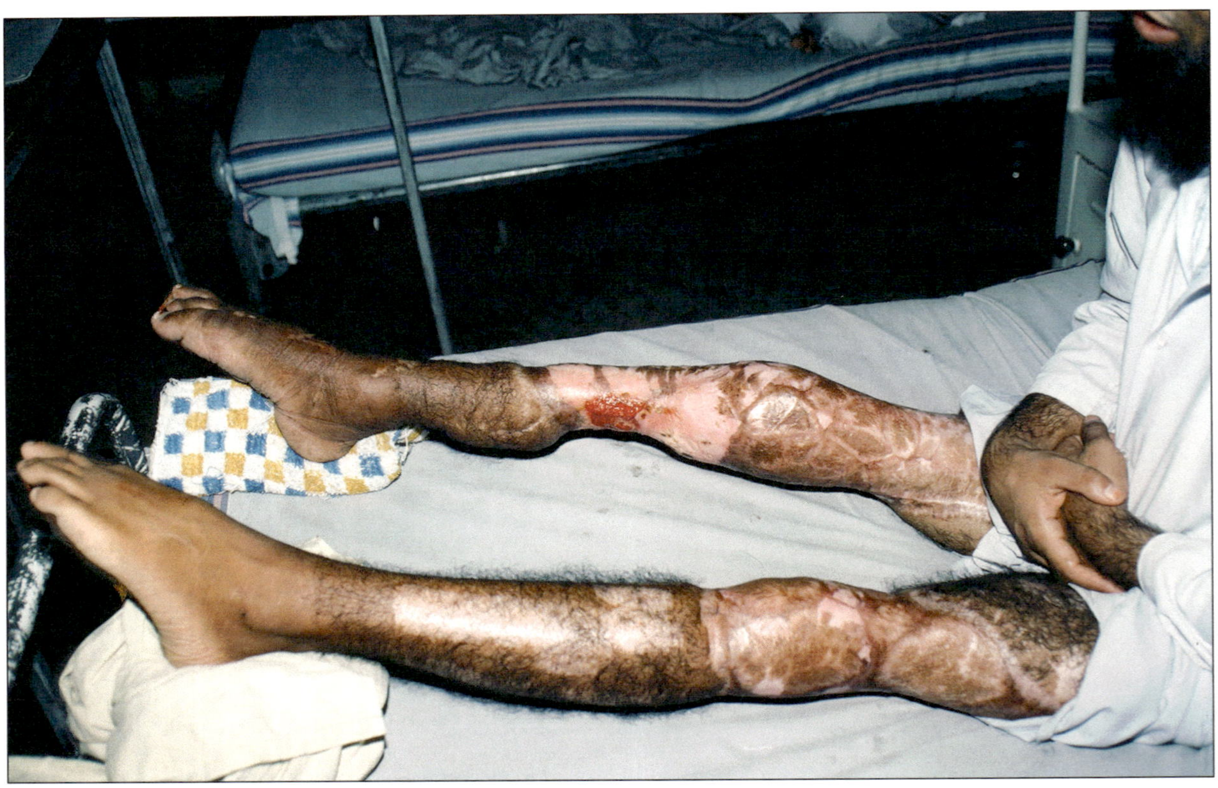

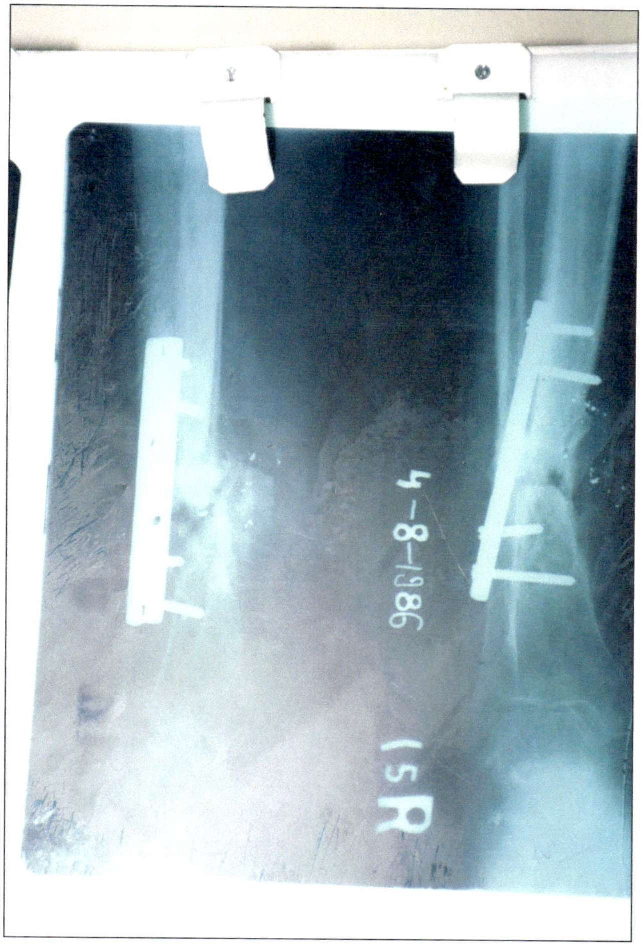

Tibial plate sticking out of skin

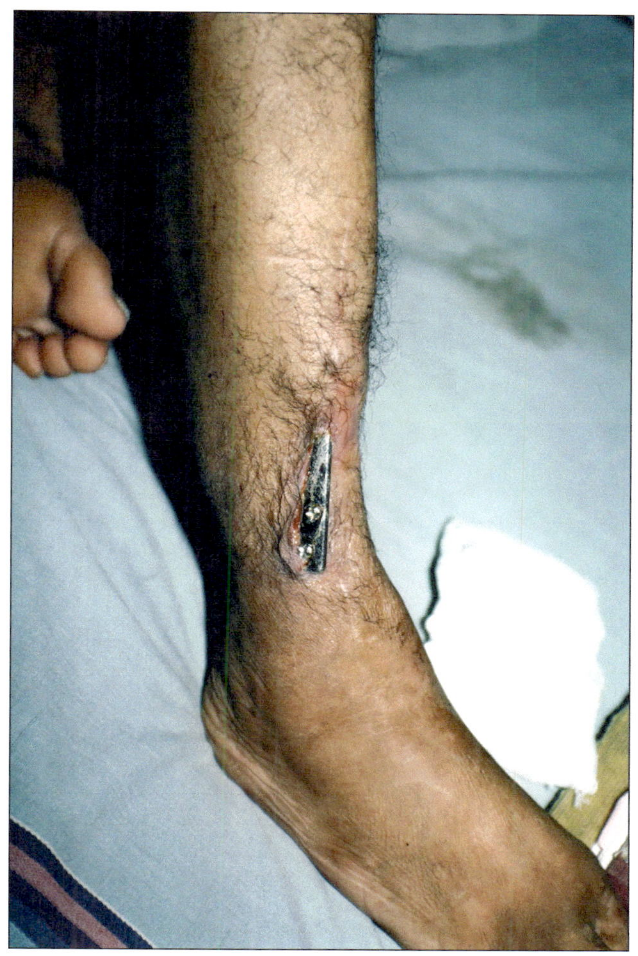

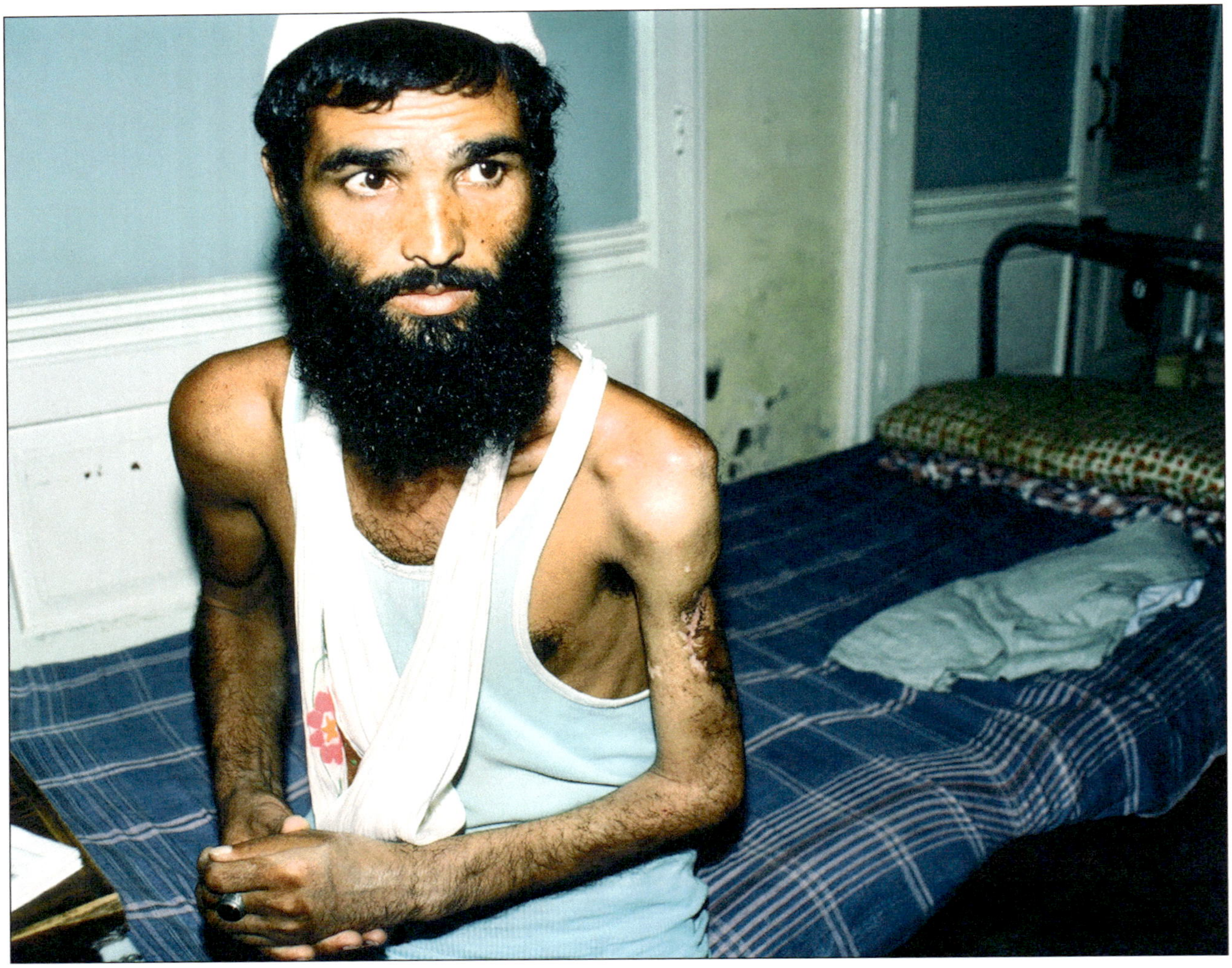

Gunshot wound to left arm with severe nerve damage

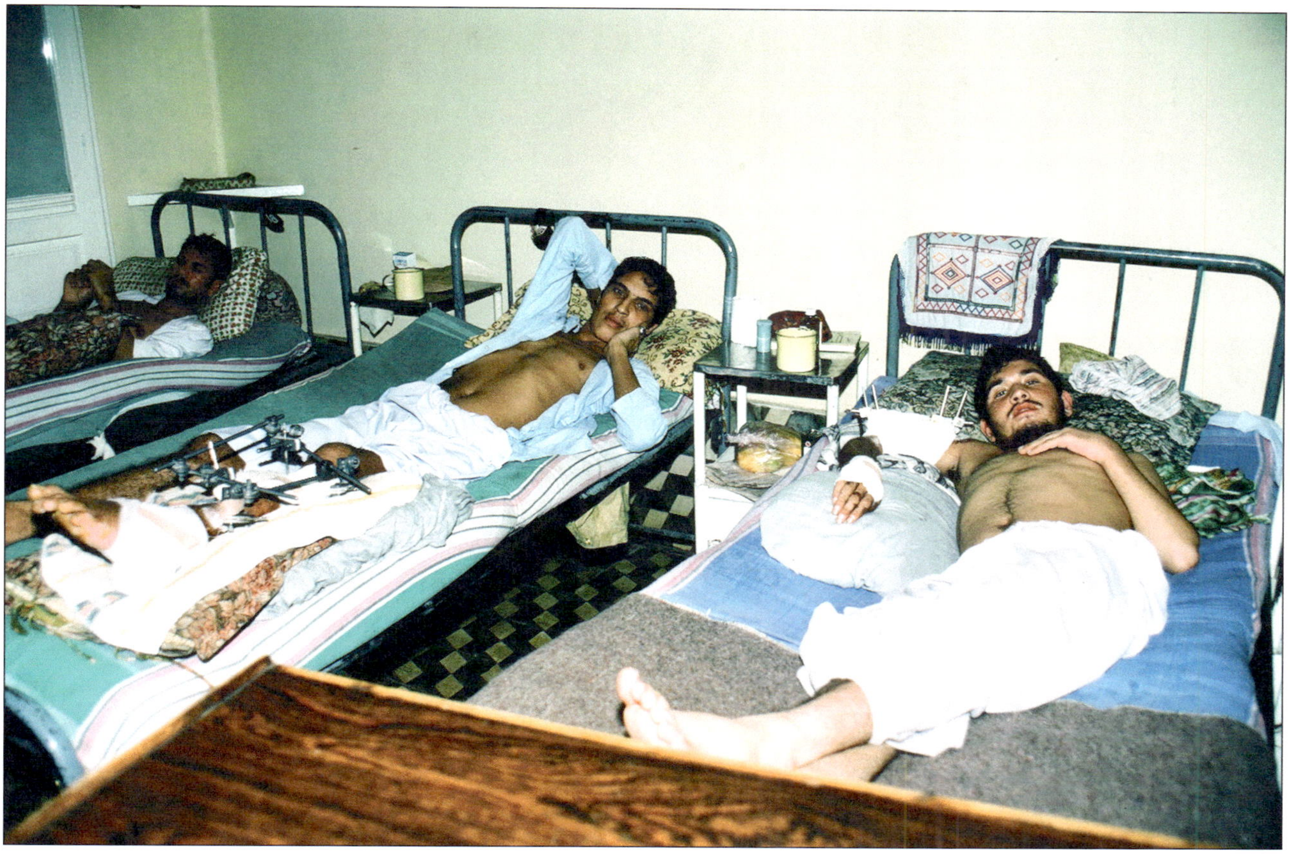

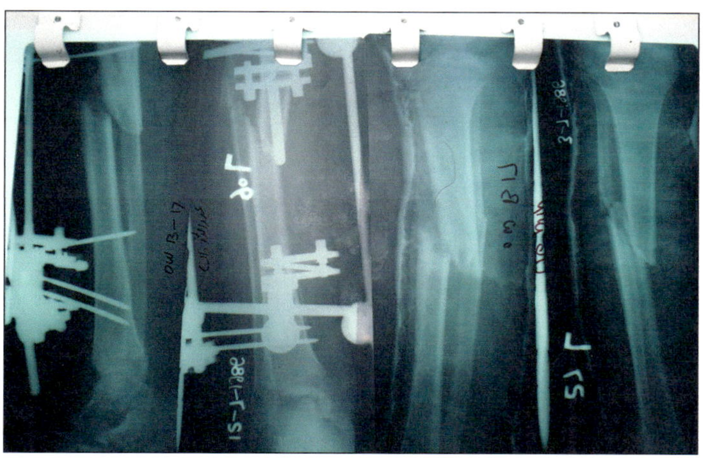

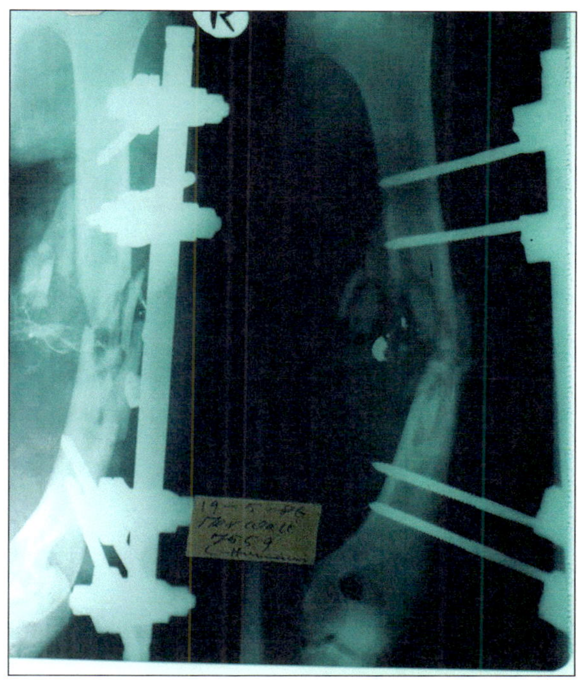

Patients with external fixators on tibia and humerus and X-rays

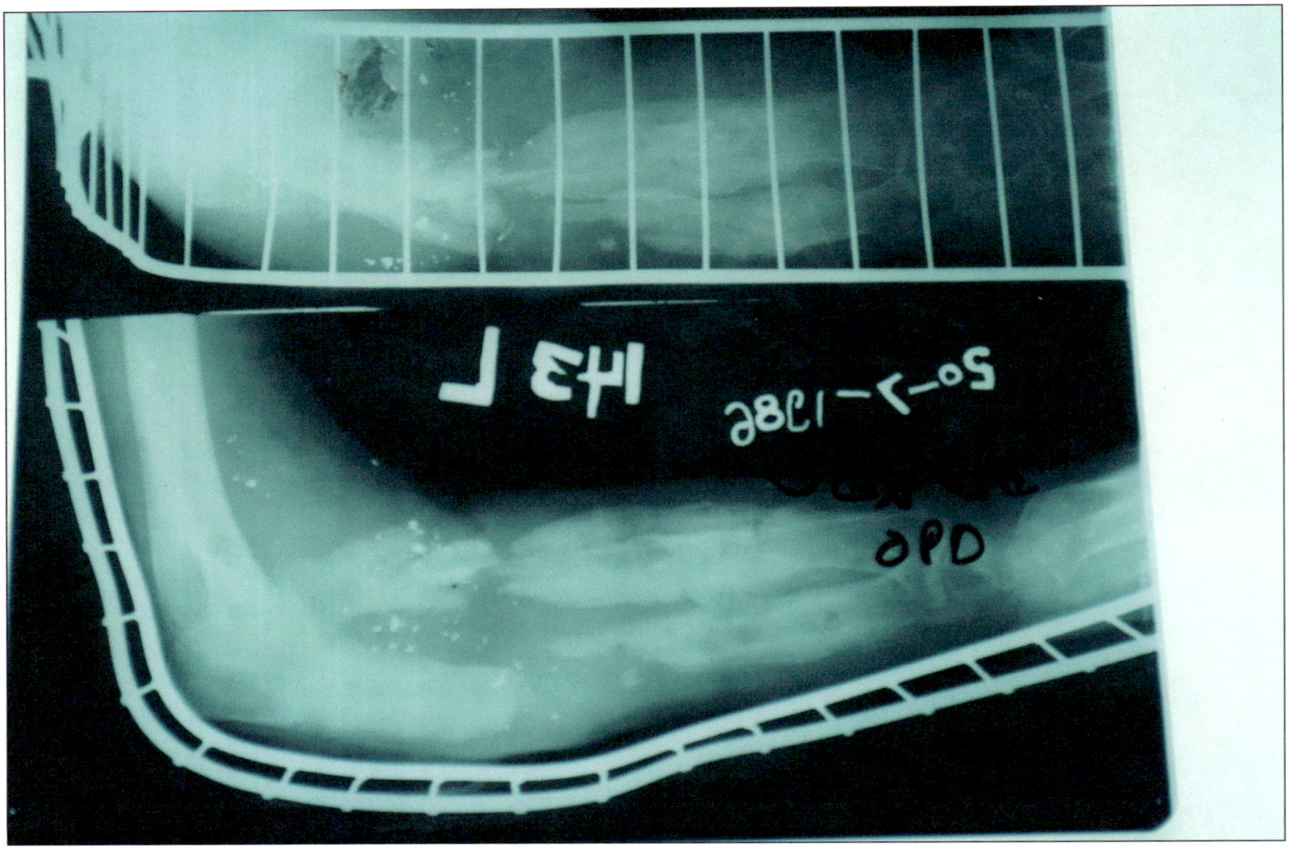

Severe bone loss of forearm

Rita presented a problem for the hospital, as women are not allowed in hospitals where men are housed. She was eventually allowed to participate but had to have her head covered at all times.

I was invited to speak at the Kuwaiti Red Crescent Hospital, but Rita was asked not to attend. I, therefore, declined the offer.

We visited one of the Afghan refugee camps where thousands of refugees were living in makeshift housing and barren surroundings. Rita attracted a huge following of children who trailed behind her during our walk through the camp. We also visited a training site for paramedics in the camp that was being run by the International Medical Corps. They were training medics to return to the battlefield and care for the injured.

We visited one of the Afghan refugee camps where thousands of refugees were living in make shift housing and baron surroundings.

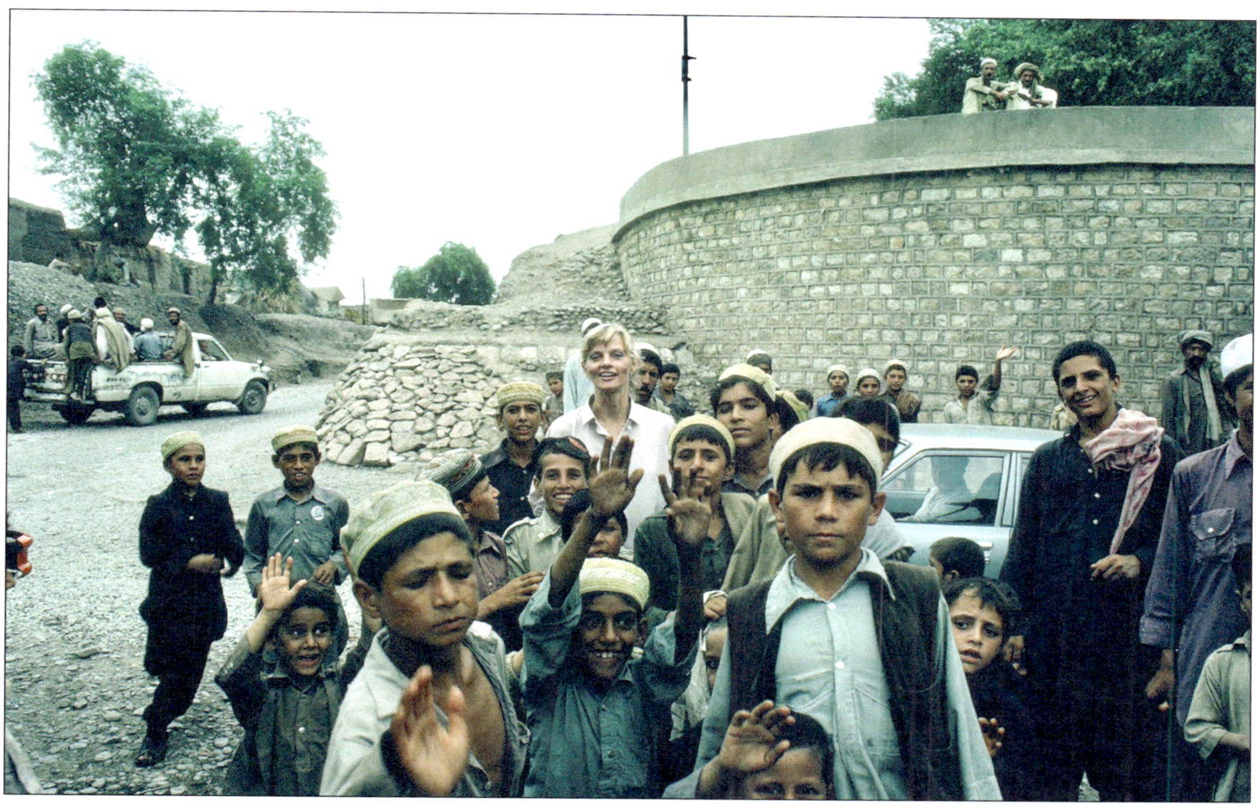

Rita's entourage

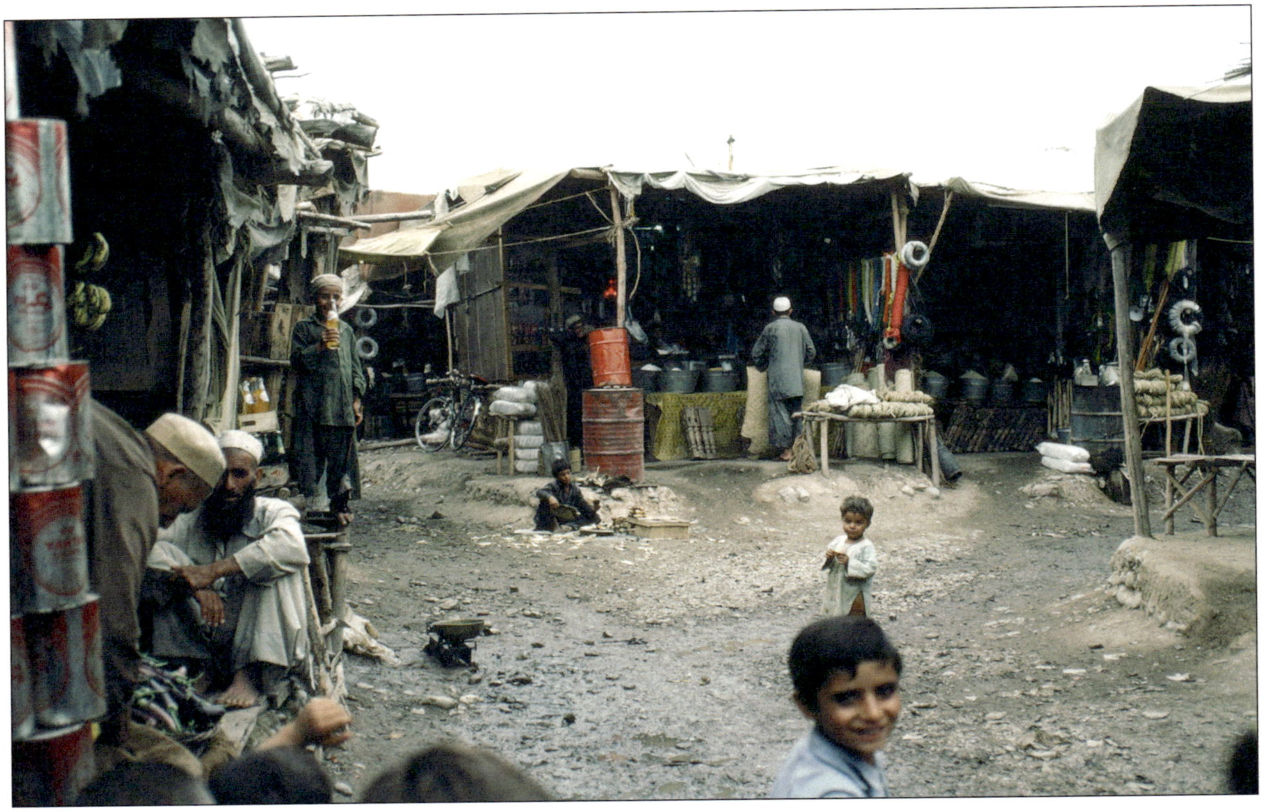

Refugee living quarters

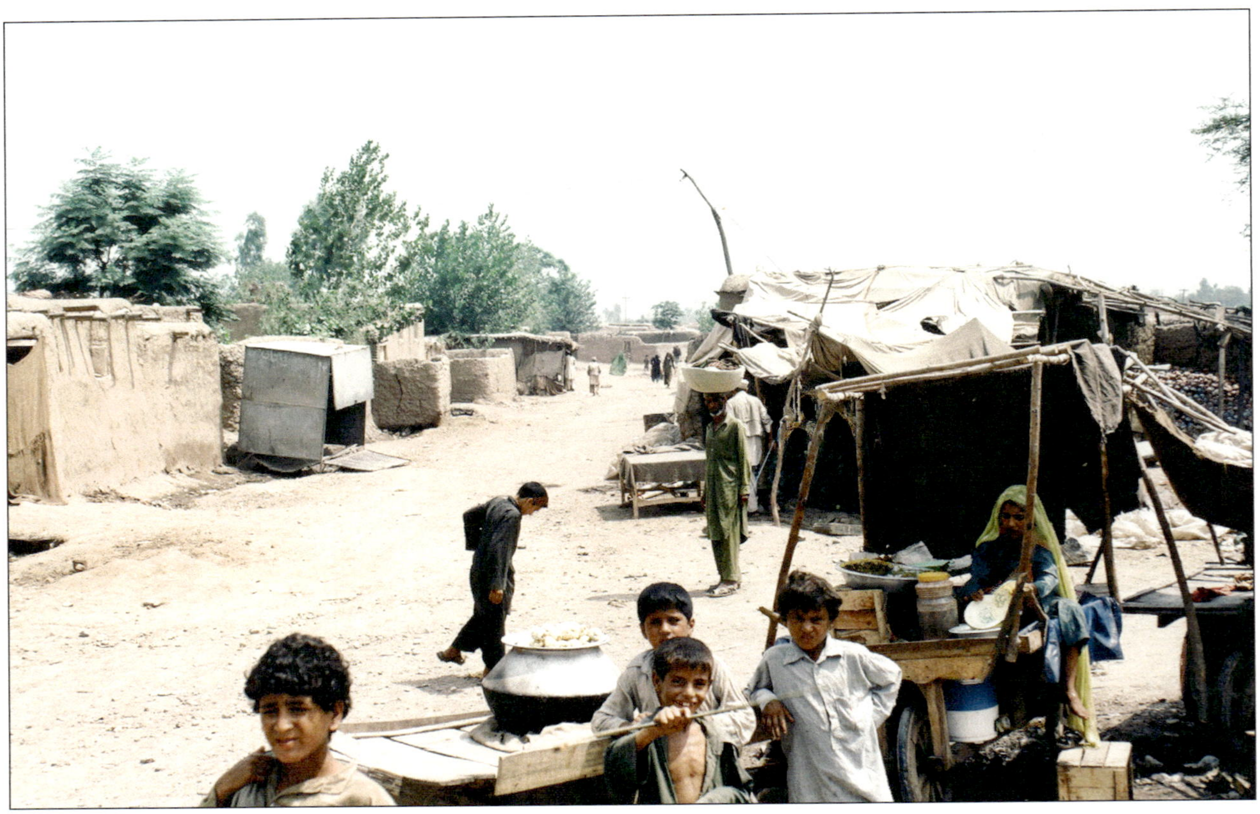

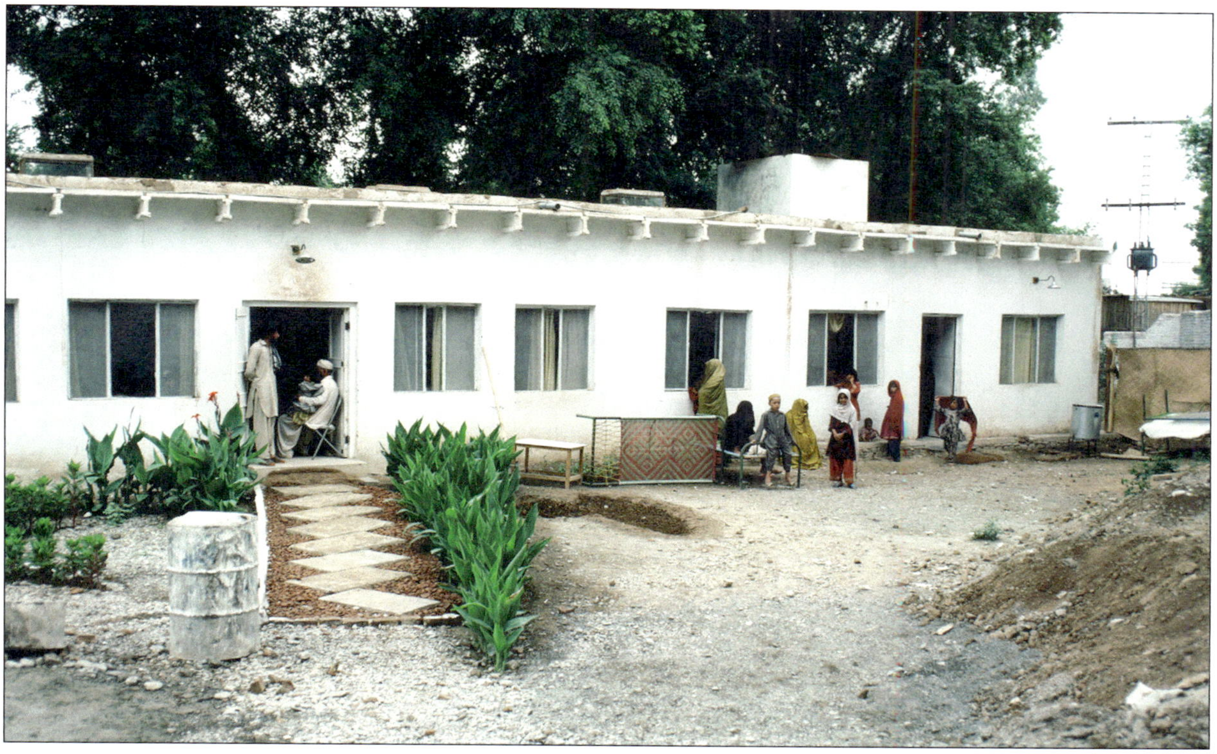

Clinic for training paramedics. Separate entrances for men and women

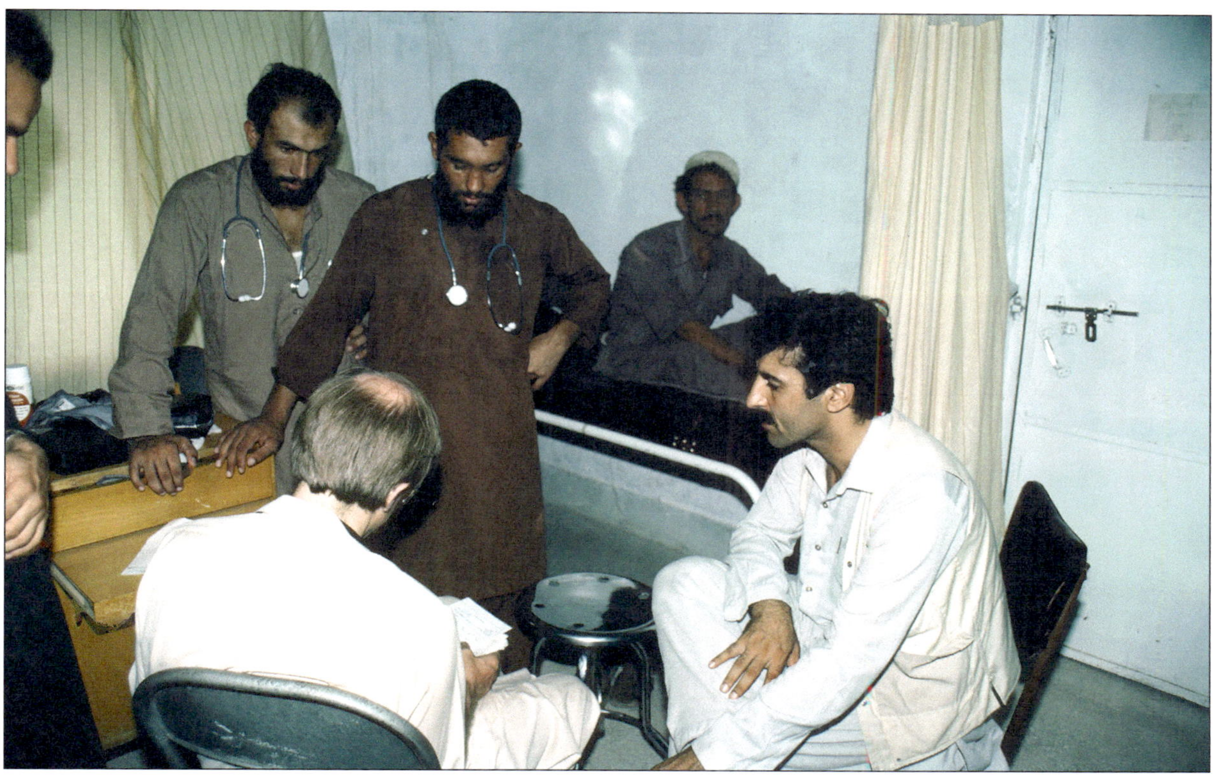

Learning how to do a history and physical exam

We were also able to meet and visit with the head of the Afghan fighting force, the Mujahideen. He was in a heavily guarded compound, a slight man, probably in his 60s and a former professor of Political Science at the University in Kabul. He was very gracious, spoke excellent English, and gave us a copy of a monograph he had published on Afghanistan history and politics.

We were also able to meet and visit with the head of the Afghan fighting force, the Mujahideen.

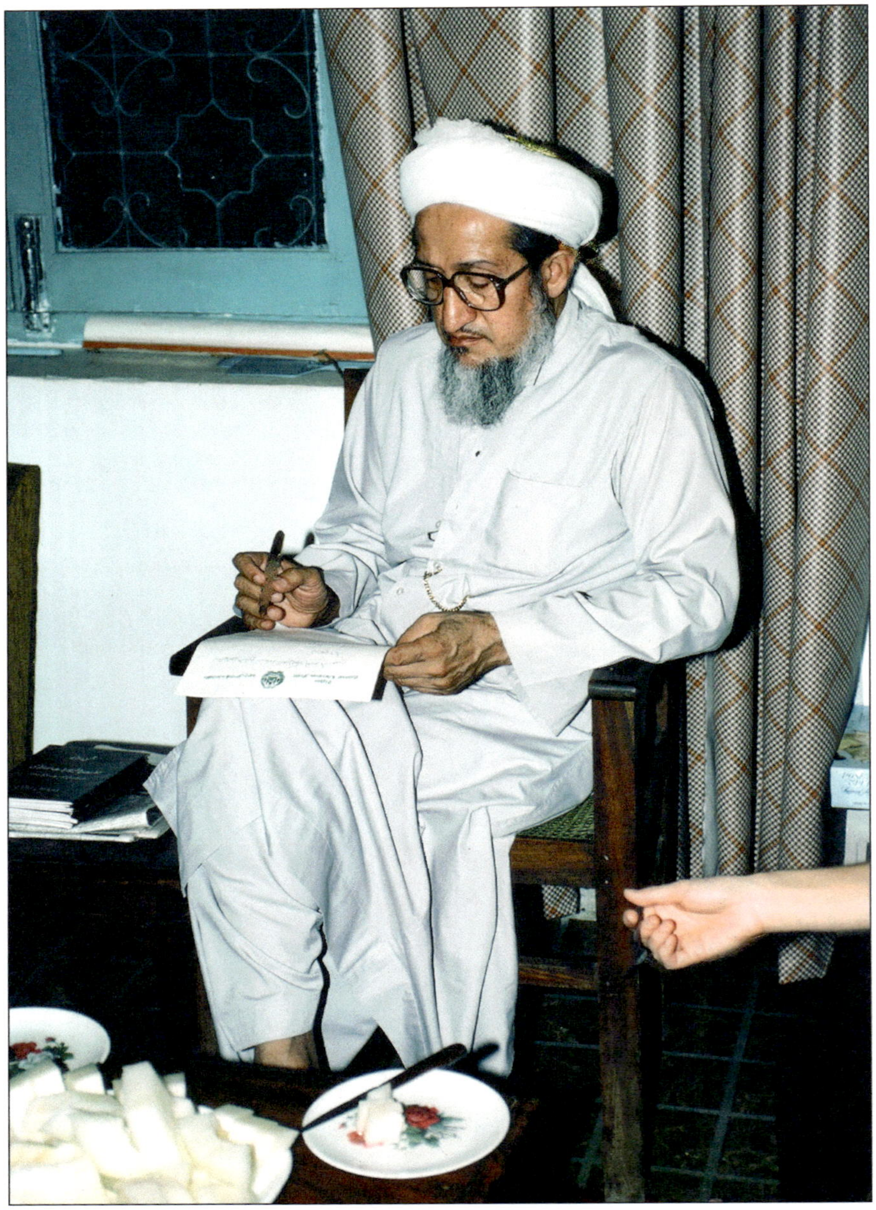

Afghan professor and Mujahideen head

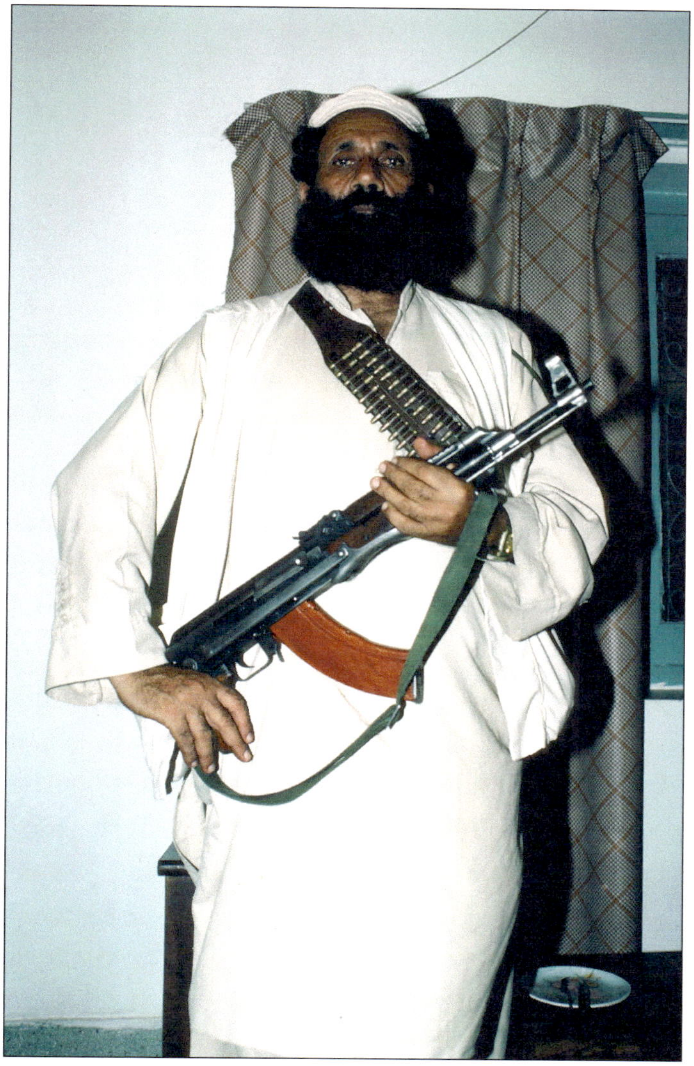

Guard at Mujahideen headquarters

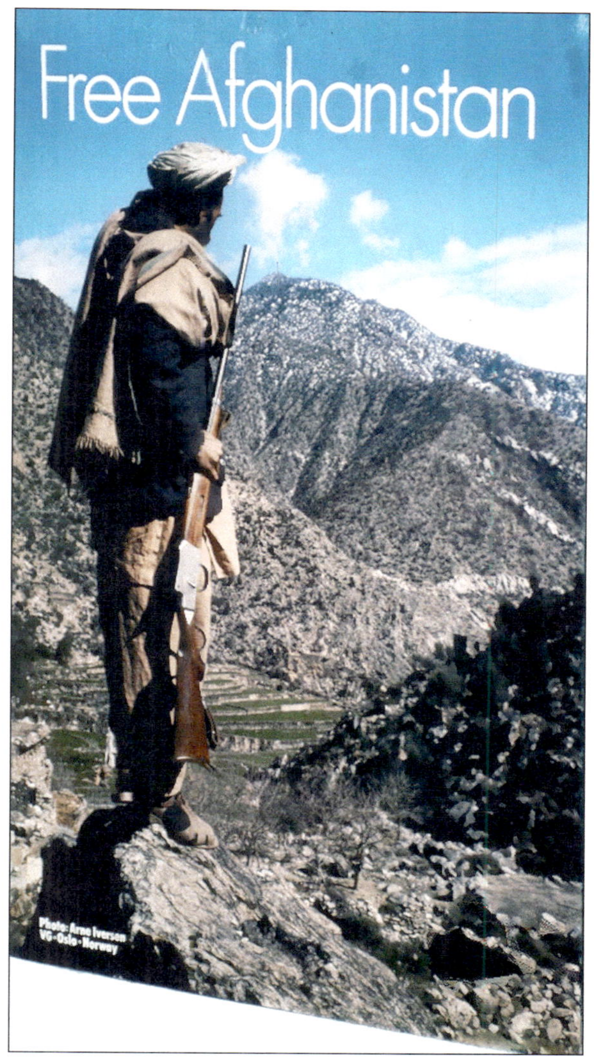

Poster on wall

Peru

> *Knee arthroscopy was a new technology in Lima, and the military possessed state-of-the-art equipment, much of which had never been used.*

The second country we visited with Orthopedics Overseas was Peru, in 1987. This was our first of five trips to that country with three different organizations. We spent time in different hospitals on this trip, the first being a large county hospital providing much trauma care. The second hospital was a military facility, where more reconstructive surgery was being performed. Knee arthroscopy was a new technology in Lima, and the military possessed state-of-the-art equipment, much of which had never been used. The City hospital had none of these devices.

The local physician contact was Dr. Gaston Barnechea, who became a good friend and with whom we worked on two other occasions. Gaston was just getting into arthroscopy and was very involved with the National Peruvian Orthopedic Organization. He arranged for us to do the first arthroscopic surgery in Arequipa, a mountainous community of more than 800,000, 580 miles from Lima. We had three days to demonstrate the new procedure, however, on day one, we did not have enough saline to use for the procedure, so it was postponed. On day two, there was not an adequate TV monitor to visualize the surgery, and, therefore, surgery was postponed once again. On day three, everything was working, and we were able to perform three surgeries. Over the years we found operating in unfamiliar environments brought unexpected challenges, which became rather routine.

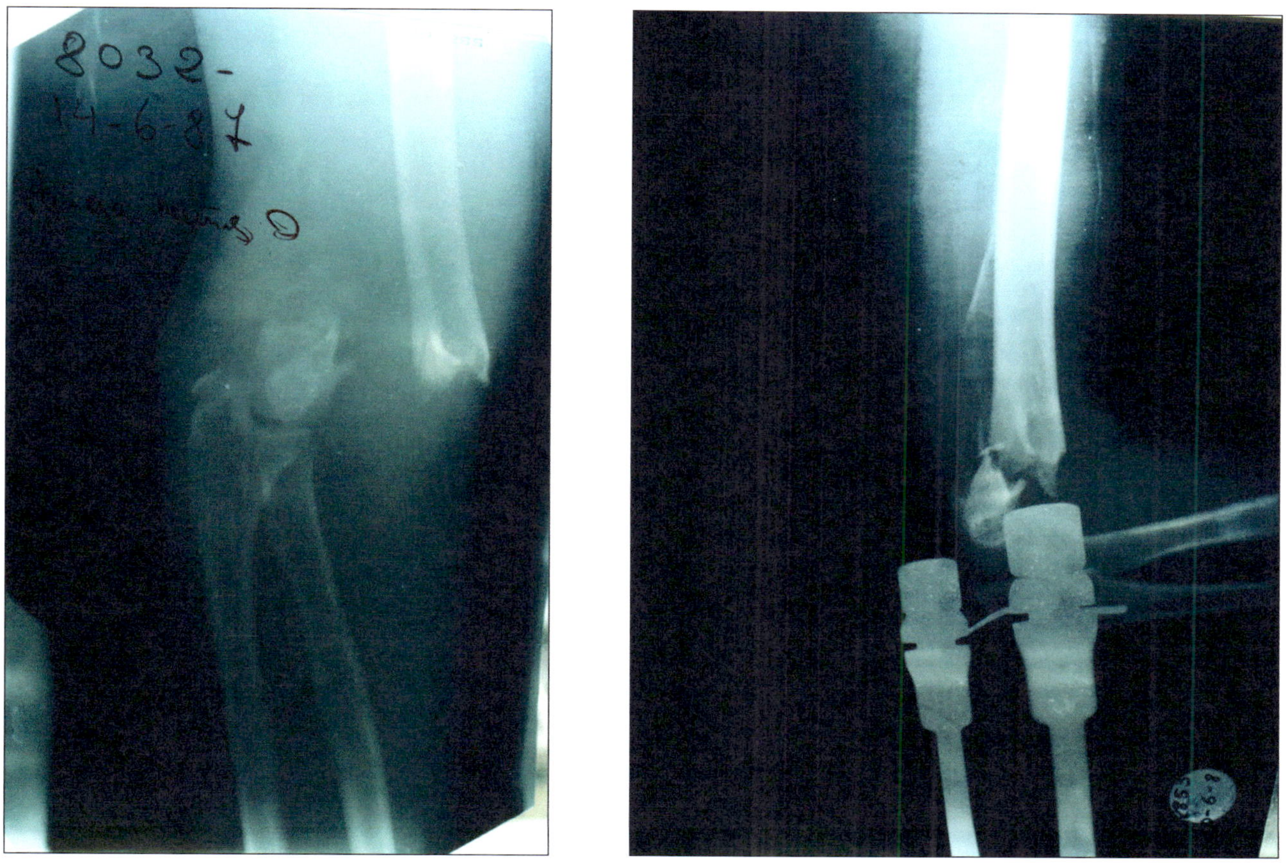

X-rays of severe elbow fracture in a child. Left is before treatment. Right is after placing arm in traction.

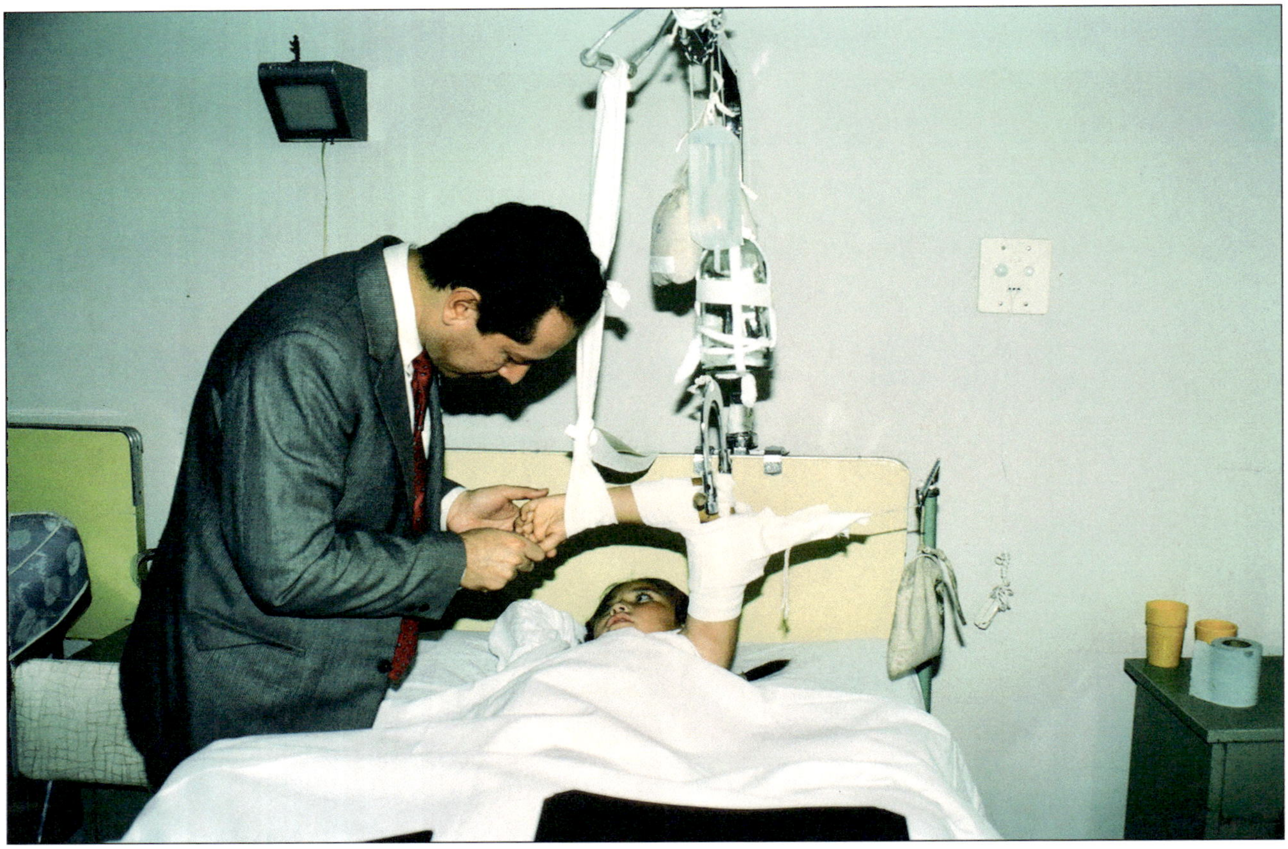

Gaston checking patient's nerve function after being placed in traction for elbow fracture

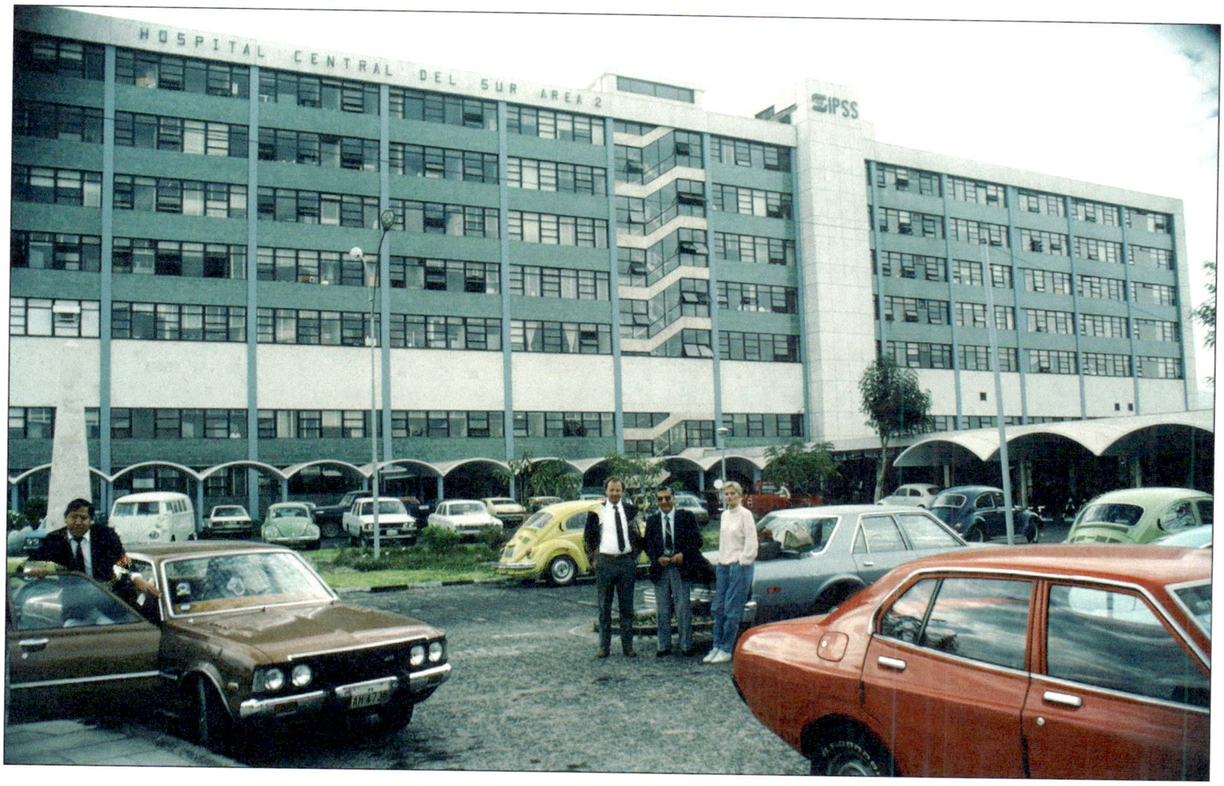

City hospital Lima

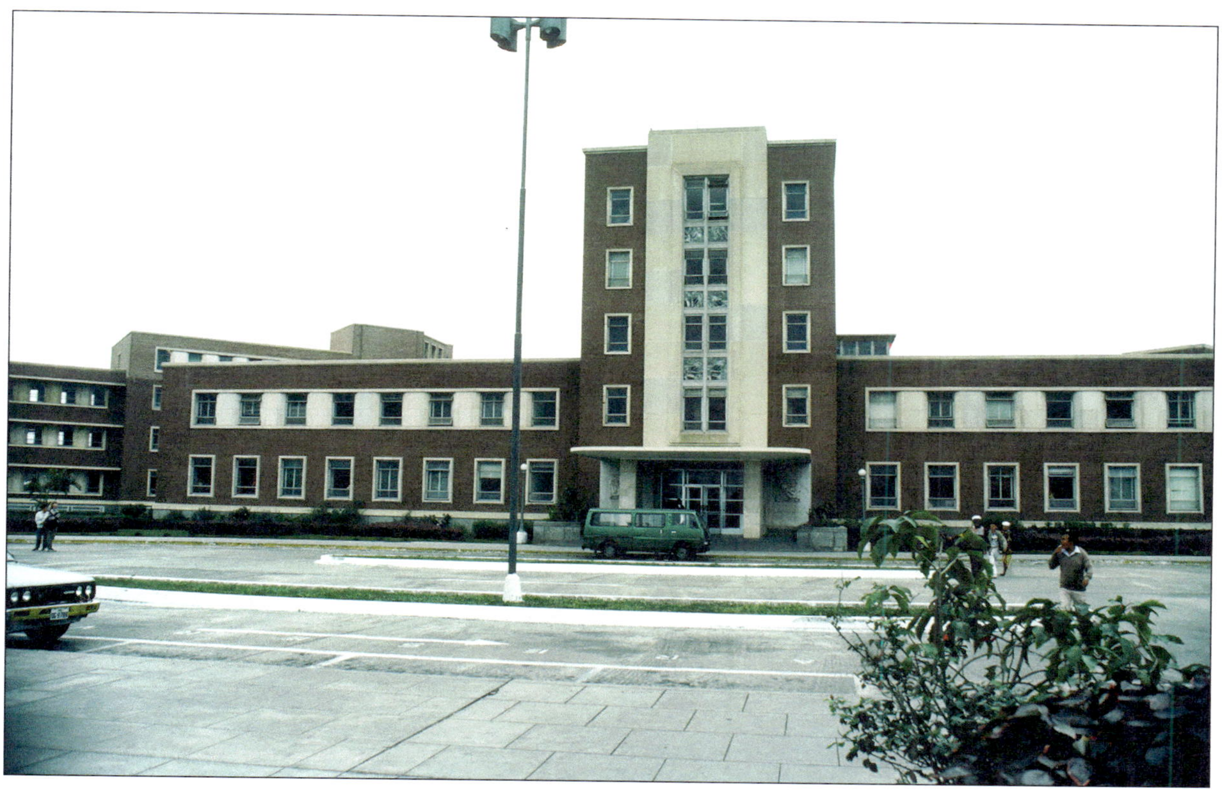

Military Hospital

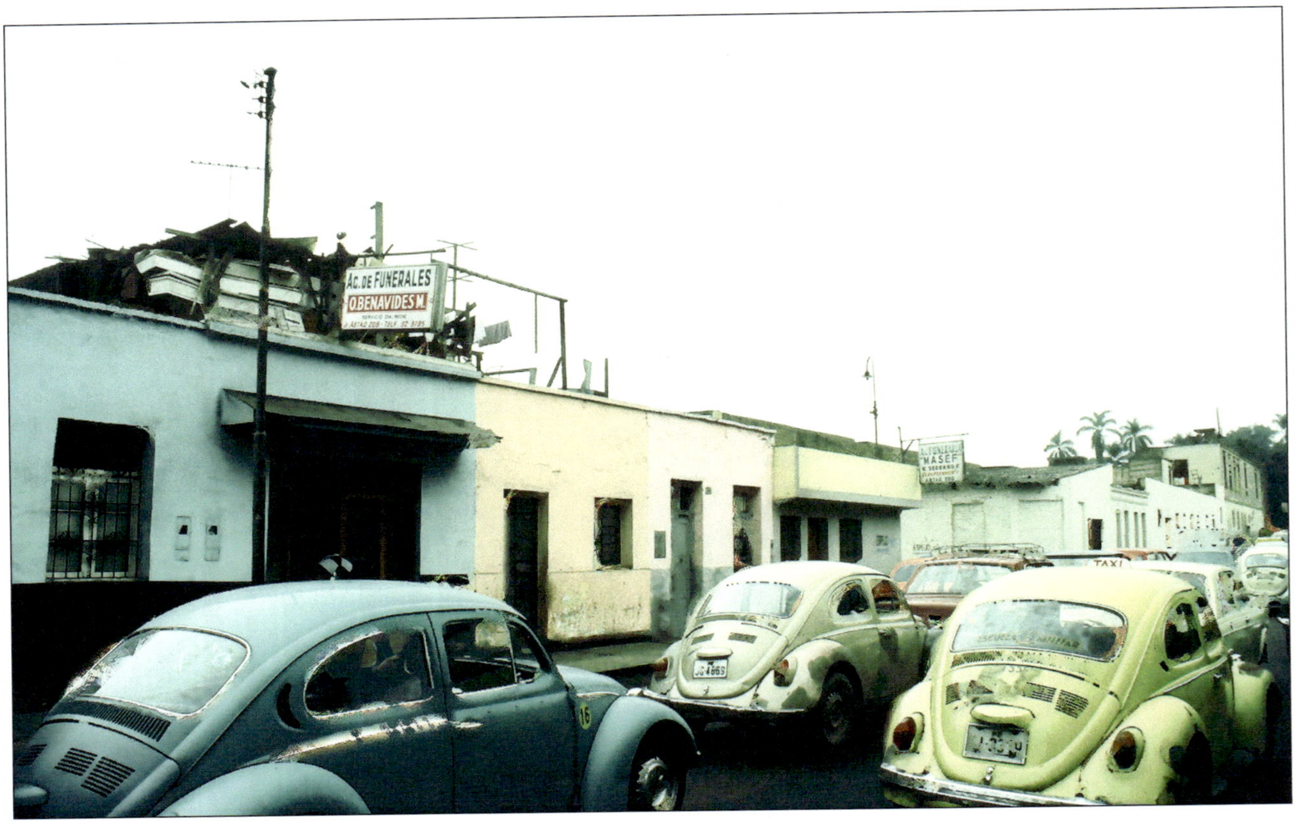

Funeral home across the street from the city hospital!!!

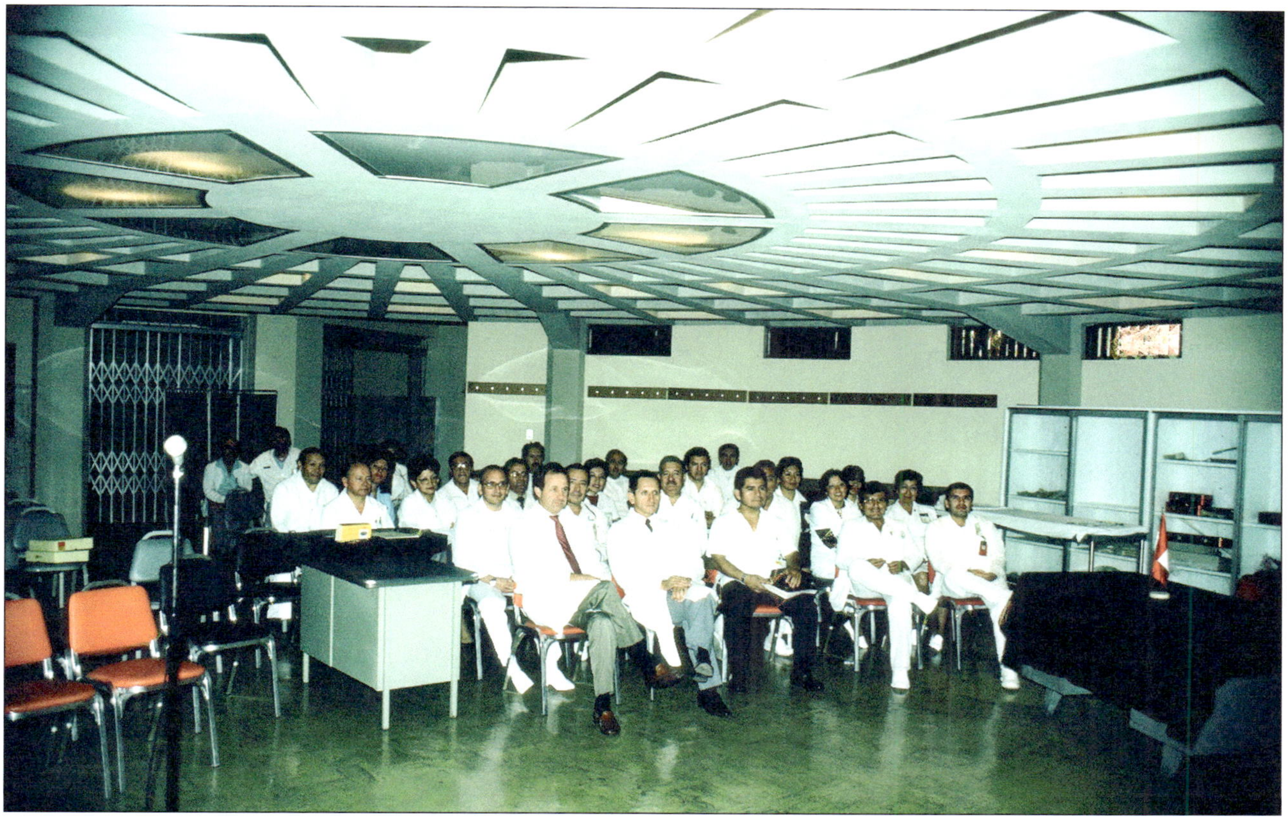

Hospital staff gathered for one of my lectures

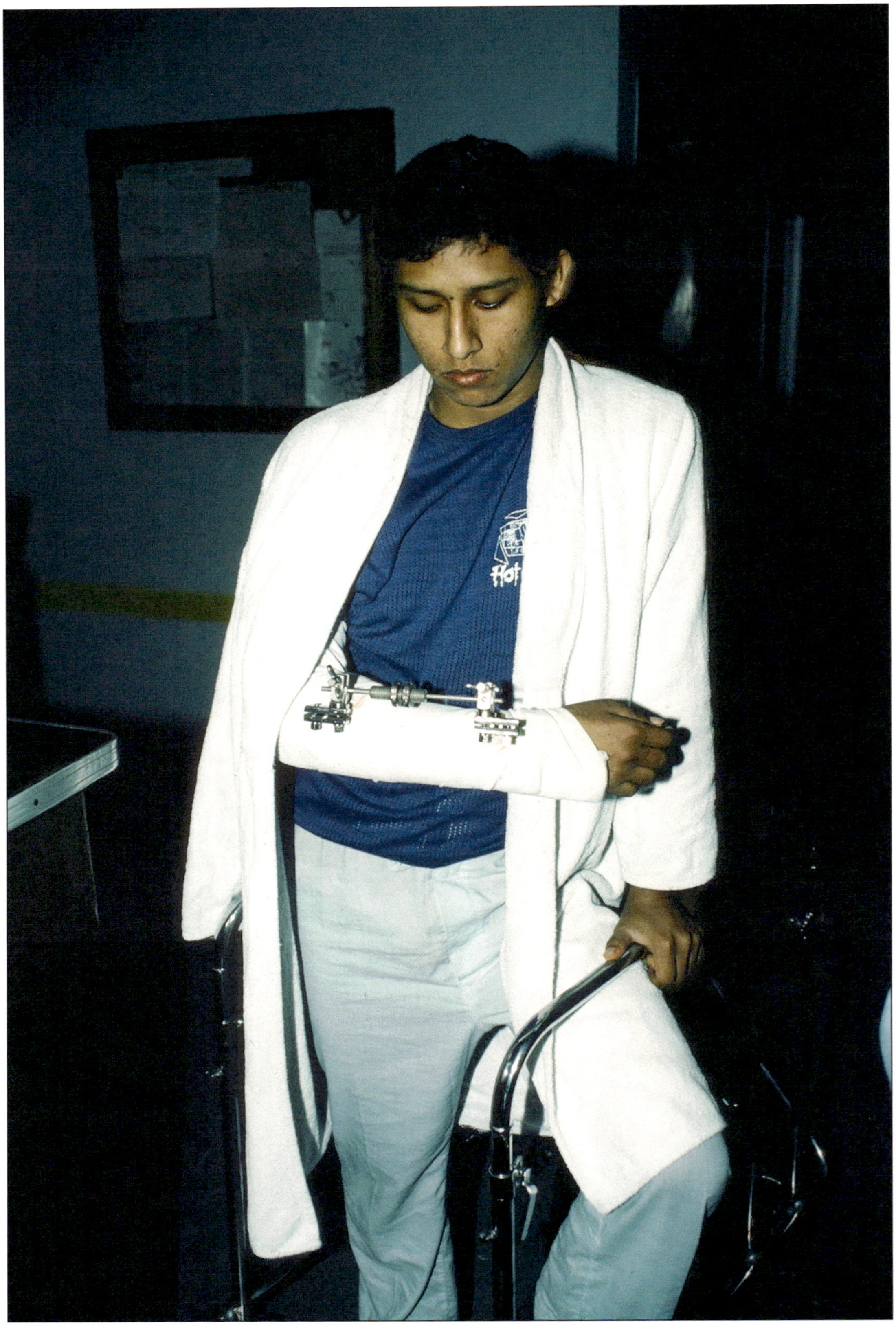

Patient with external fixator awaiting large bone grafting of forearm

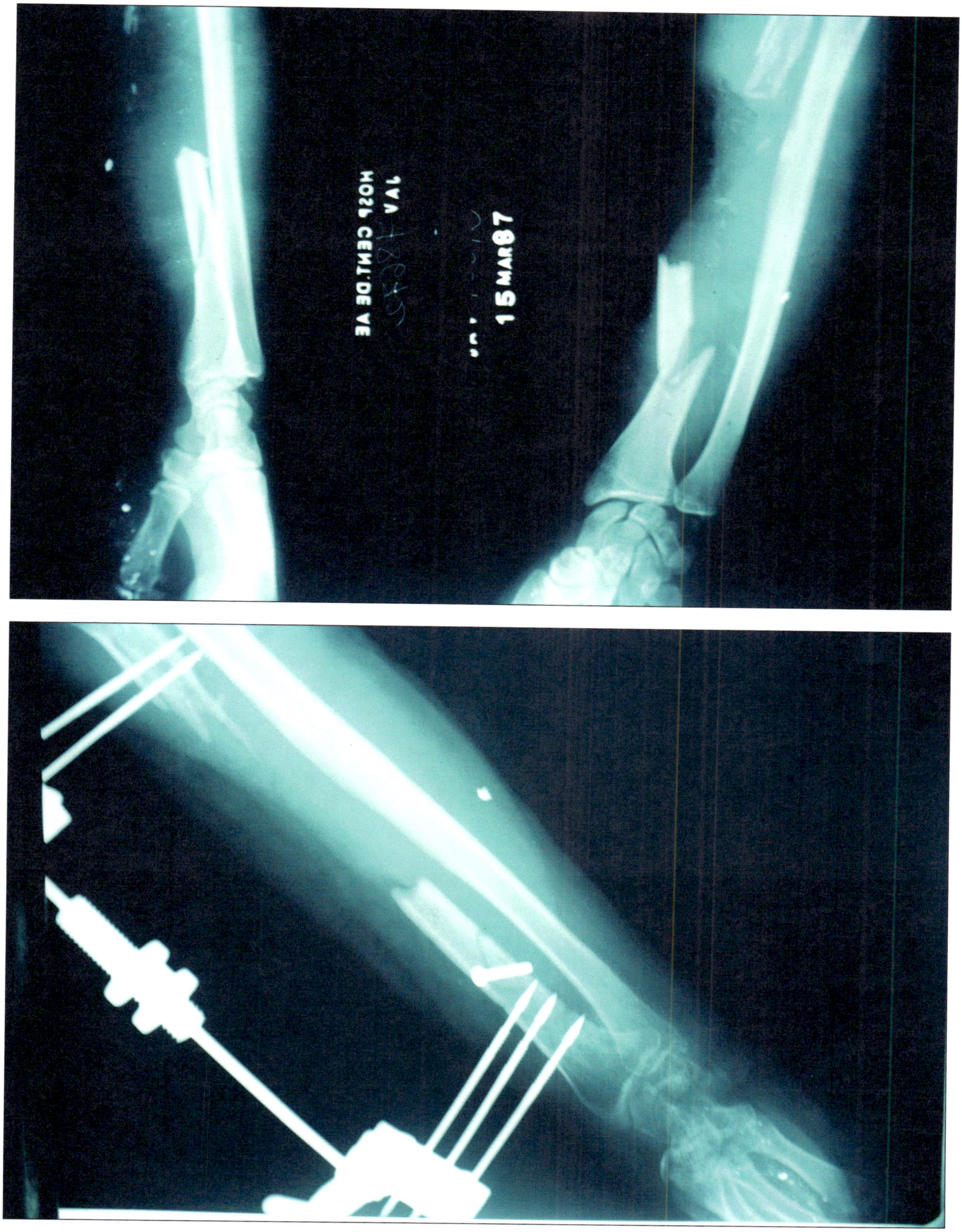

Large segmental bone loss of forearm

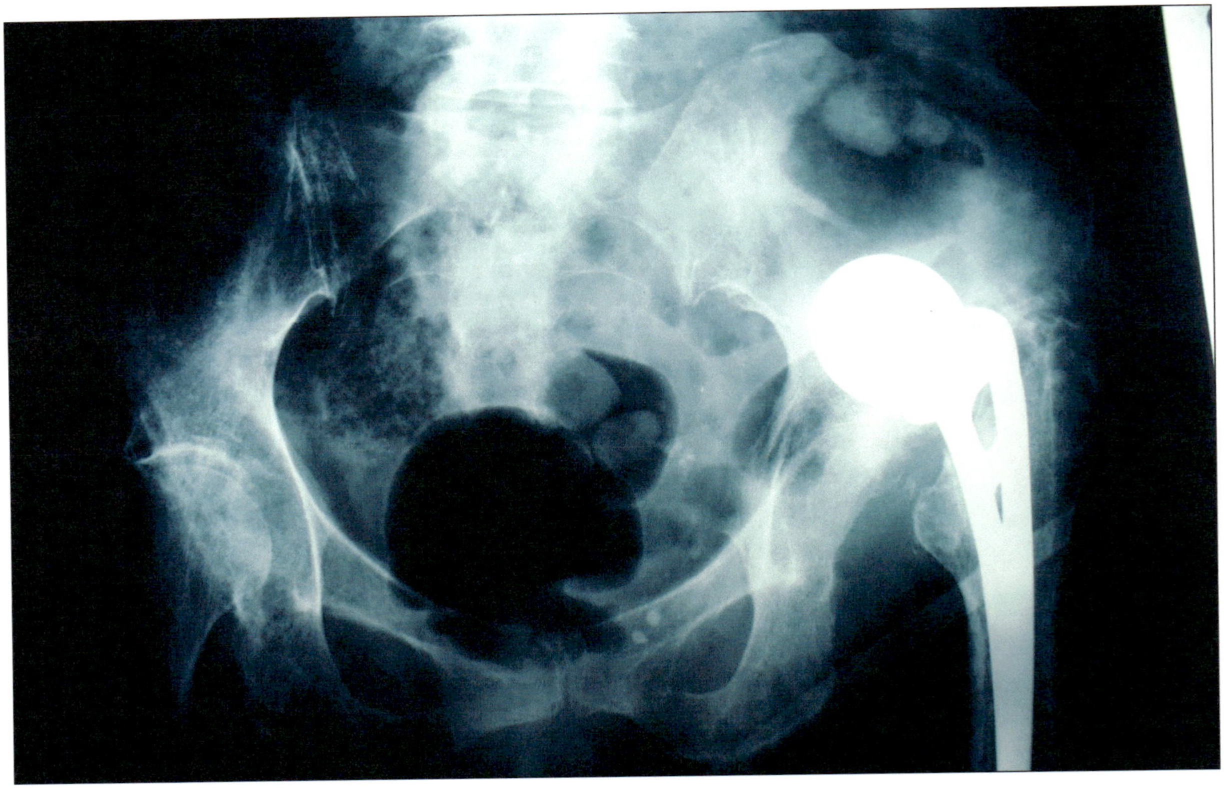

Dislocated hip prosthesis

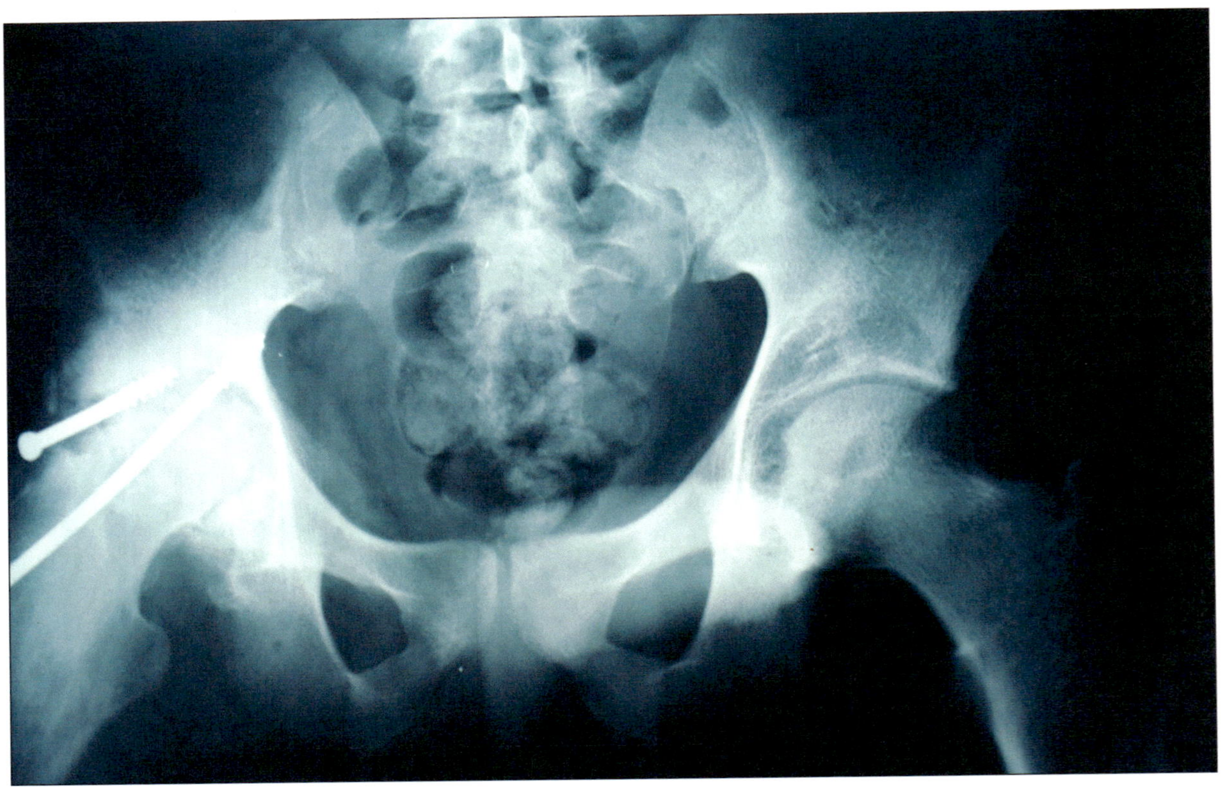

Hip pinning gone awry: Pins across the joint

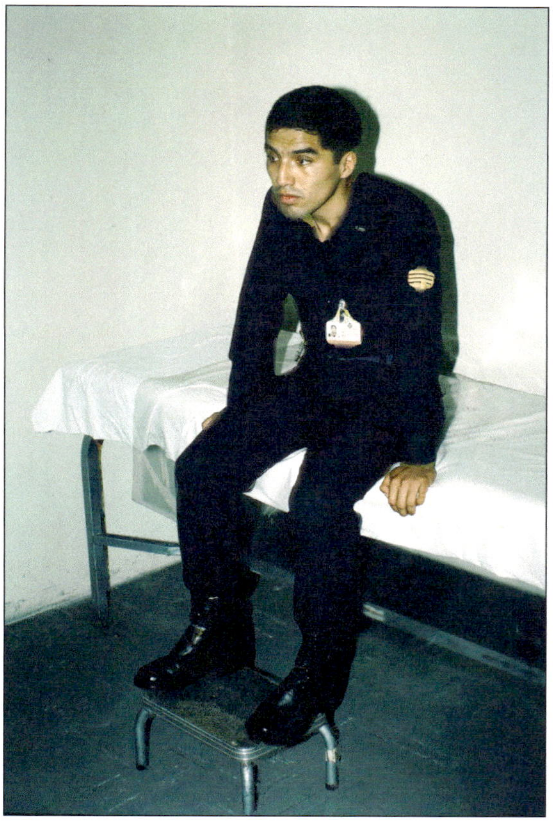

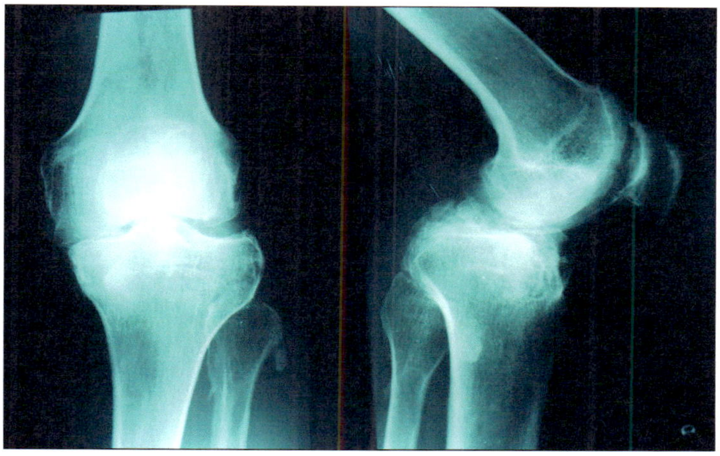

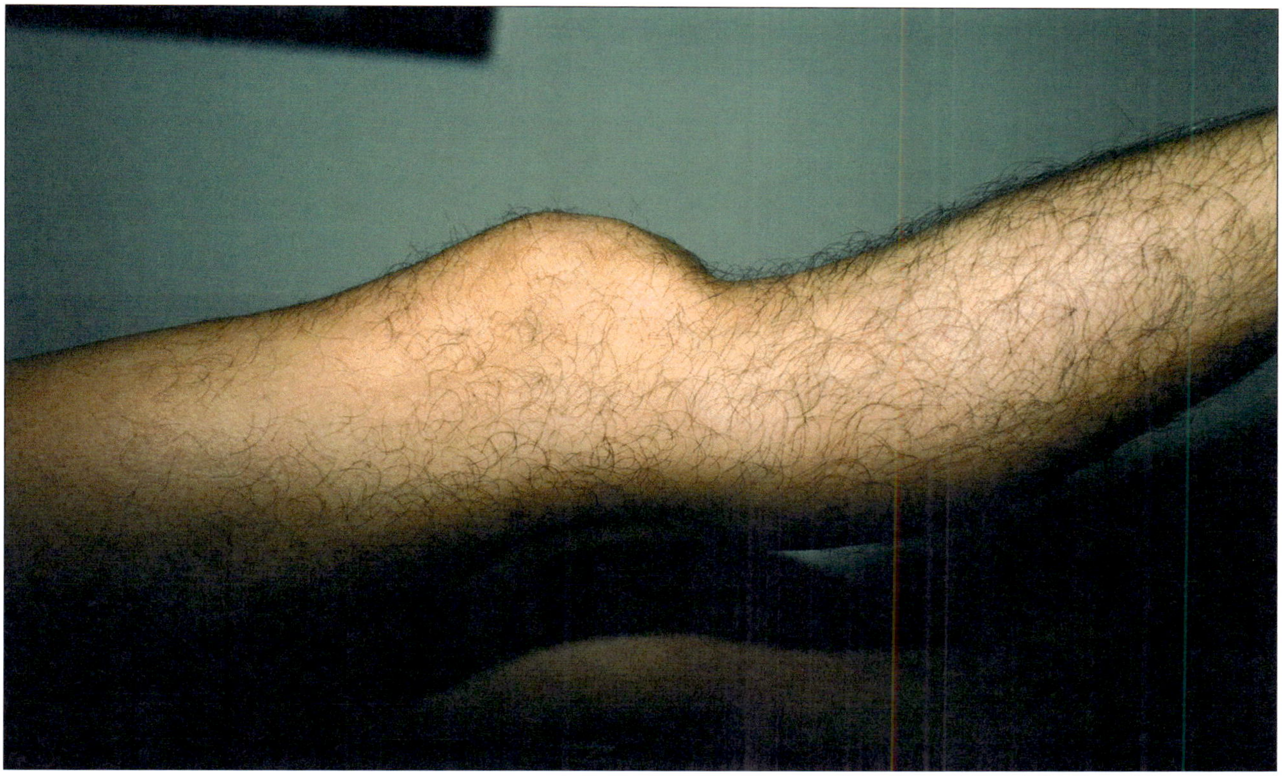

Soldier with a partially dislocated knee

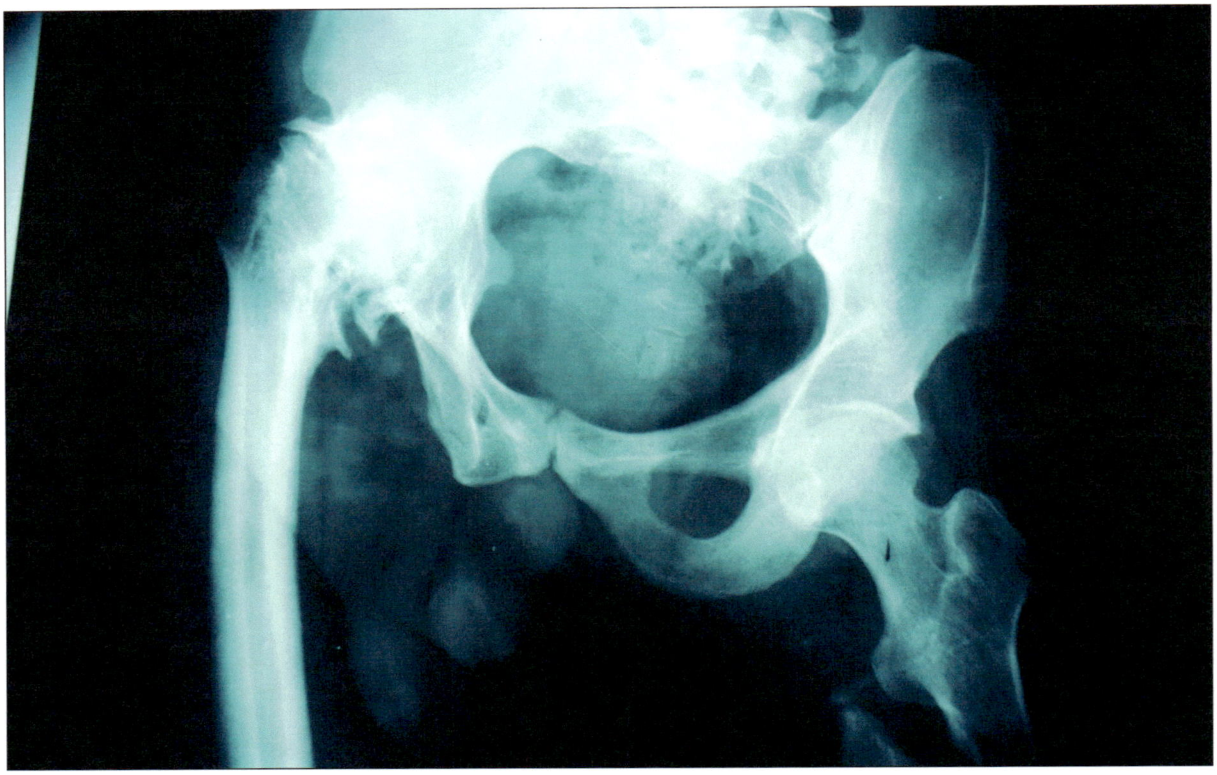

Severely destroyed and dislocated right hip joint

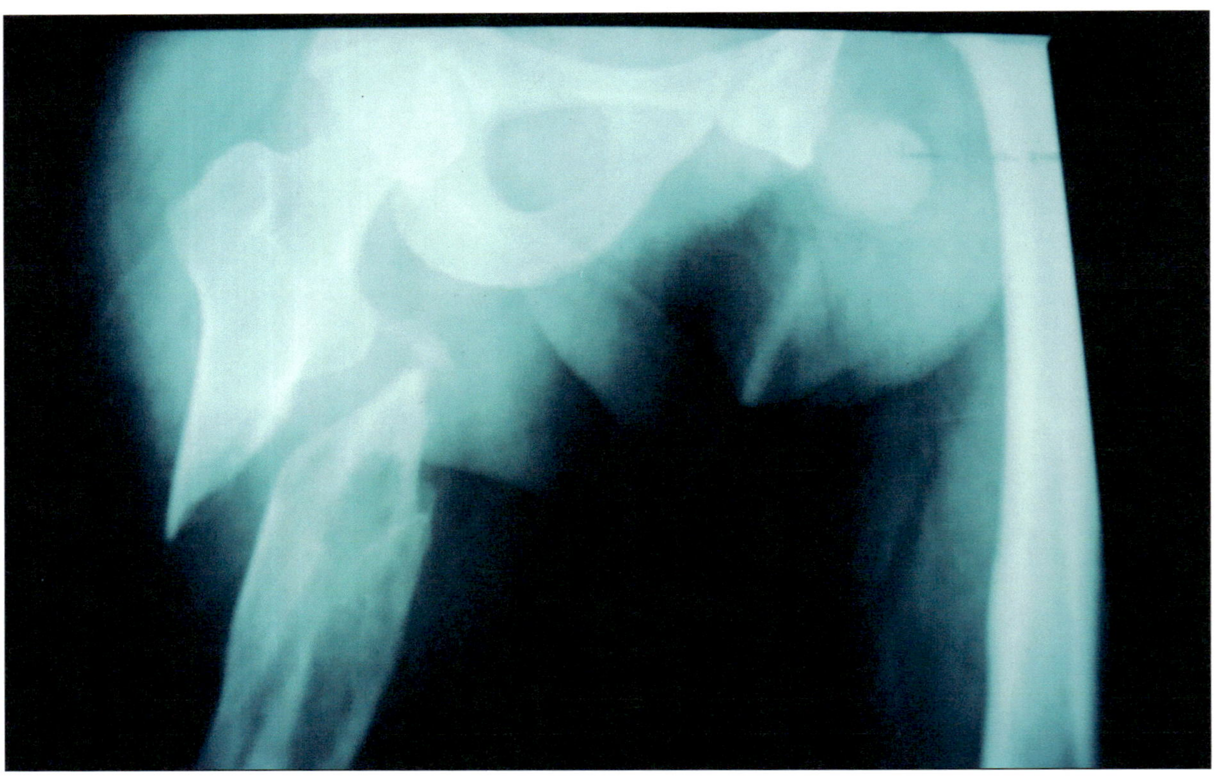

Untreated upper femur fracture

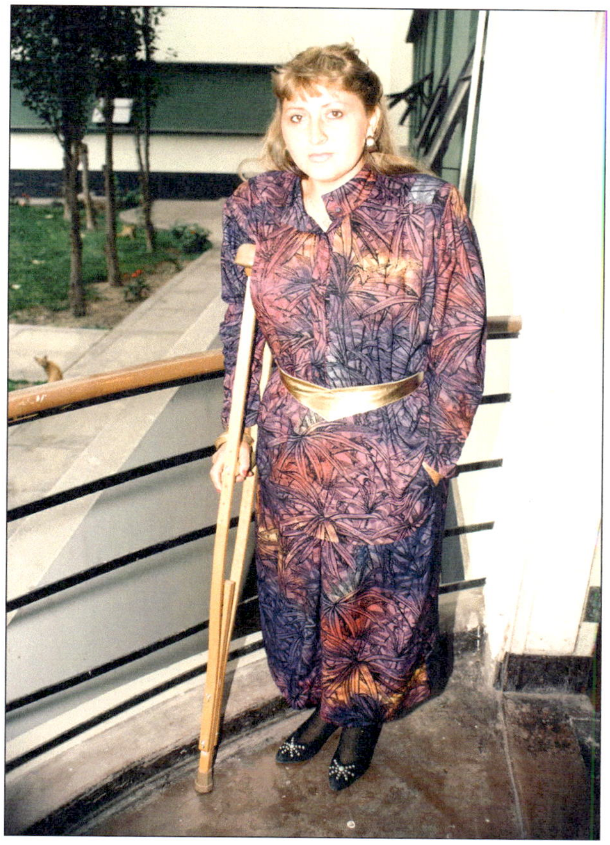

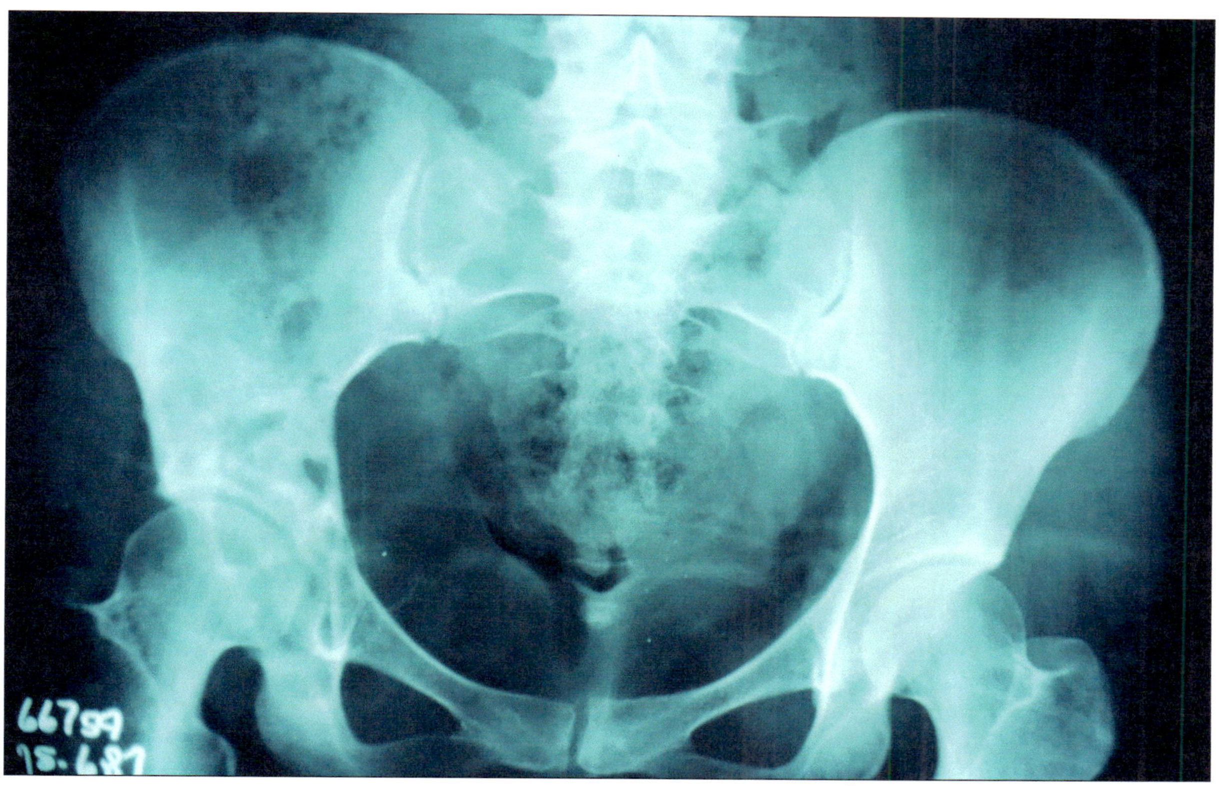

Young woman with severe hip arthritis. Needs total hip replacement, but it was too expensive

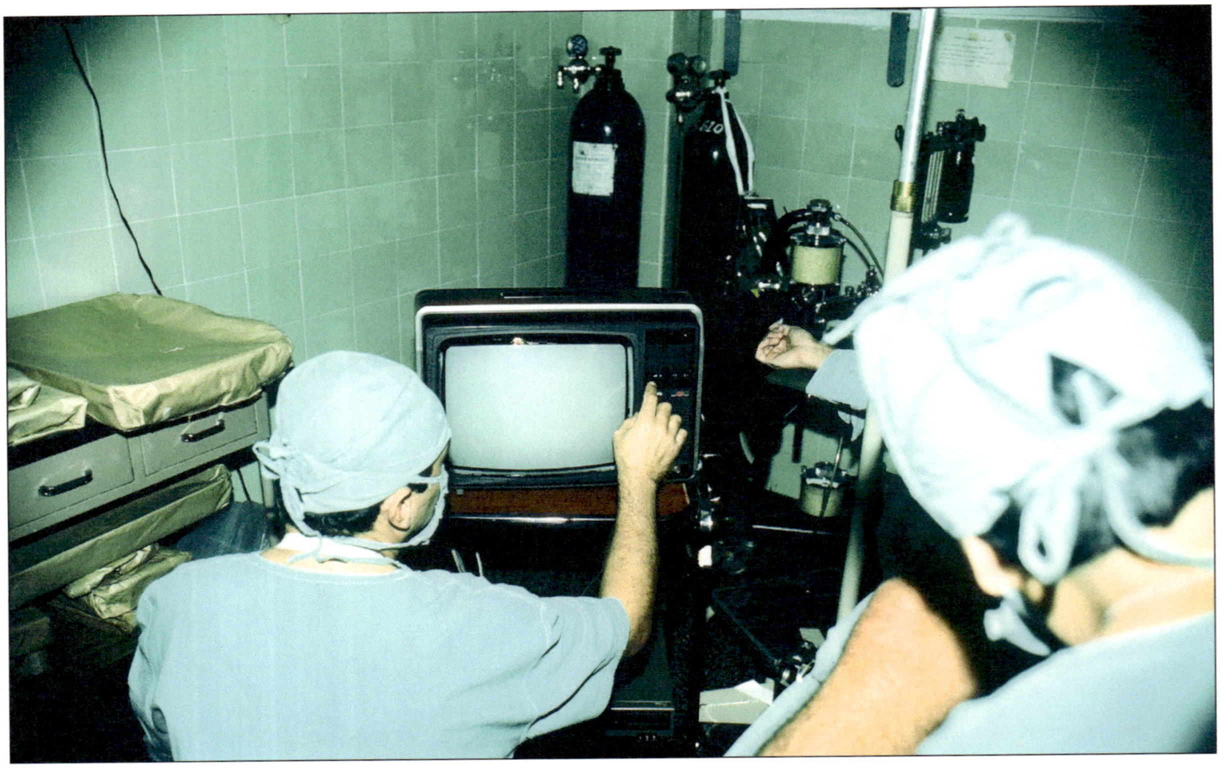

Trying to get TV to work as a monitor for arthroscopy in Arequipa

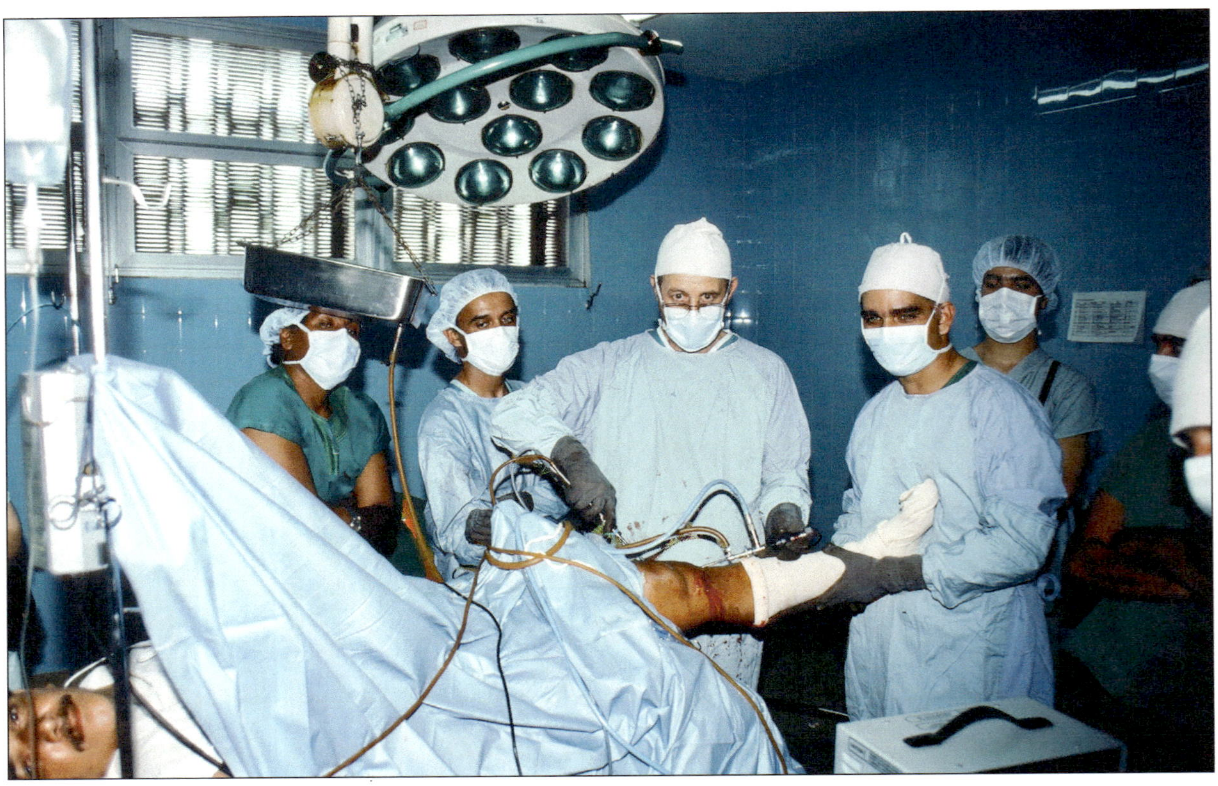

Finally doing arthroscopy in Arequipa

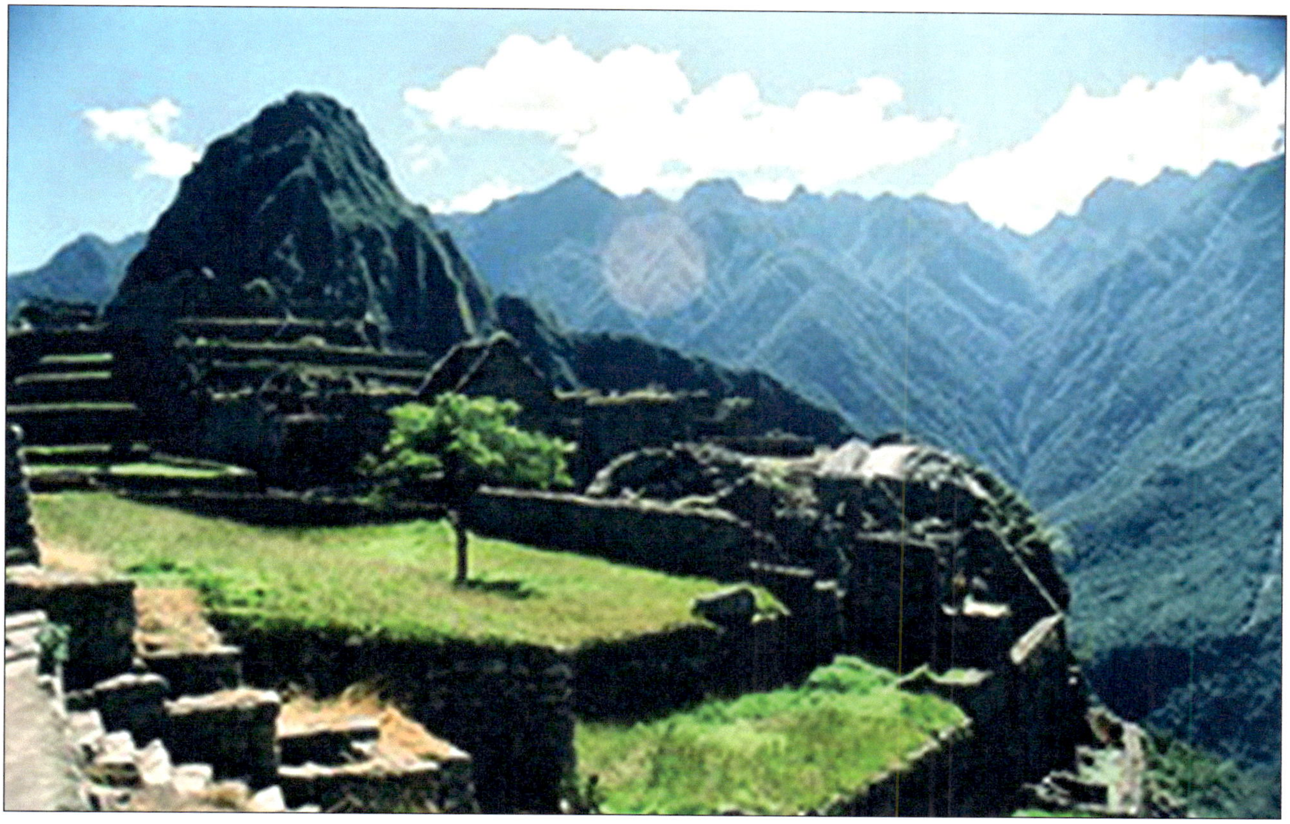

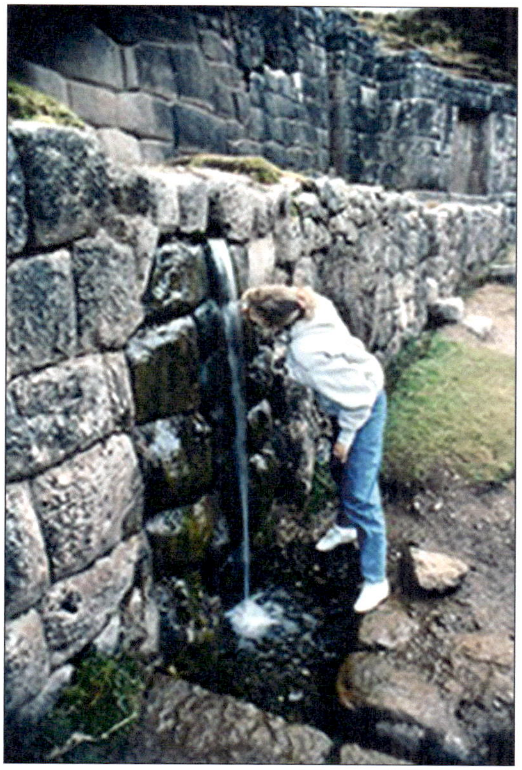

At the end of our stay in Lima, we flew to Cuzco and visited the surrounding sites as well as Machu Picchu, a memorable experience.

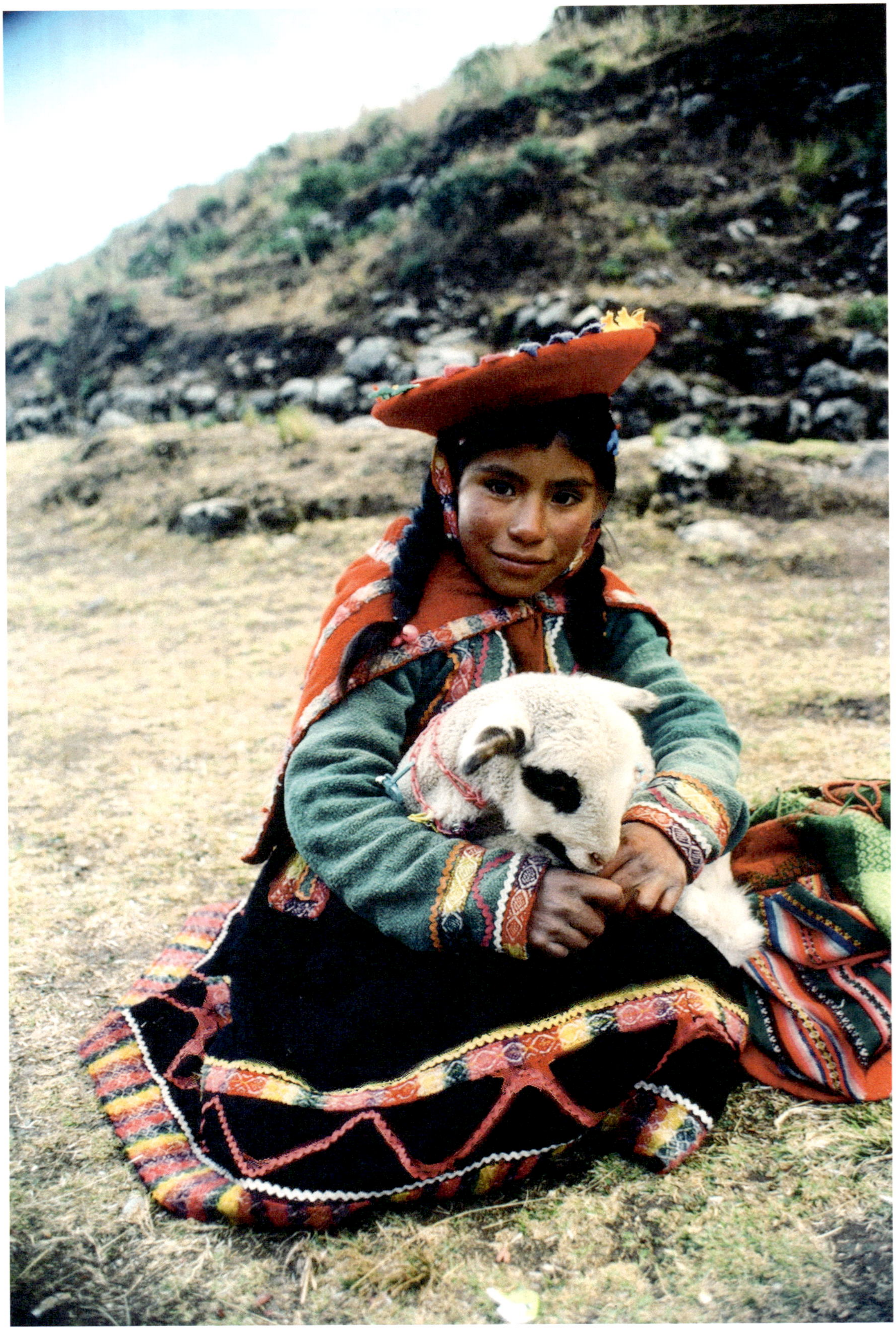

We made two trips to Caras, Peru, with Dr. Raul Osorio, a Peruvian gynecologist in Mesa who would take medical teams every couple of years to his hometown in the Peruvian mountains, a community of fewer than 20,000 people approximately 300 miles northeast of Lima — an eight-hour-plus bus ride. The hospital has four operating rooms, and the team consisted of orthopedic, general surgeons, gynecology surgeons, plus three or four general practitioners who ran daily clinics while the surgeons operated. Again we carried our own supplies, usually surpassing twenty filled trunks. On one of our journeys after landing in Lima on a Saturday, customs stated they needed to examine every item brought into the country, which could not be completed in one day. On Sunday, they were short staffed and could not complete the evaluation, and Monday was a holiday! We stayed in Lima Saturday, and finally, Raul was able to contact a friend in the government, and the supplies were released on Sunday. In addition to the doctors, we were accompanied by nurses and scrub techs, for a total of up to twenty people.

On one of our journeys after landing in Lima on a Saturday, customs stated they needed to examine every item brought into the country, which could not be completed in one day.

One patient I sadly remember was a six-month-old child with a clubfoot who would not normally receive treatment in the mountains of Peru. I recommended surgical repair, but the mother stated she had three other children she had left at her village, which was a short distance from Caras. She deliberated for a few hours but then left for home. I think she was apprehensive about the child having surgery. Hopefully she has received treatment, but it is unlikely.

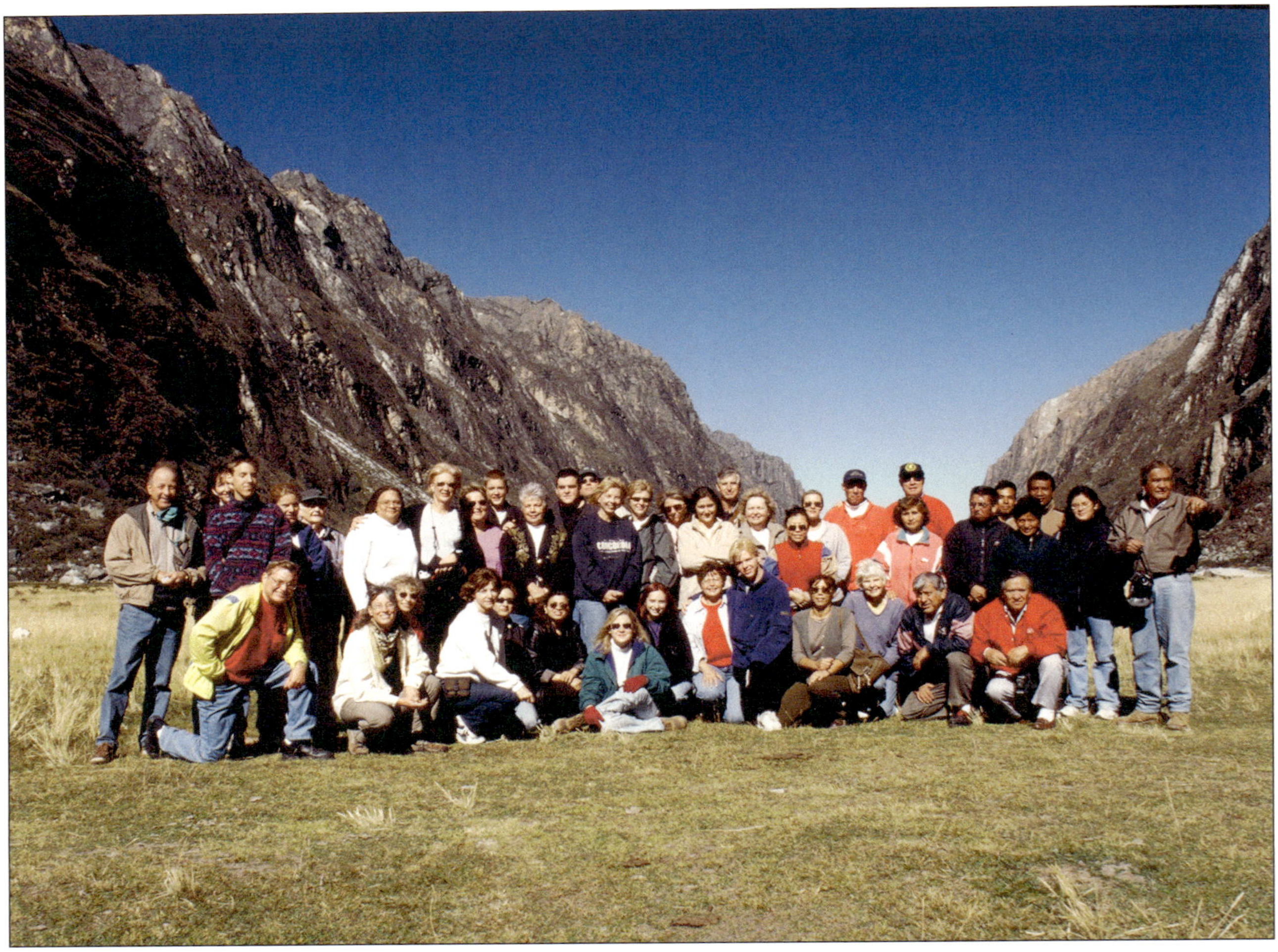

Caras team and hospital personnel

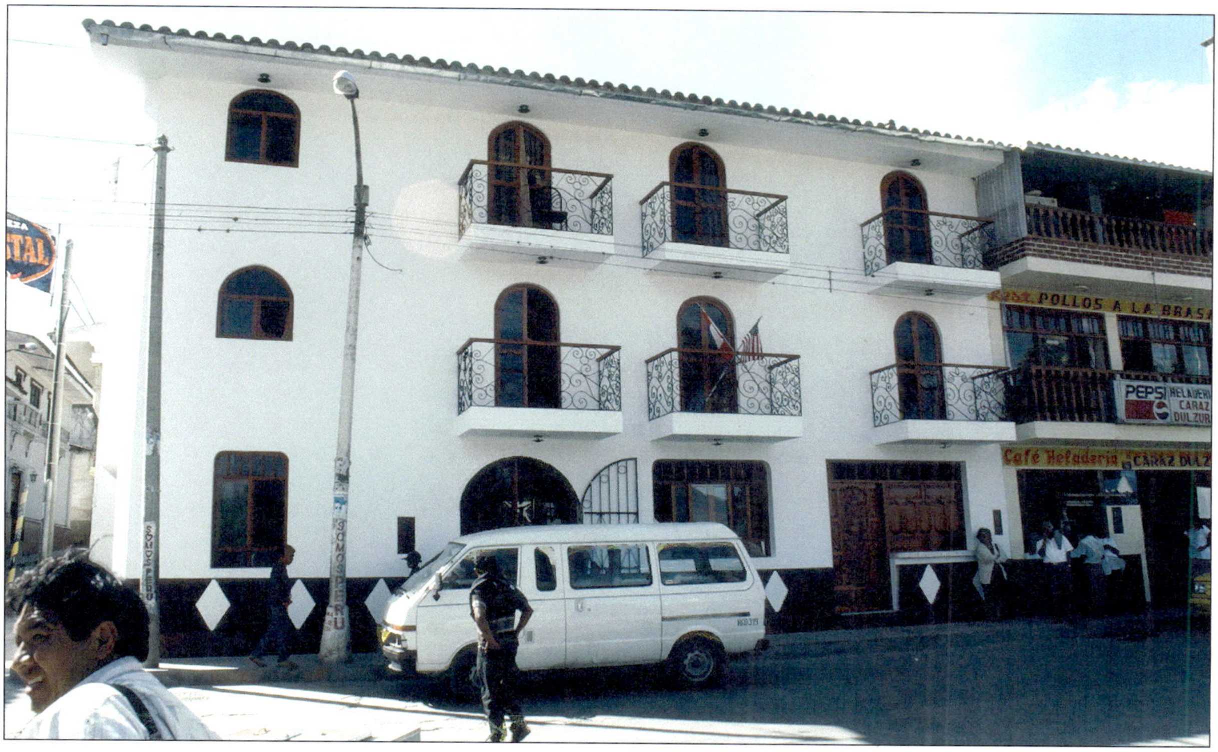

Hotel in Caras

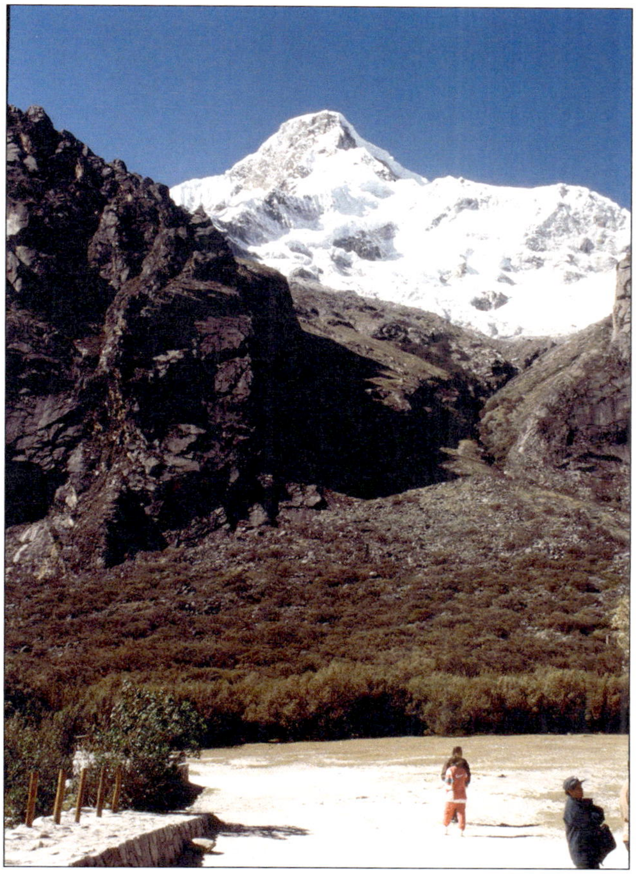

Mountain view outside Caras

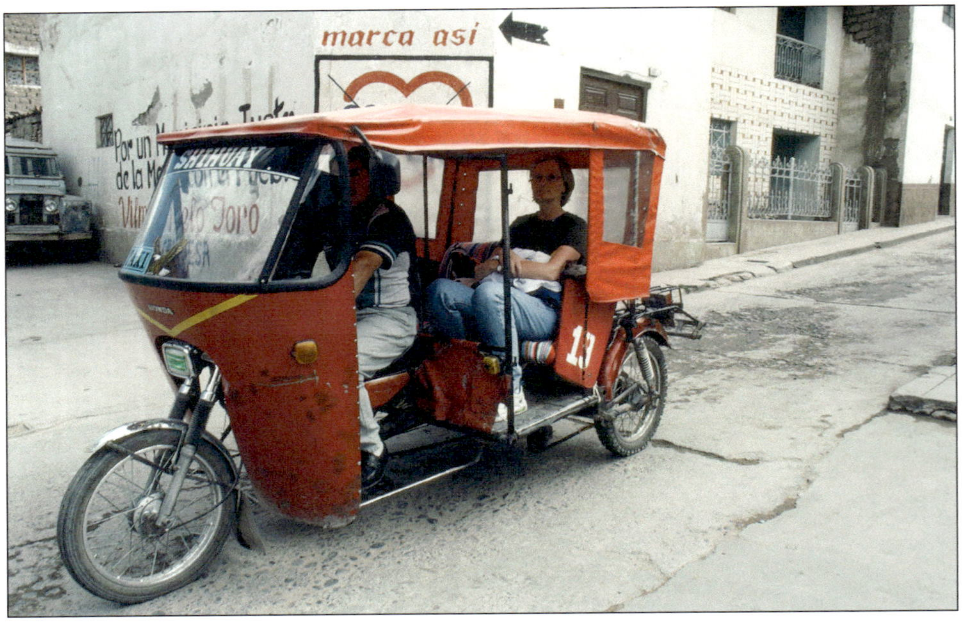

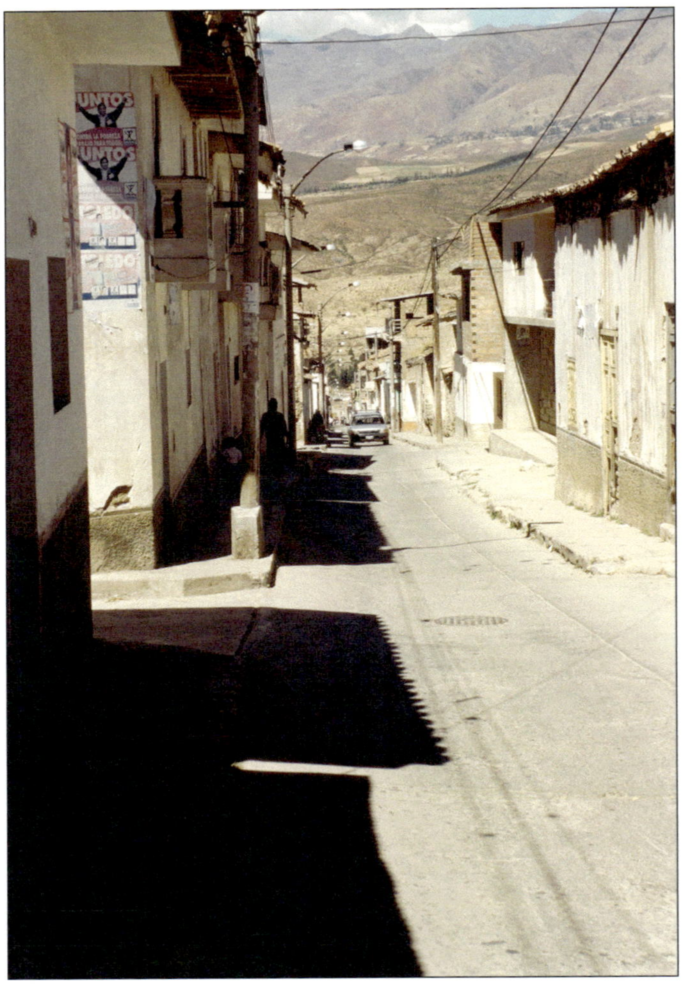

Caras taxi/street

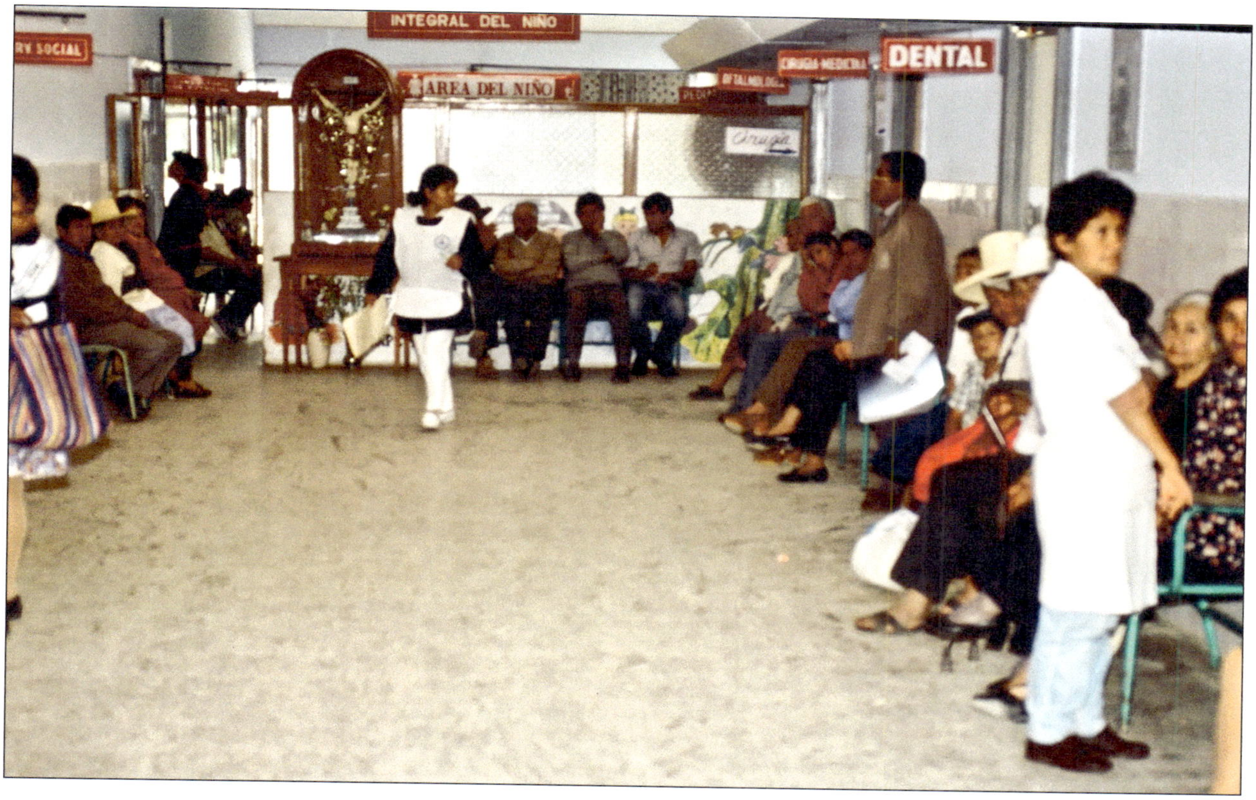

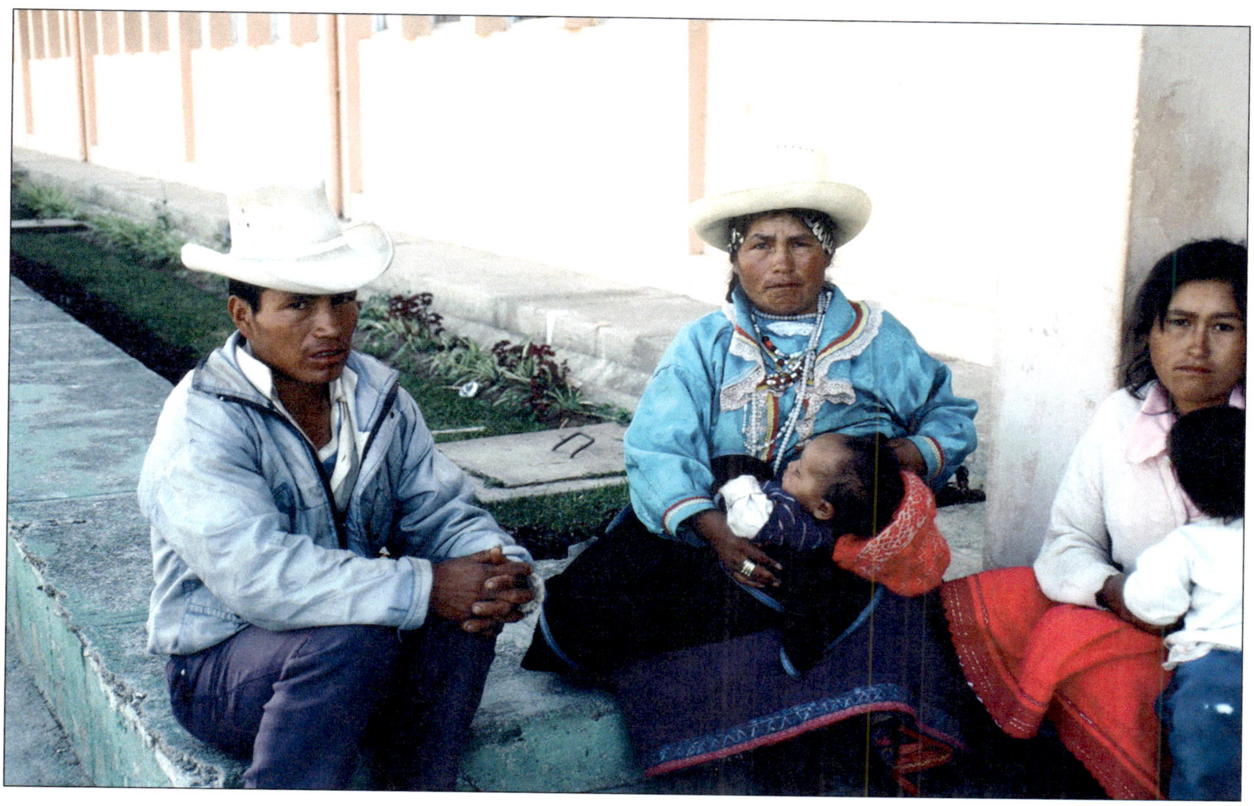

Patients waiting to be seen

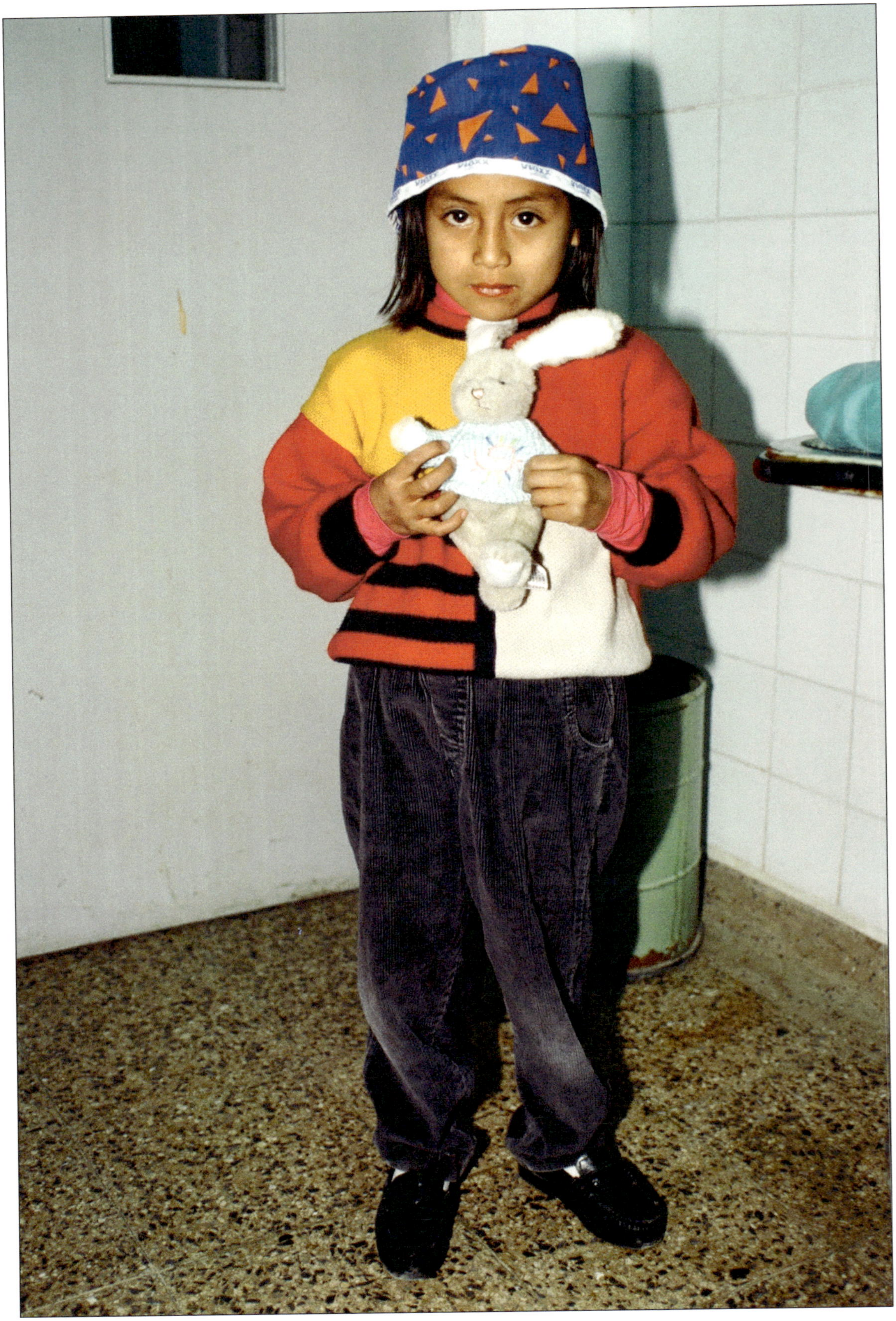

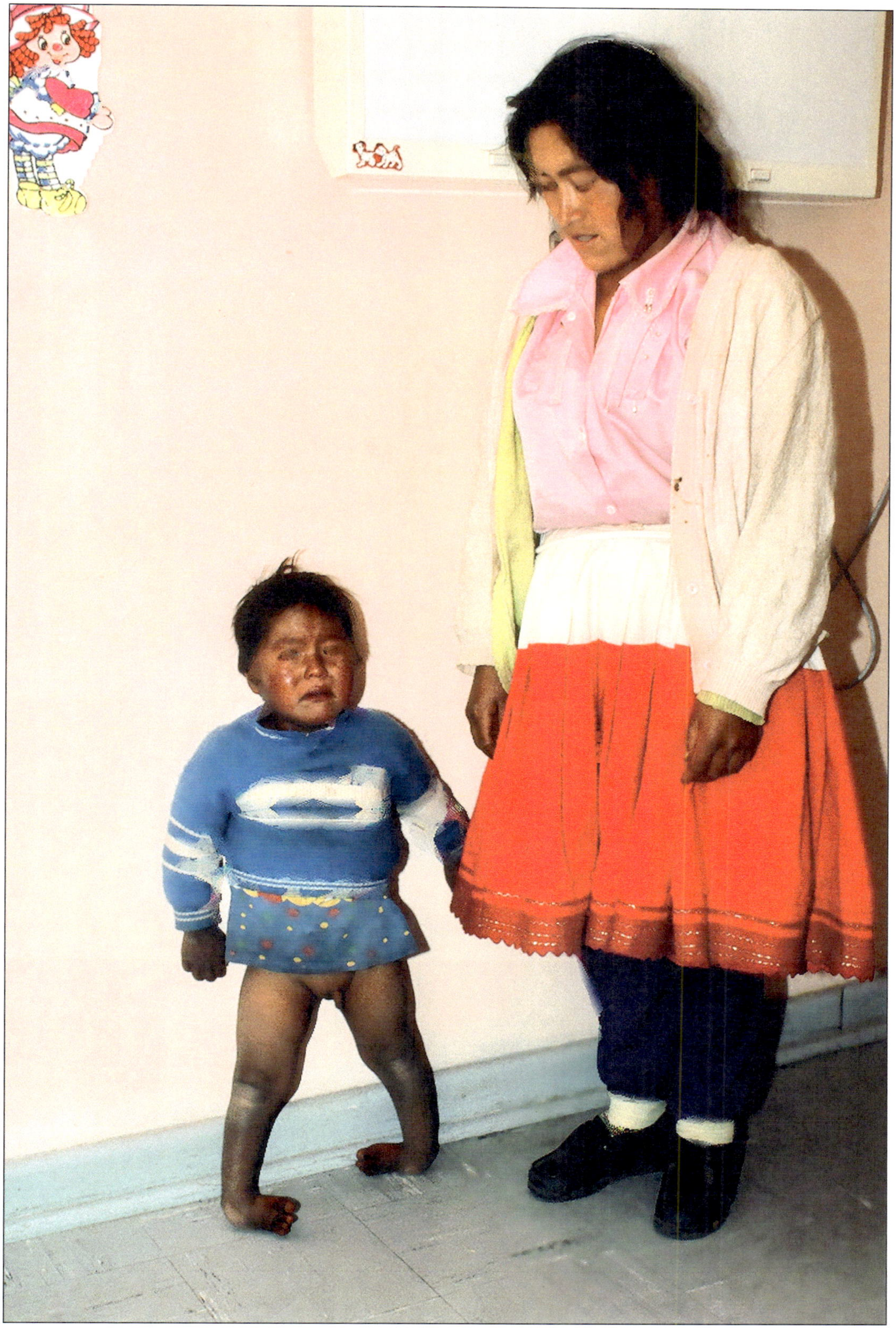

Bilateral clubfeet

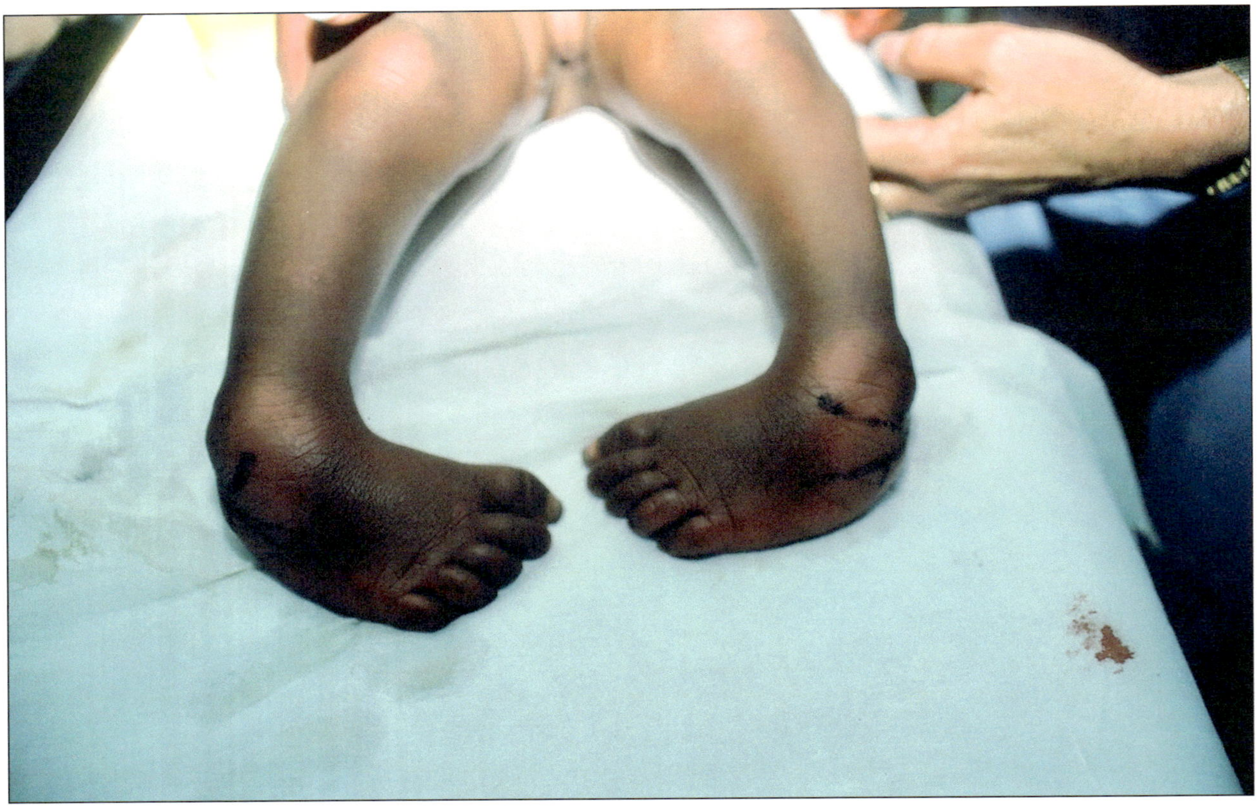

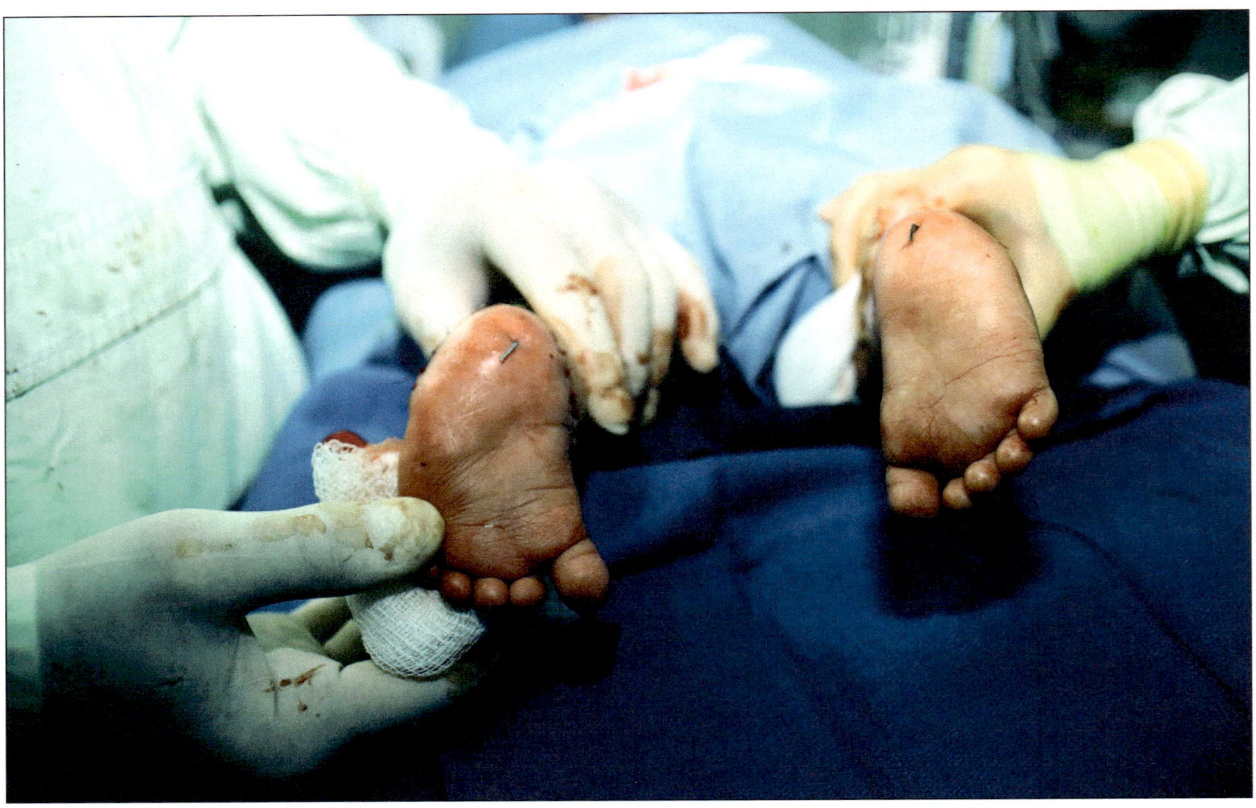

After surgery

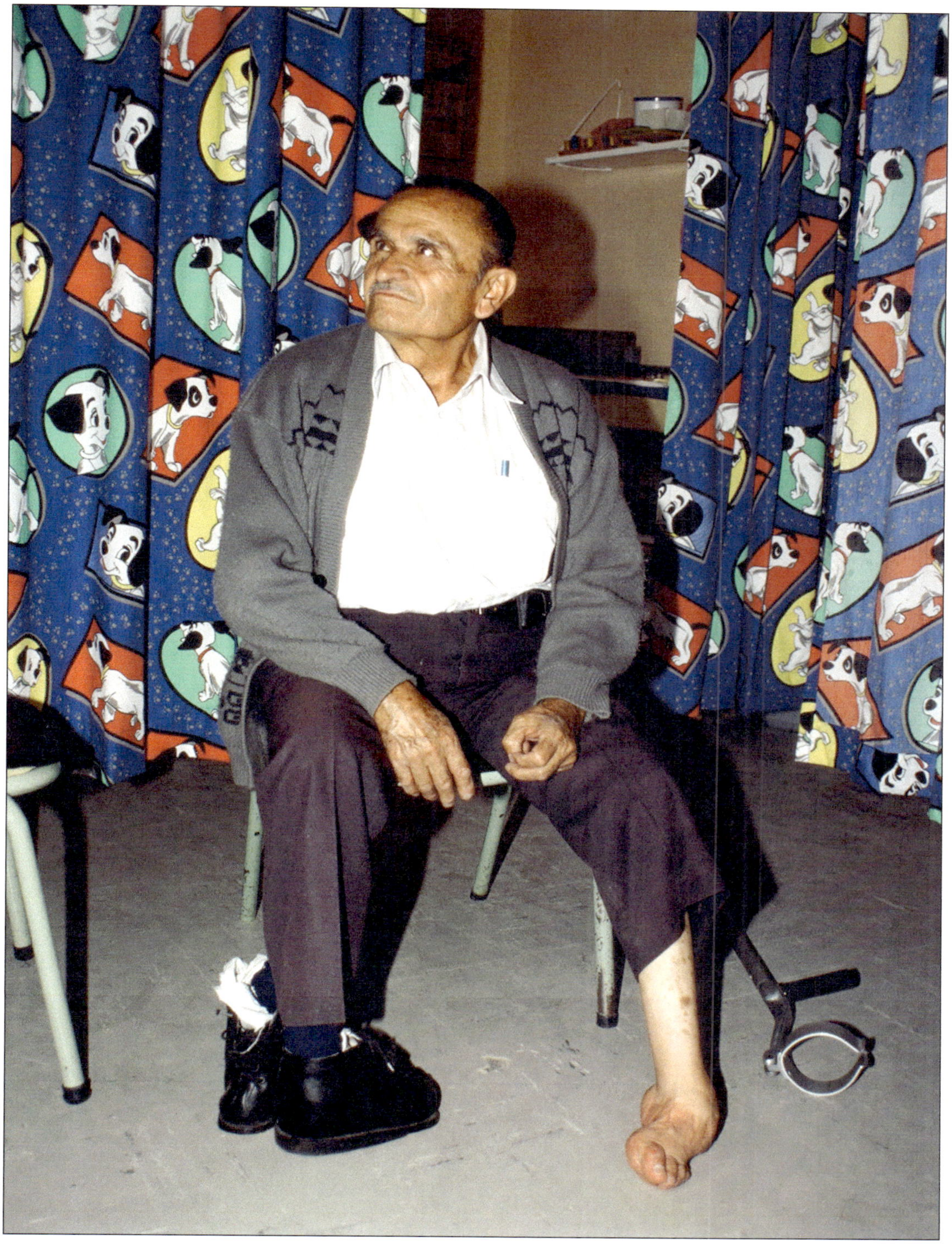

Older man with clubfoot. Too old to operate

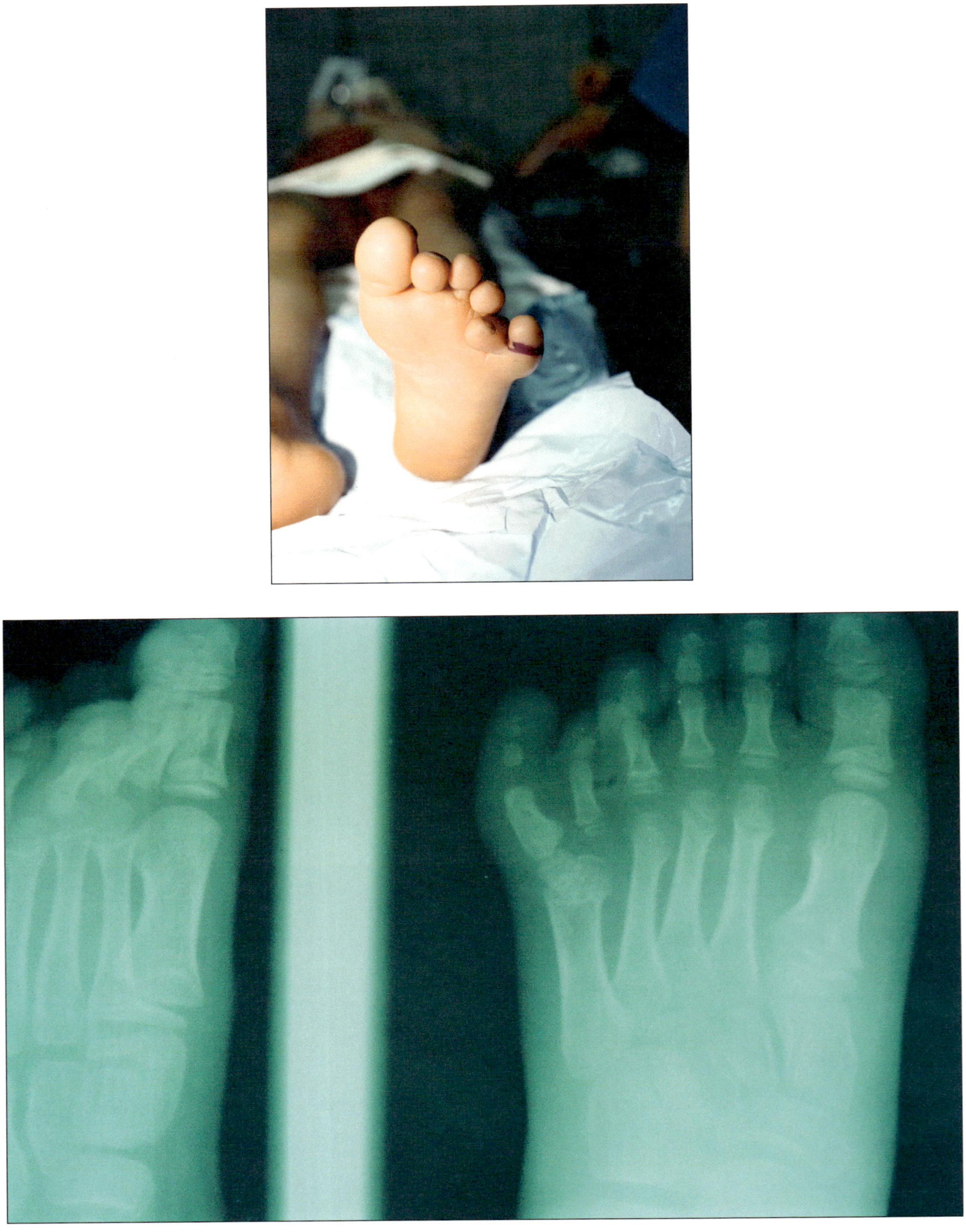

Adolescent with extra 5th toe

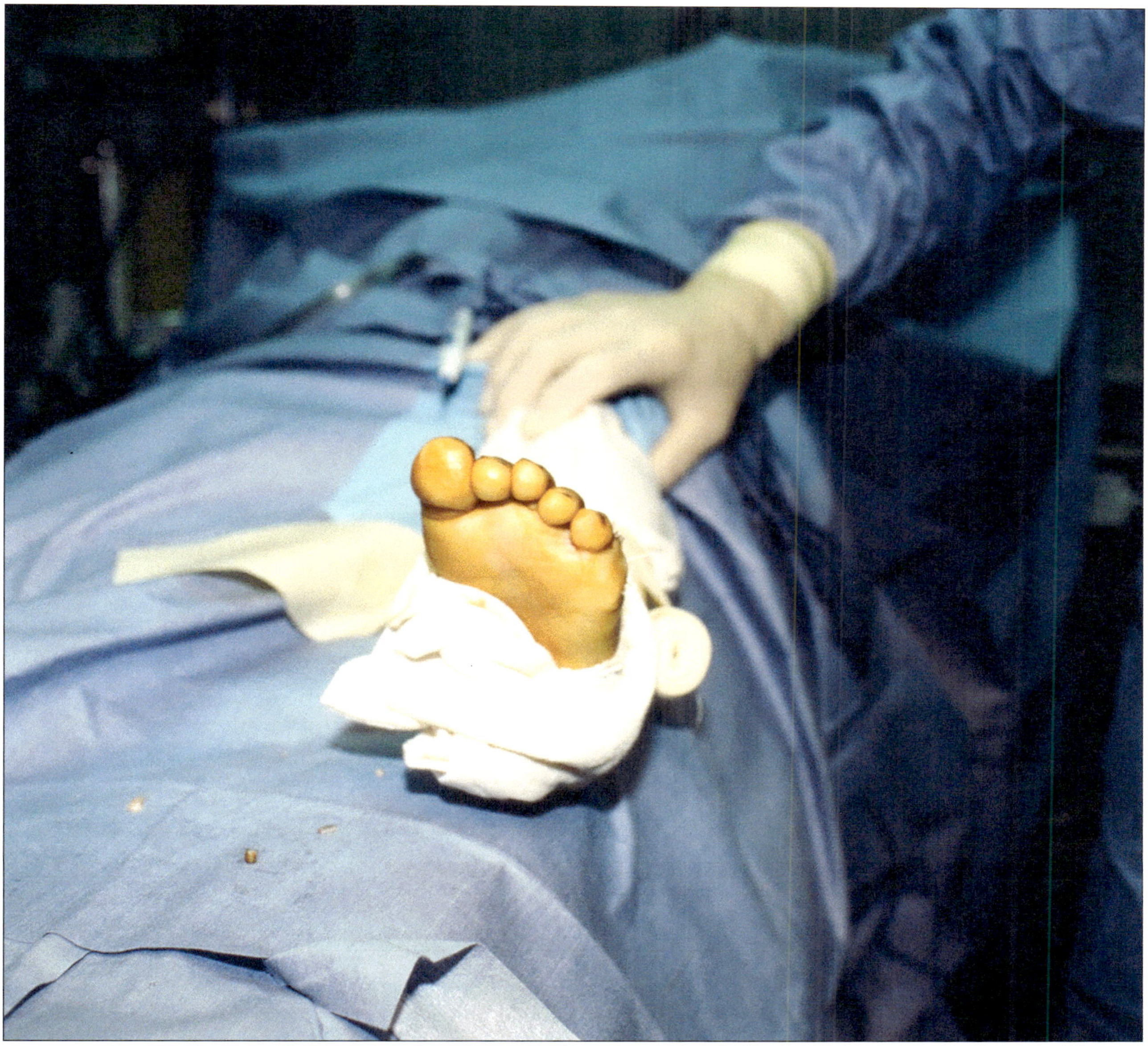

After surgery

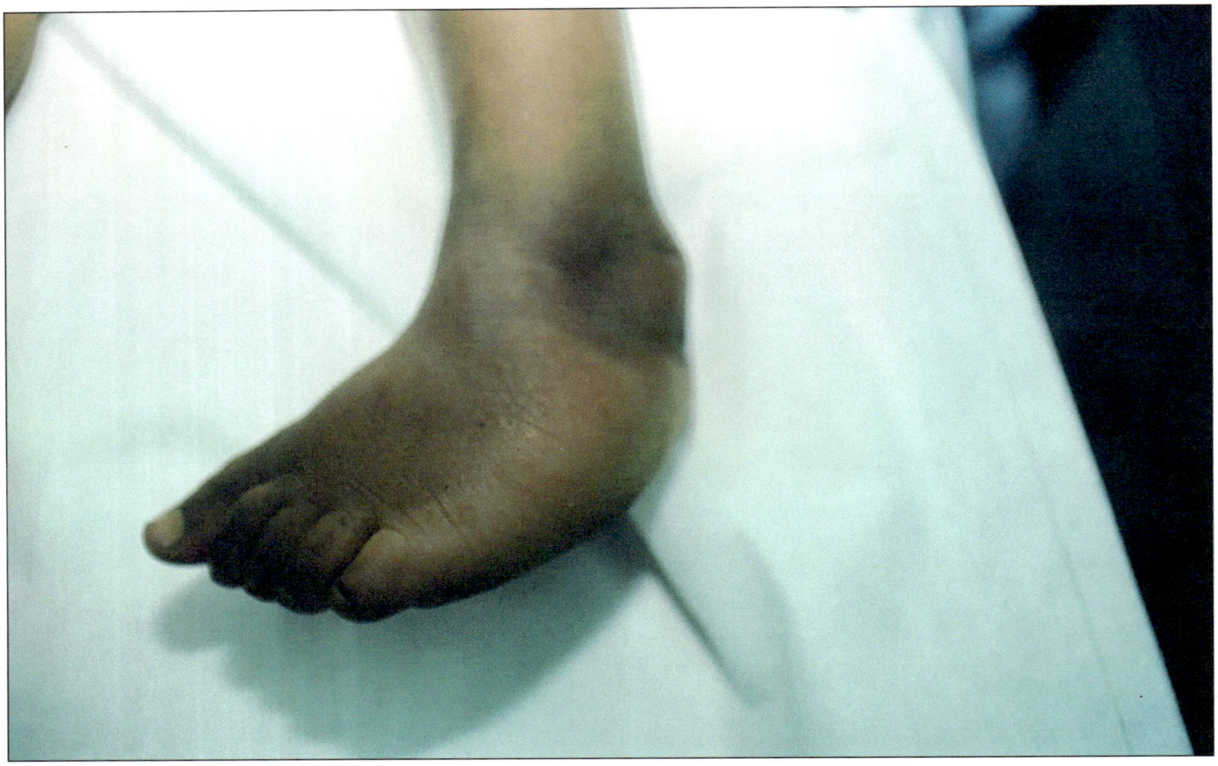

Left-foot deformity

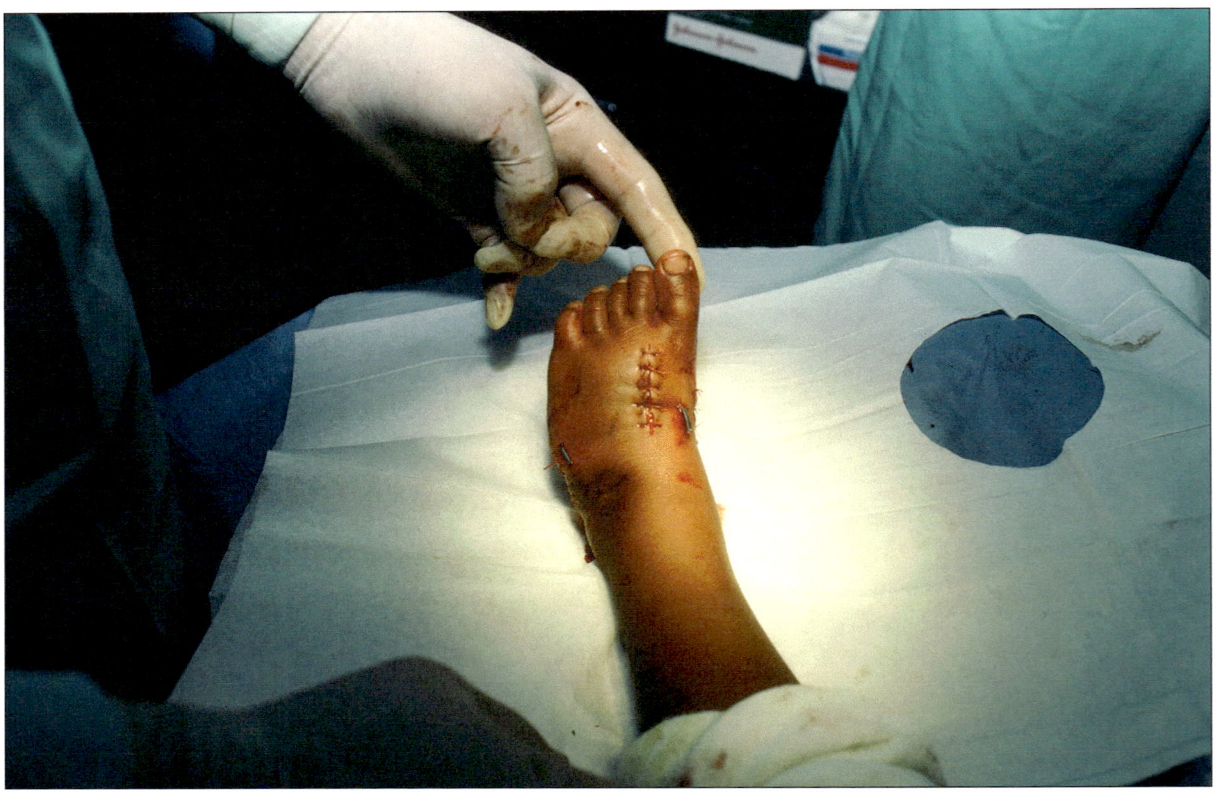

After correction

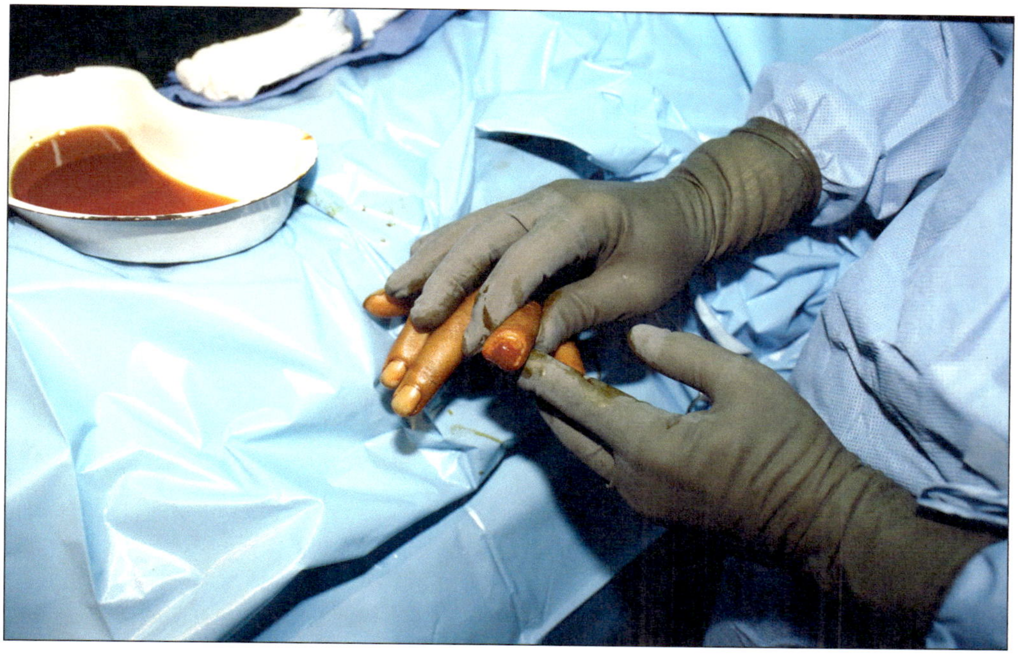

Fingertip amputation

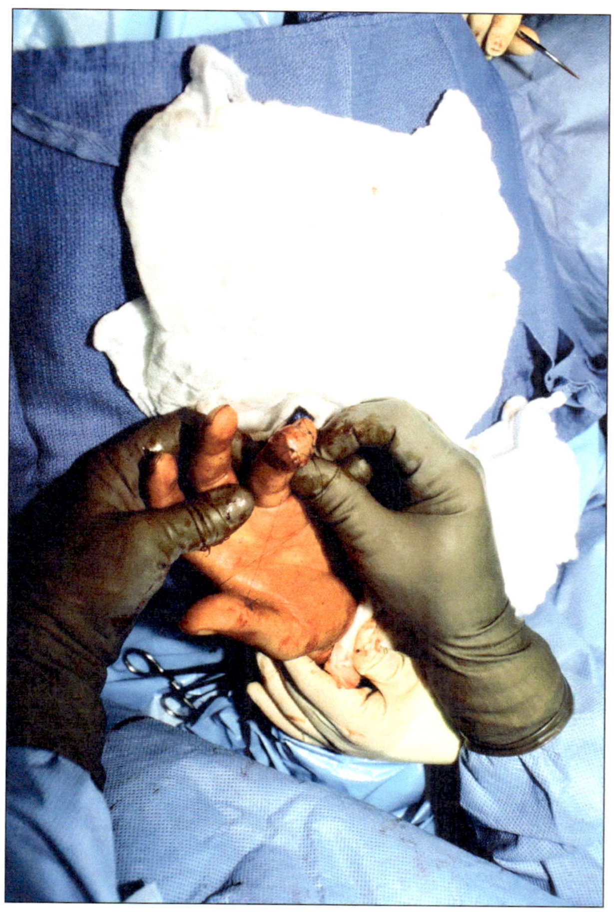

After graft applied to tip

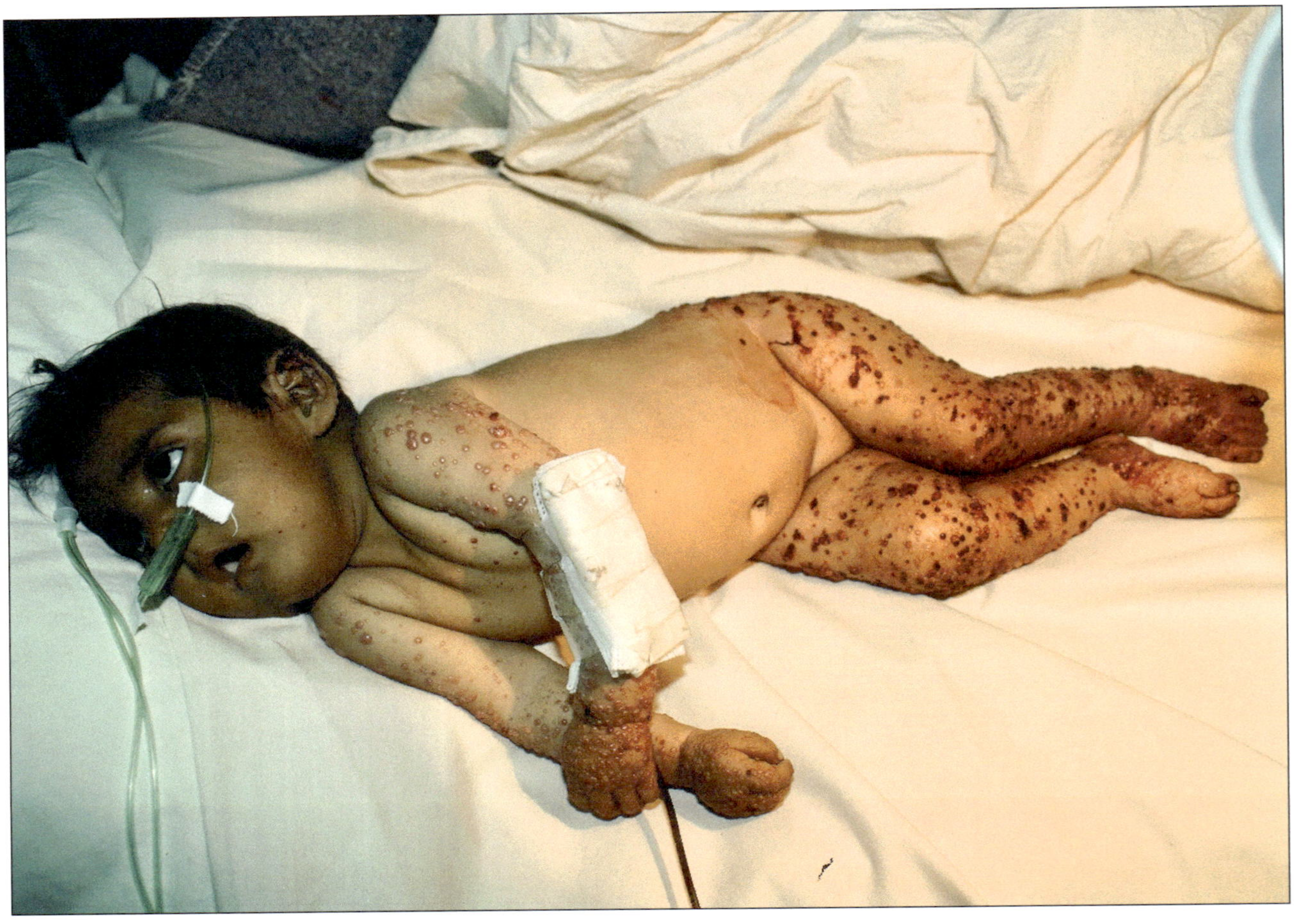

Child with viral rash

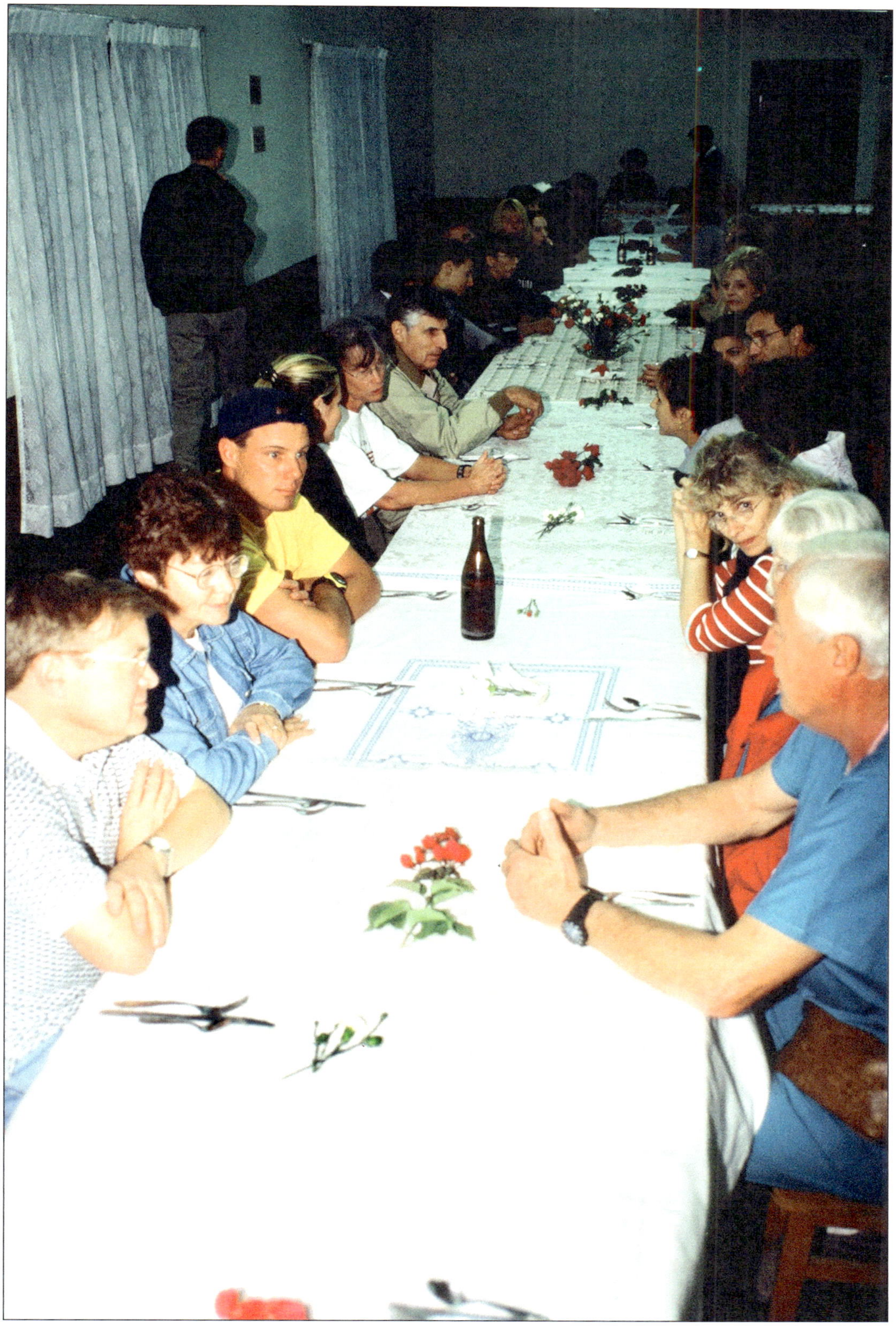

Ceremonial dinner with locals

We made two other trips to Peru, one to Trujillo (2004), and another to Lima (2008). These were with Operation Walk, an organization founded and run by a longtime friend and fellow Iowan, Dr. Larry Dorr. Larry and I have known each other since middle school, played football against one another in college, and attended medical school together at the University of Iowa. Larry became a preeminent orthopedic surgeon in the field of hip and knee replacement and has recently retired as the chief of joint-replacement surgery at USC Medical Center. He has published multiple papers and a book. He travels the country lecturing on hip and knee joint replacement.

With the fruits of his success, he founded Operation Walk in 1996. The organization takes surgical teams consisting of six to eight orthopedists, physical therapists, scrub techs, internists, nurses, and anesthesiologists as well as more than $1M in donated prosthetic devices to Third World countries, teaching techniques to the local physicians and operating on individuals who would not have access to such treatment otherwise. The trips last usually one week and are rigidly structured and arranged by Larry's girl Friday, Jeri Ward. Upon arrival, the non-surgeons go about setting up and organizing the surgical supplies while the surgeons screen patients. A conference follows, in which each doctor presents his patients for group discussion and the surgical schedule is constructed for the next three to four days. Fifty to sixty patients are operated on, giving them a new lease on life, free of pain.

Fifty to sixty patients are operated on, giving them a new lease on life, free of pain.

During the Trujillo trip, I operated on a patient sent by Gaston Barnechea from Lima. Gloria Prado was a 60-year-old with severe arthritis of her right hip. She also happened to be a poet and a non-stop talker, but a delight. After my return to the US, she sent me some of her poetry as well as some Peruvian trinkets for Christmas. Upon our return to Lima in 2008, she came to see me in follow-up and presented me with some beautiful Peruvian artifacts and a picture that hangs in my den today. Unfortunately, the artifacts were confiscated at the airport by the authorities, who claimed that these were possessions of the State and could not leave the country.

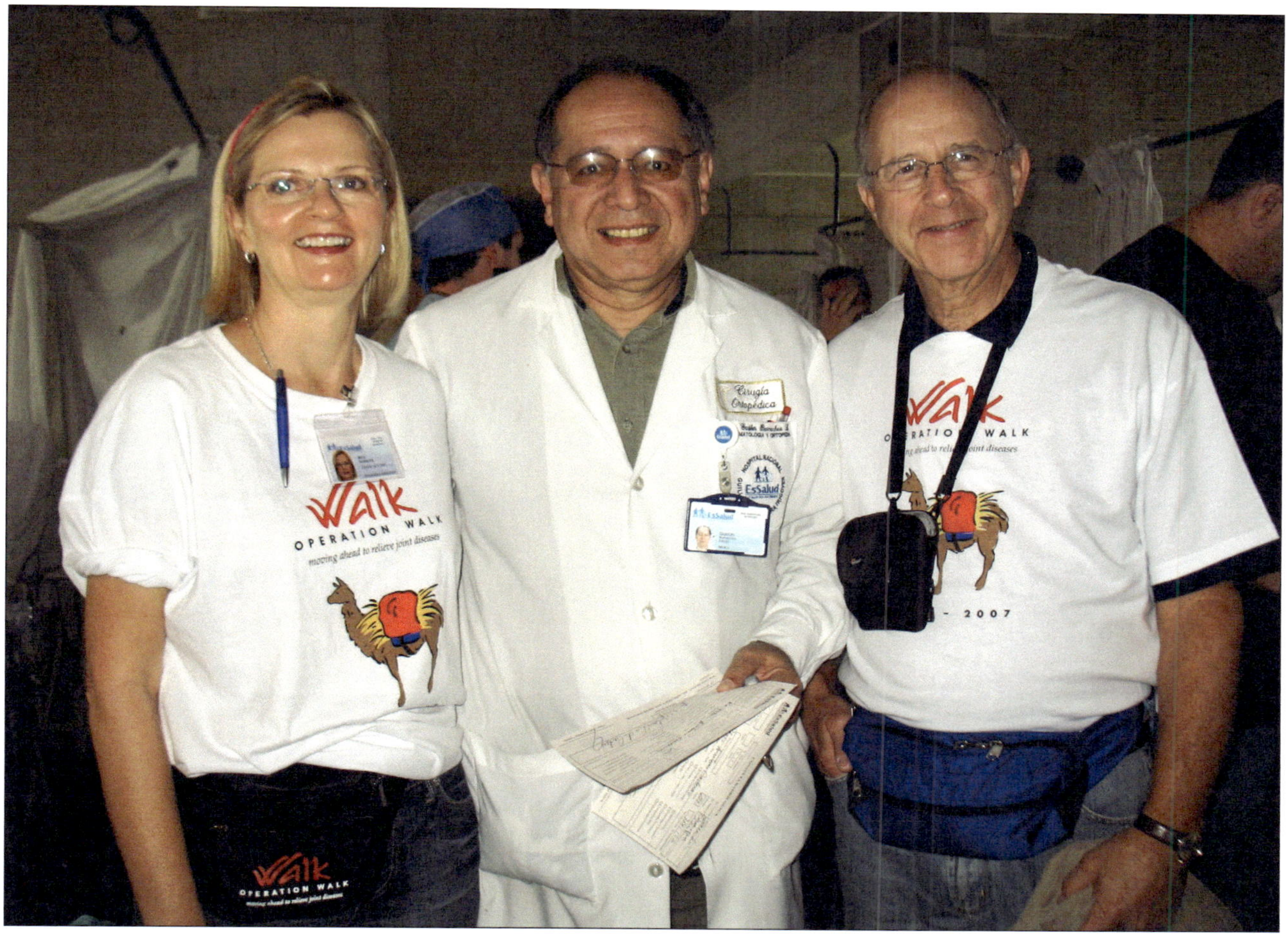

Rita, Gaston, and me in 2008

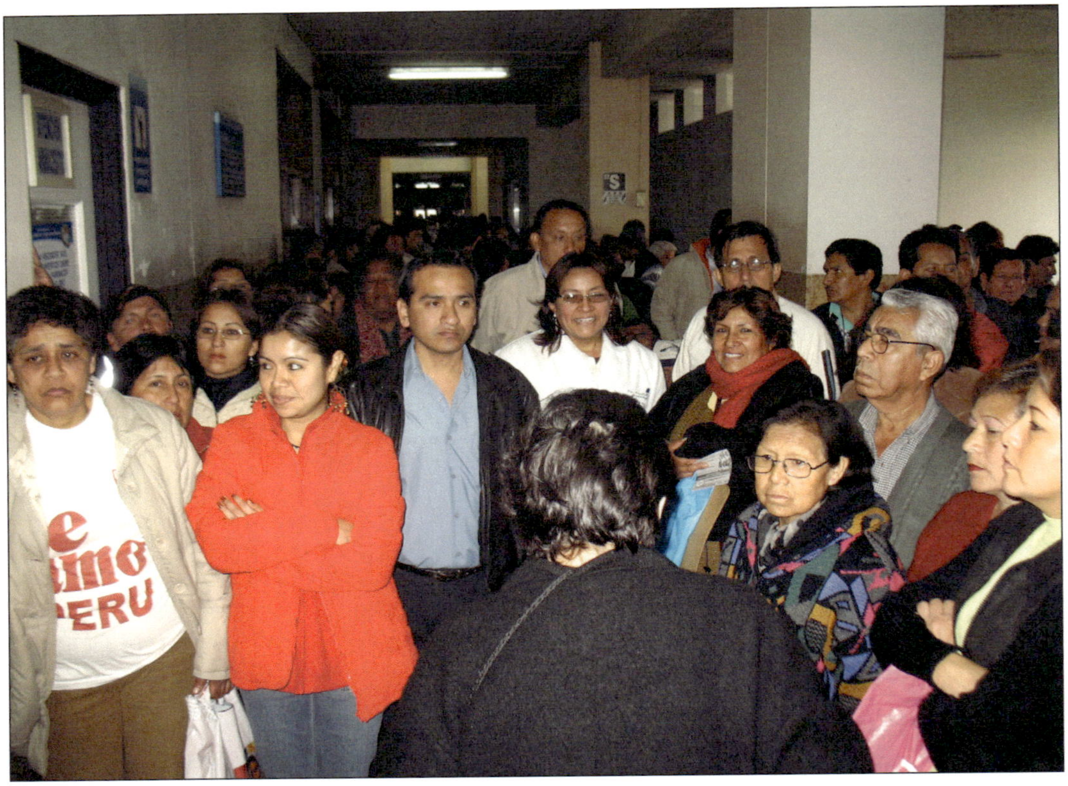

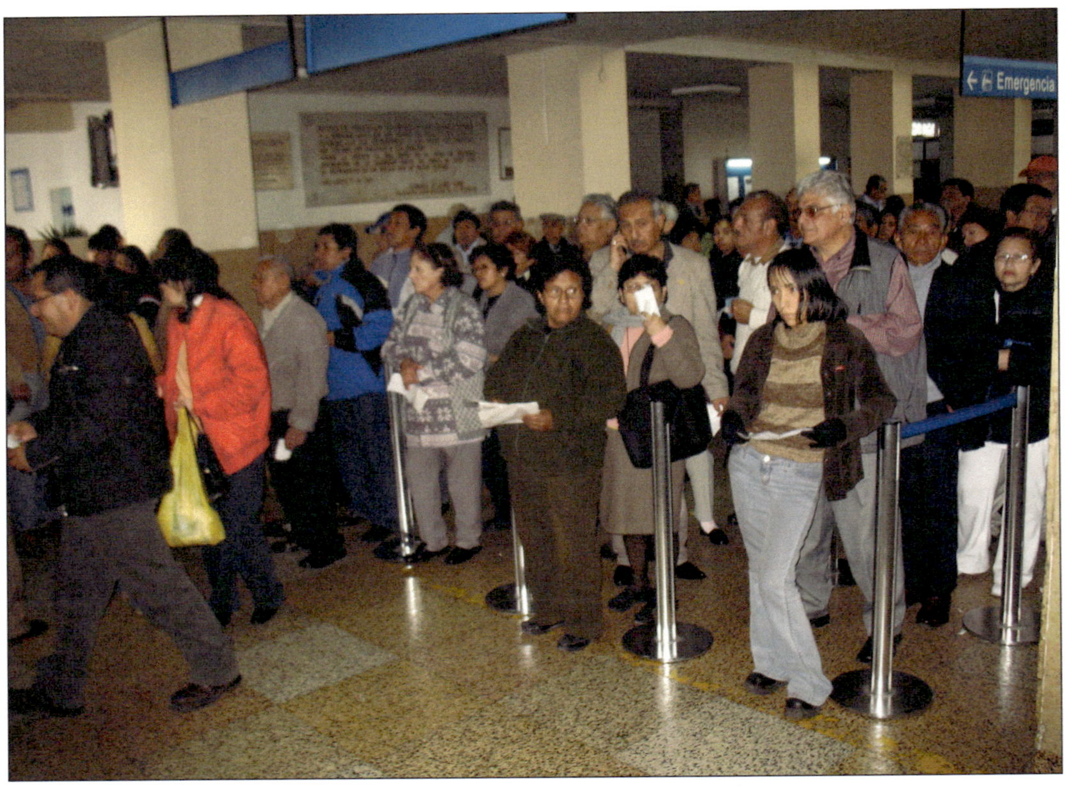

Patients and families wanting to be seen for joint replacements

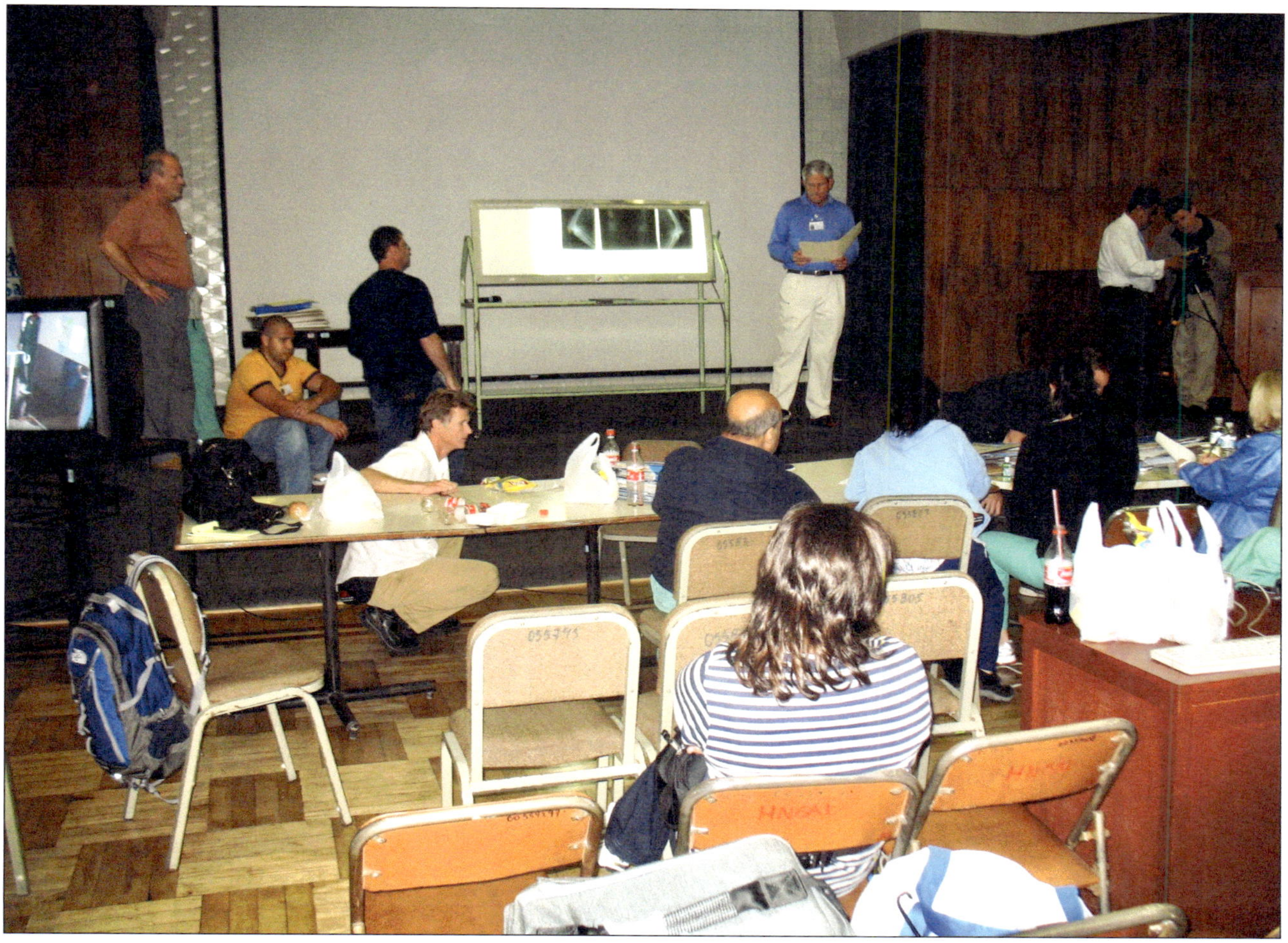

Pre-op conference

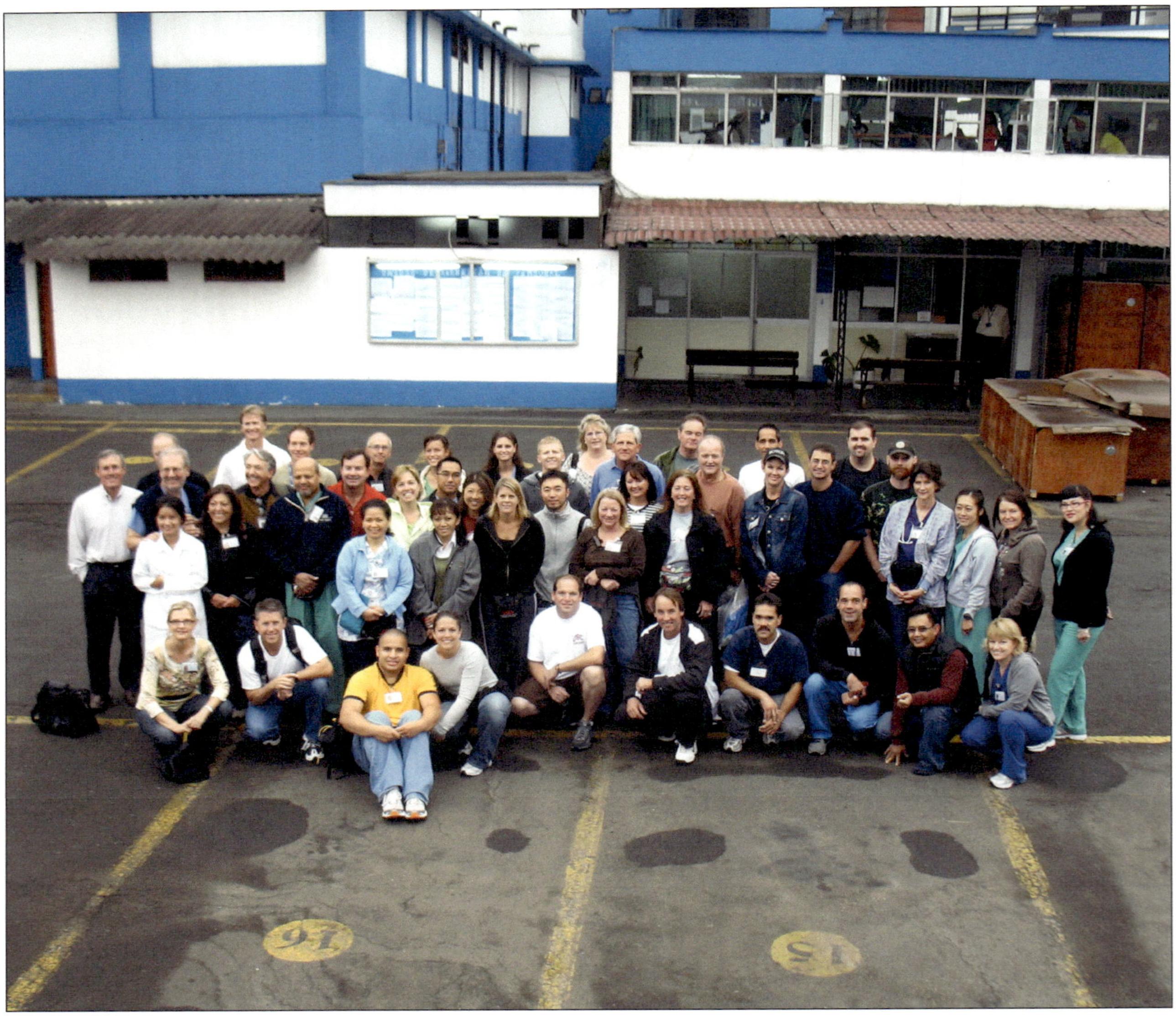

Operation Walk Team '08

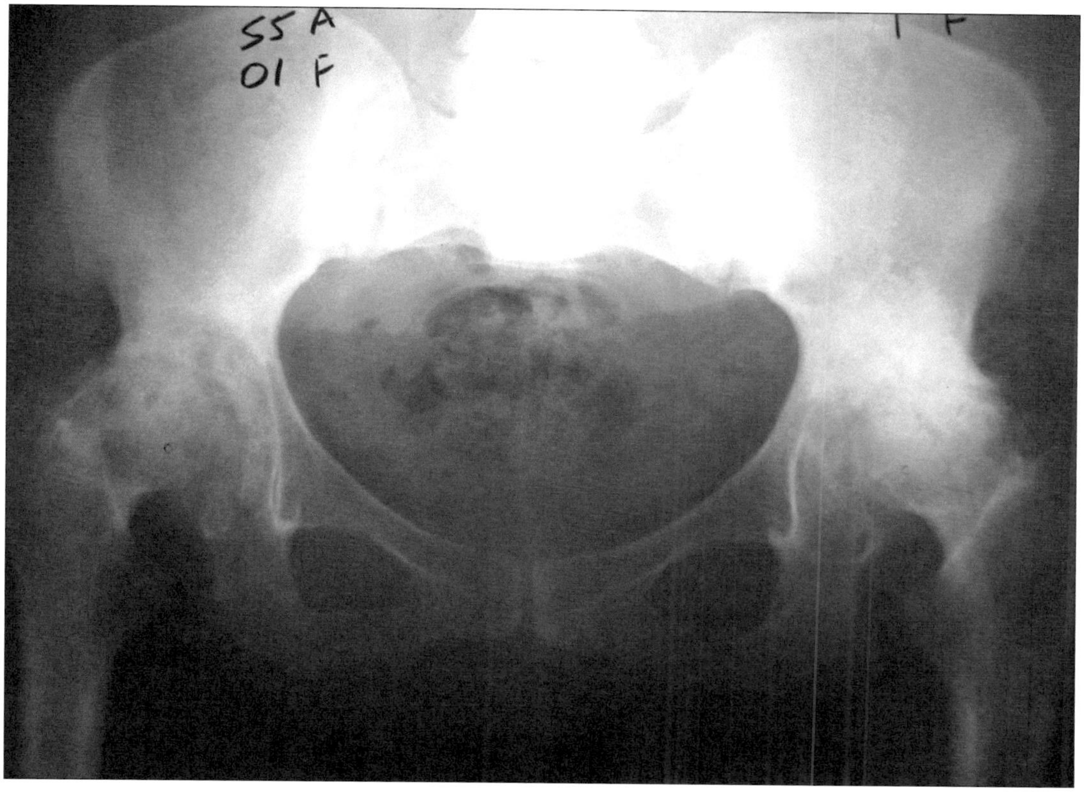

Severe arthritis both hips

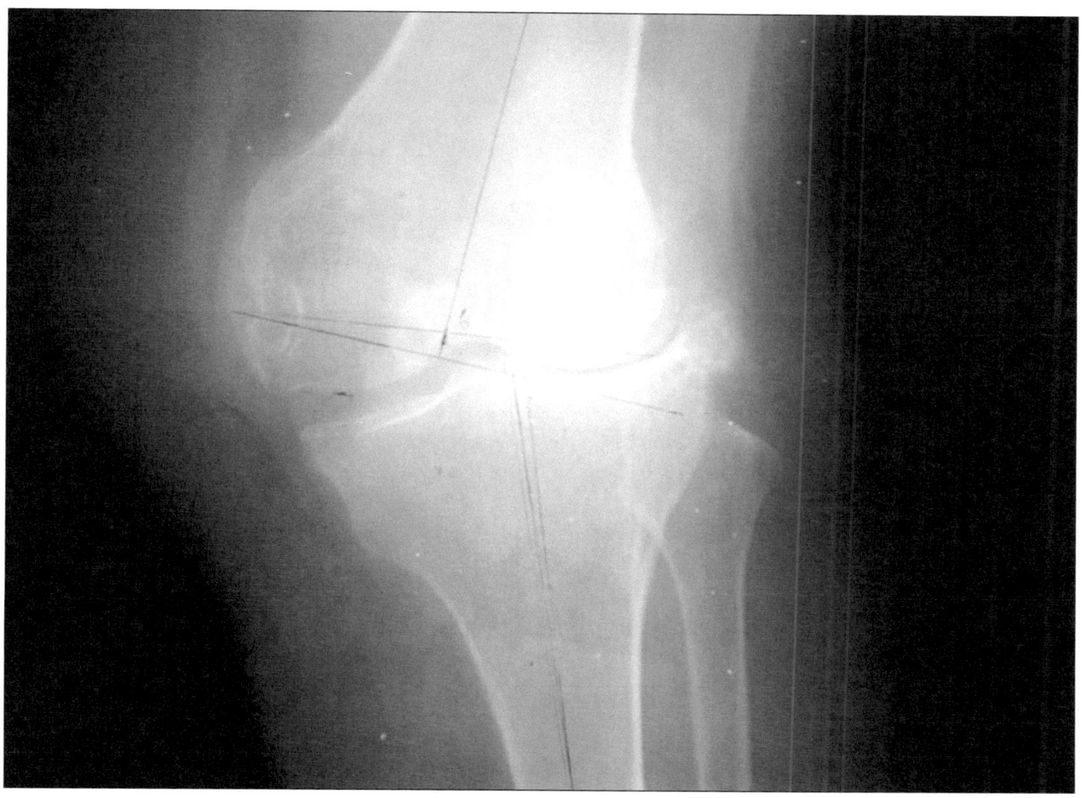

Arthritic deformity, left knee

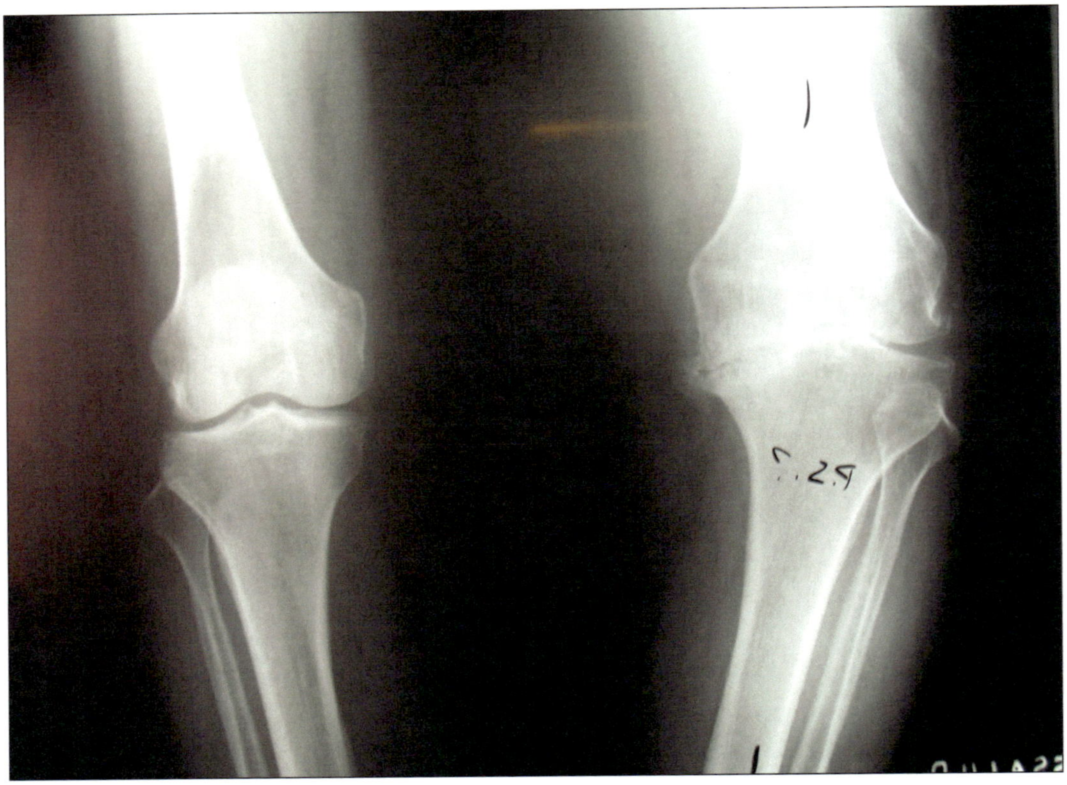

Left knee arthritis with deformity

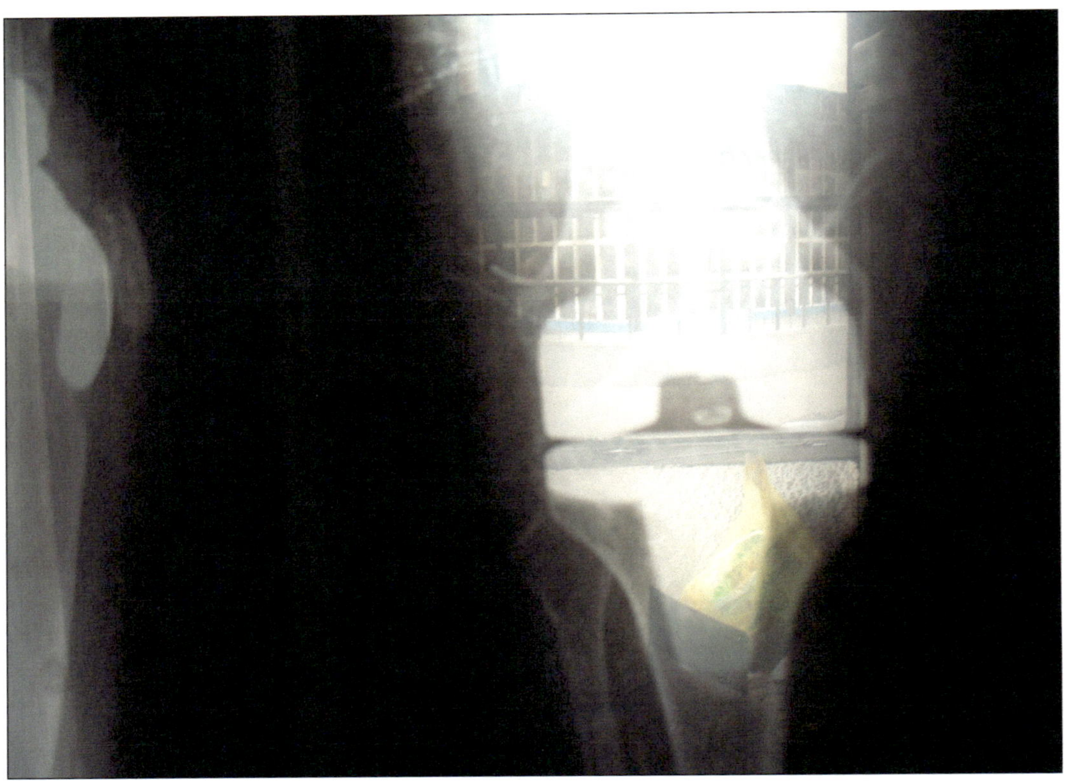

After replacement

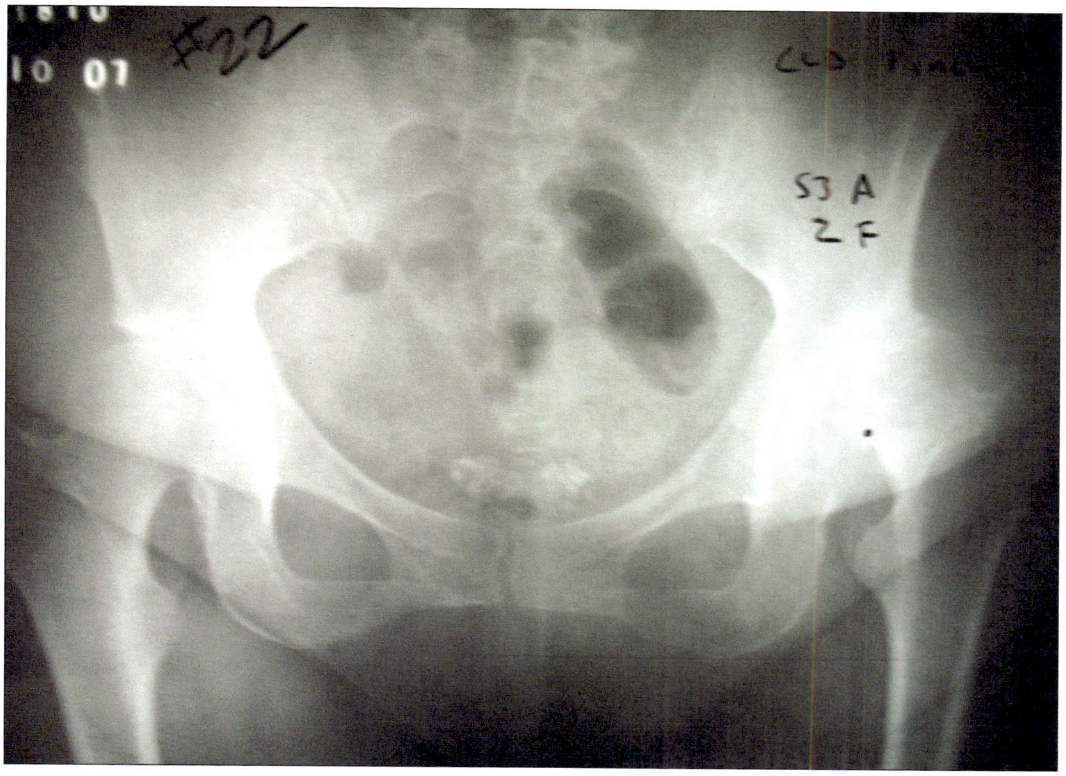

Arthritis left hip

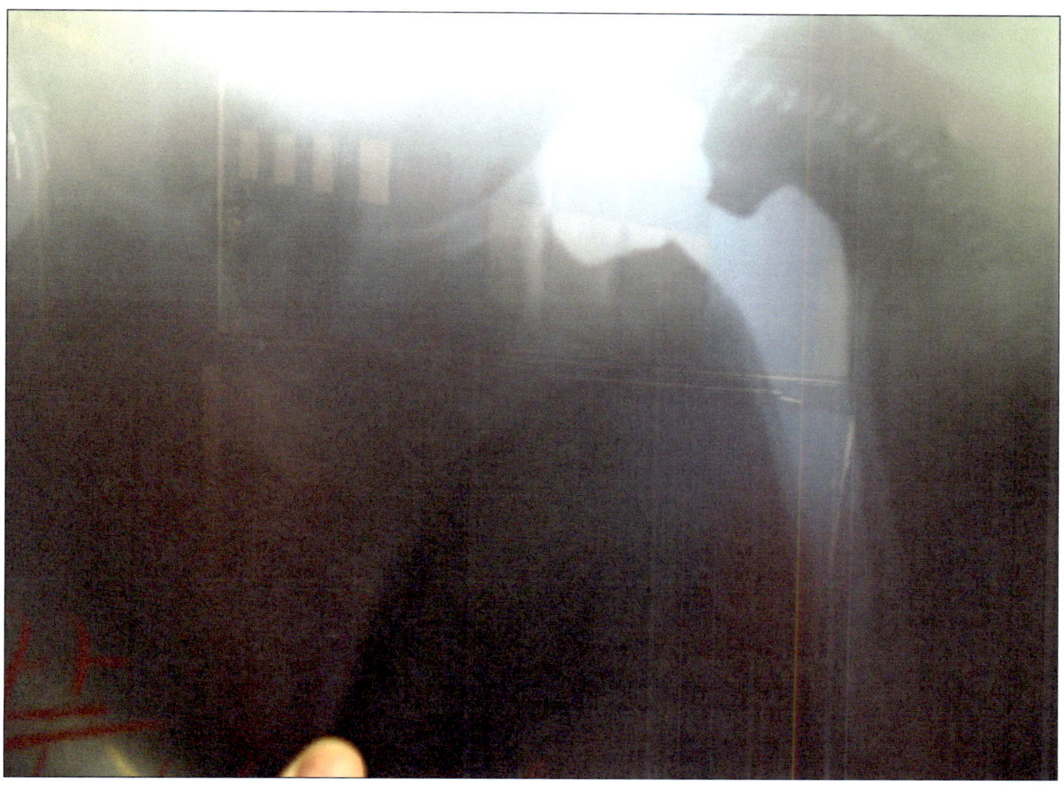

After replacement

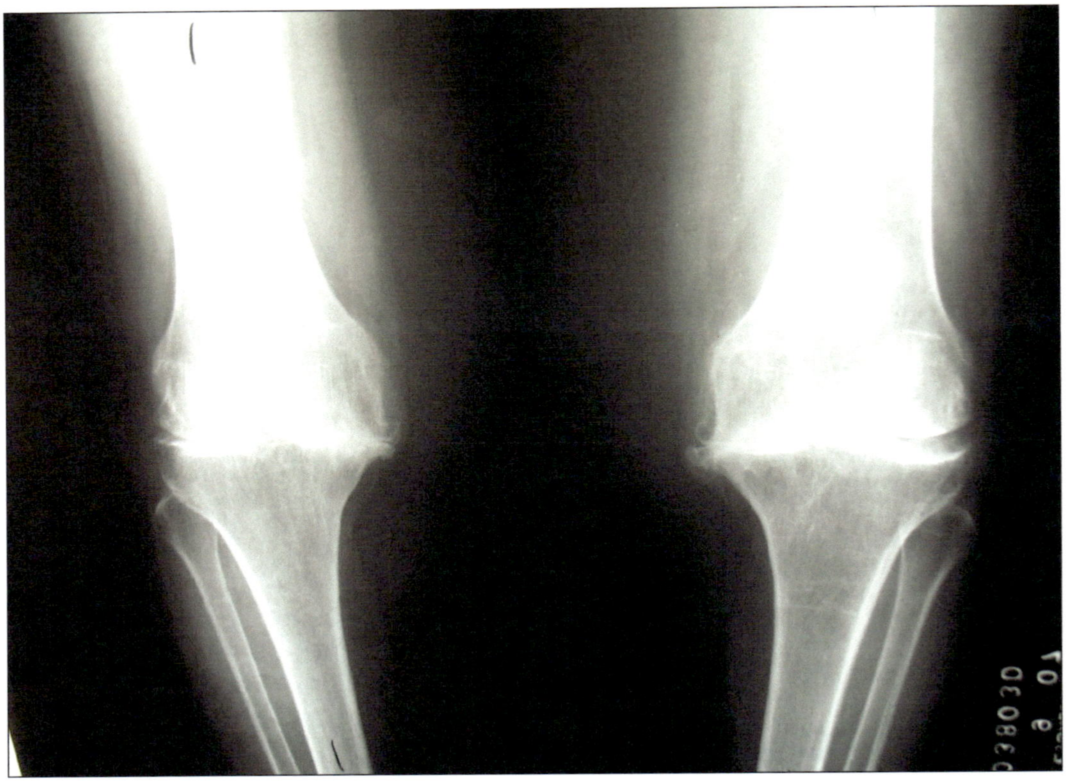

Arthritis both knees

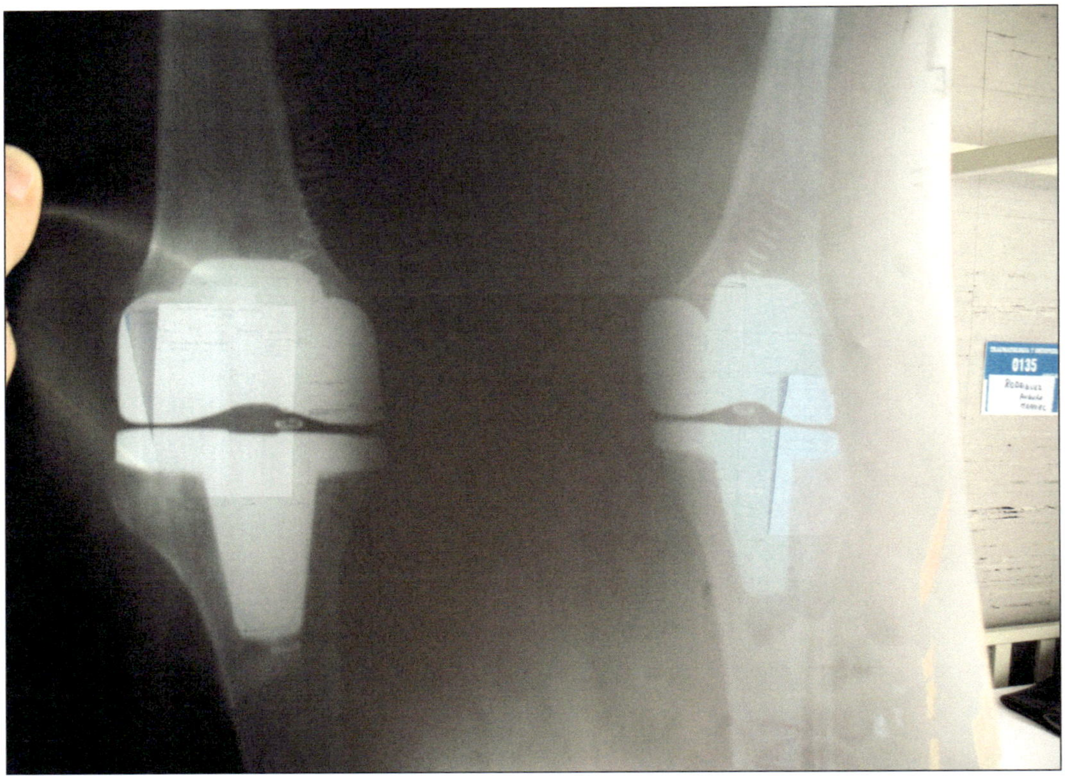

After replacement

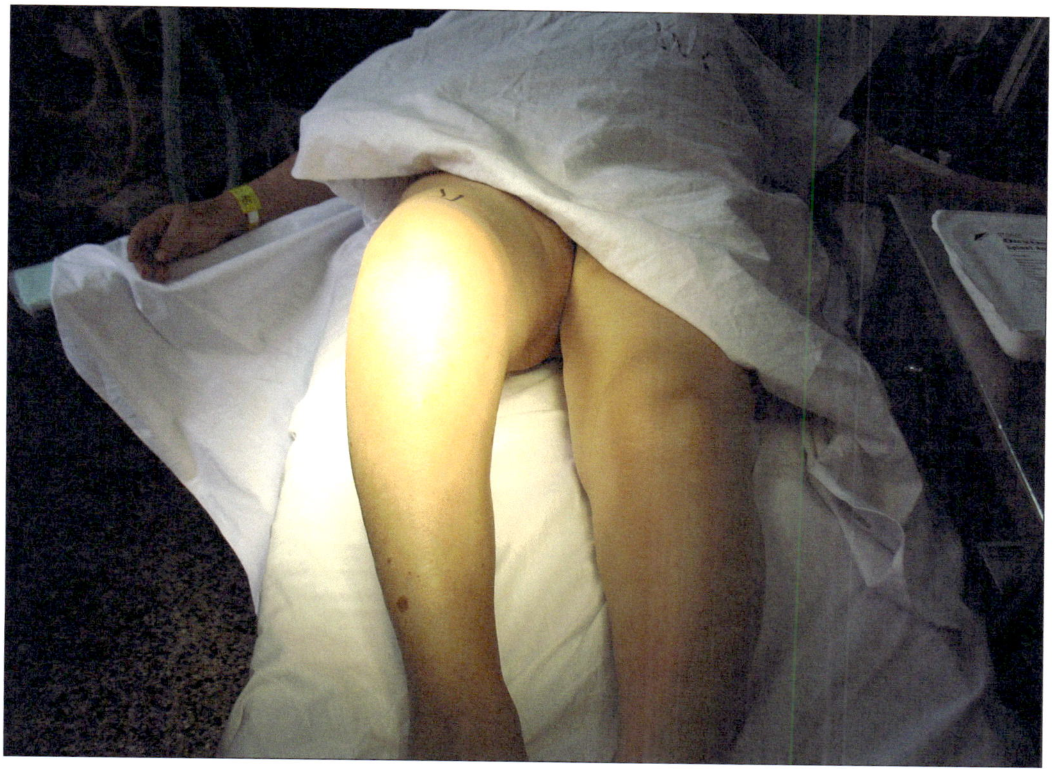

Deformed arthritic knee

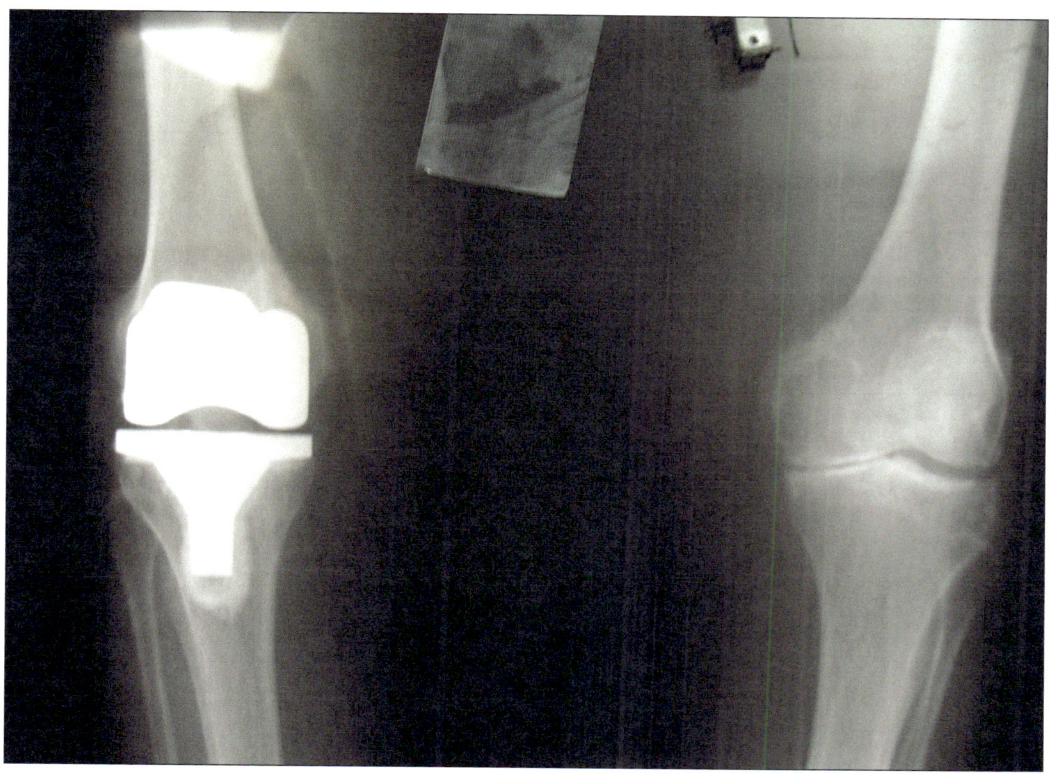

Post-op X-ray

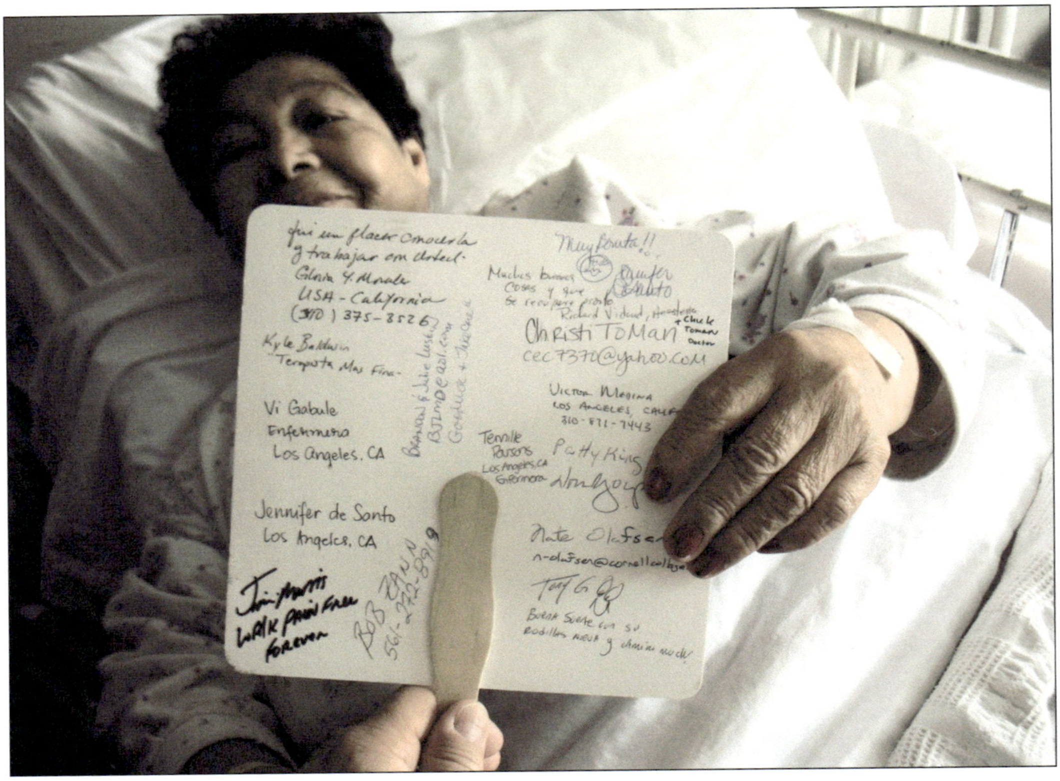

Patient requesting contact information of doctors and nurses

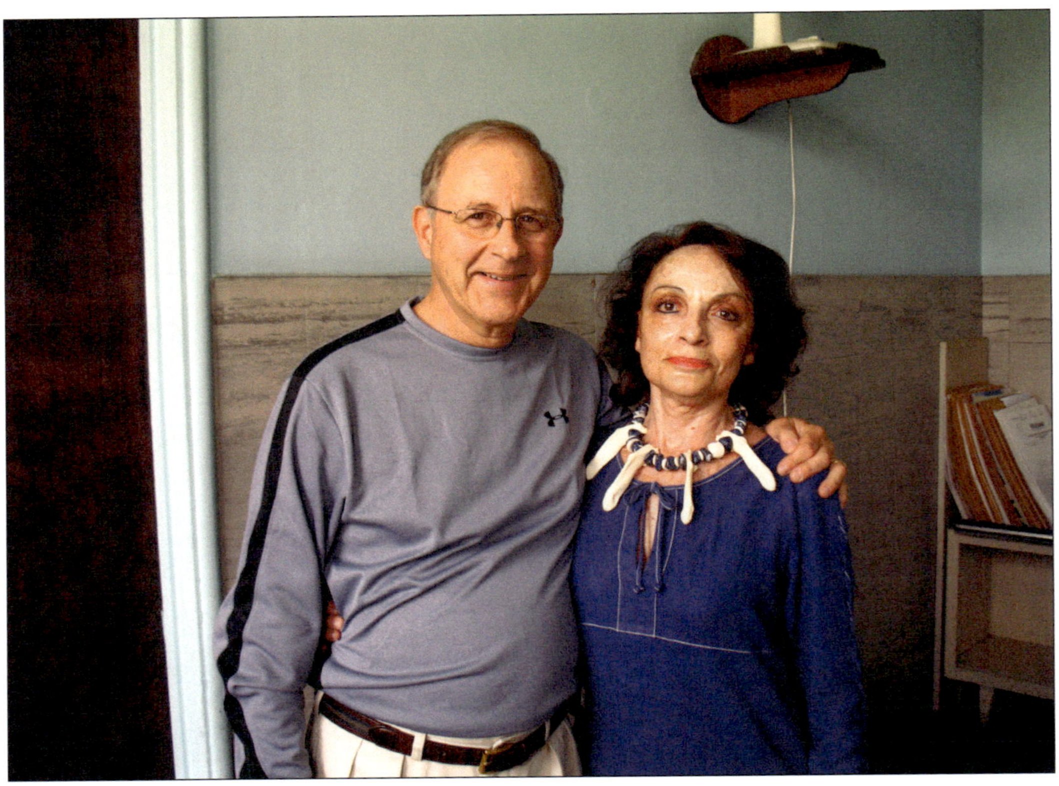

With patient Gloria Prado

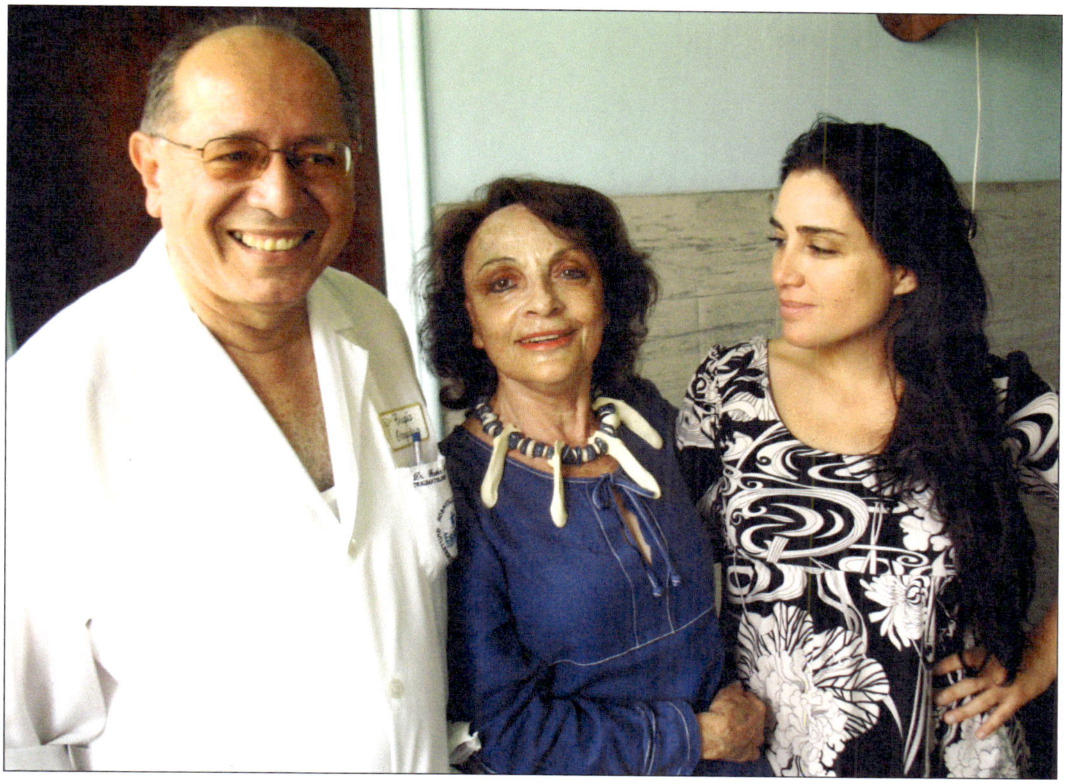

Gaston, Gloria, and her daughter

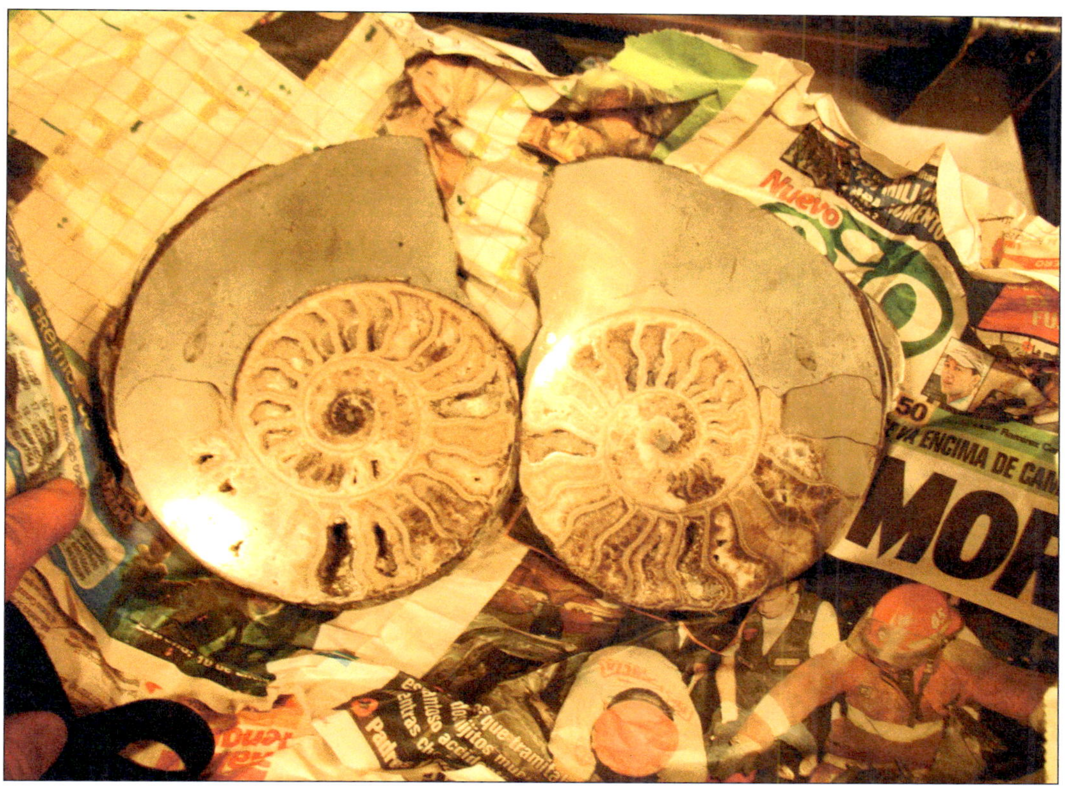

Confiscated artifact

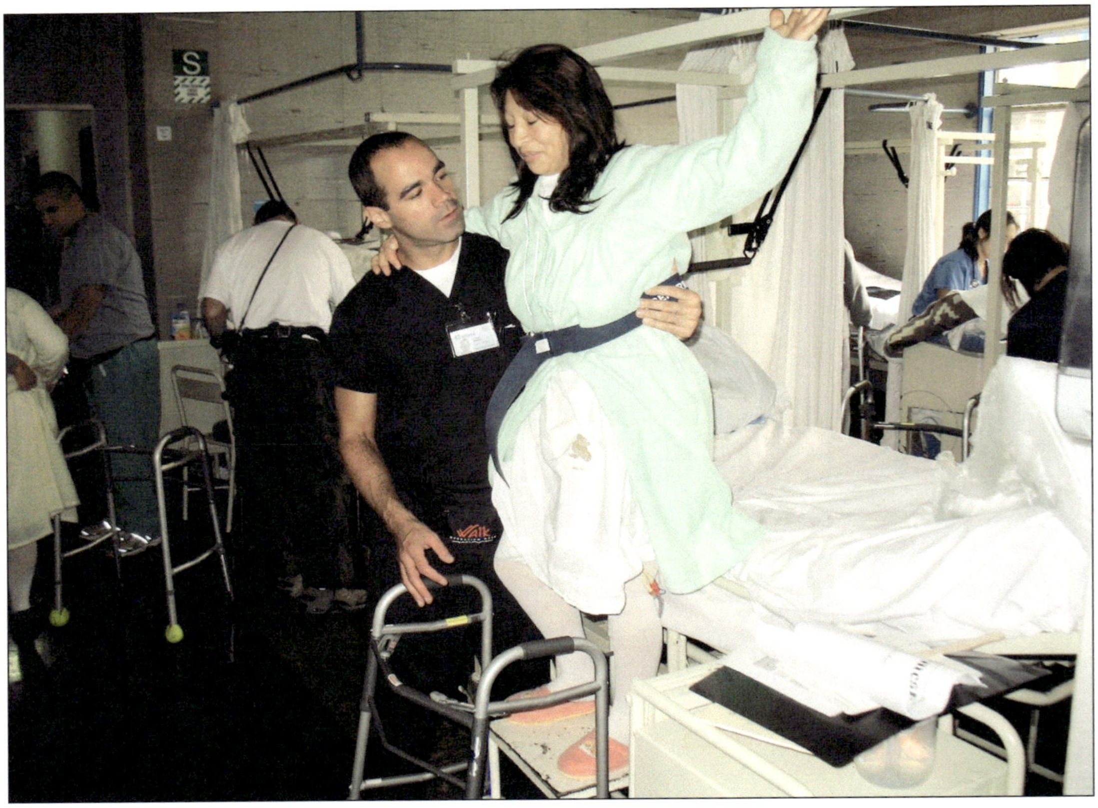

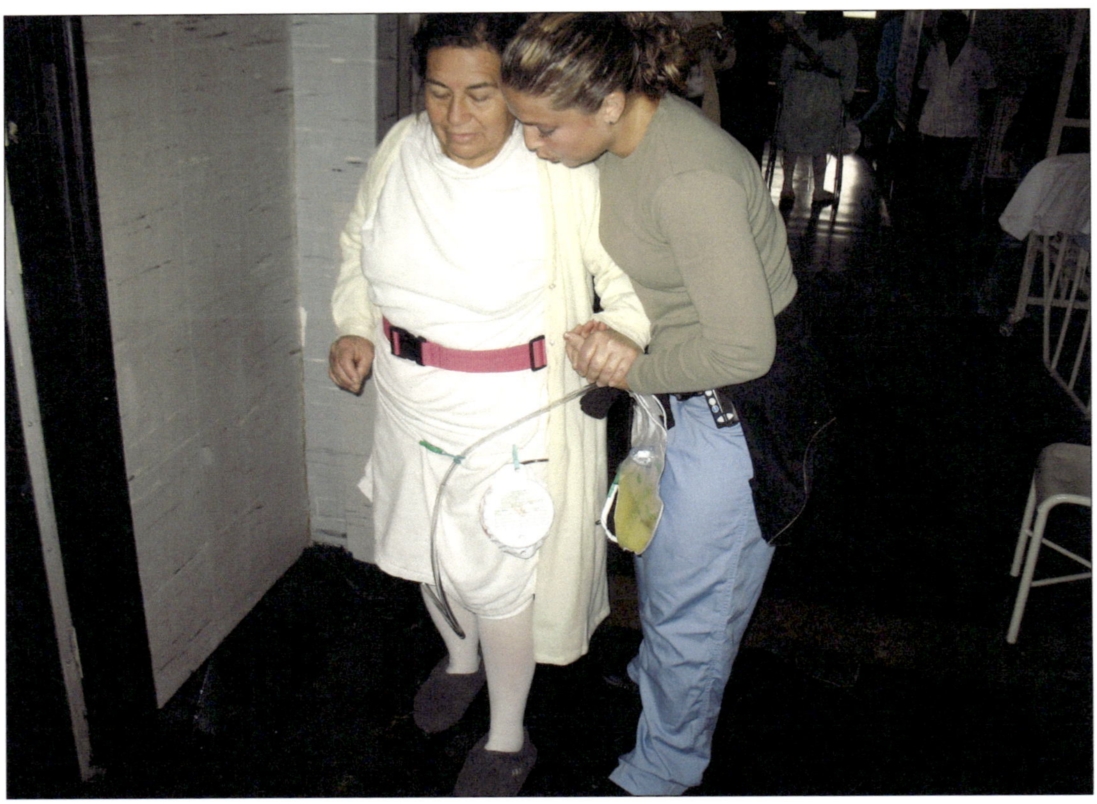

Patients being mobilized after surgery by physical therapy

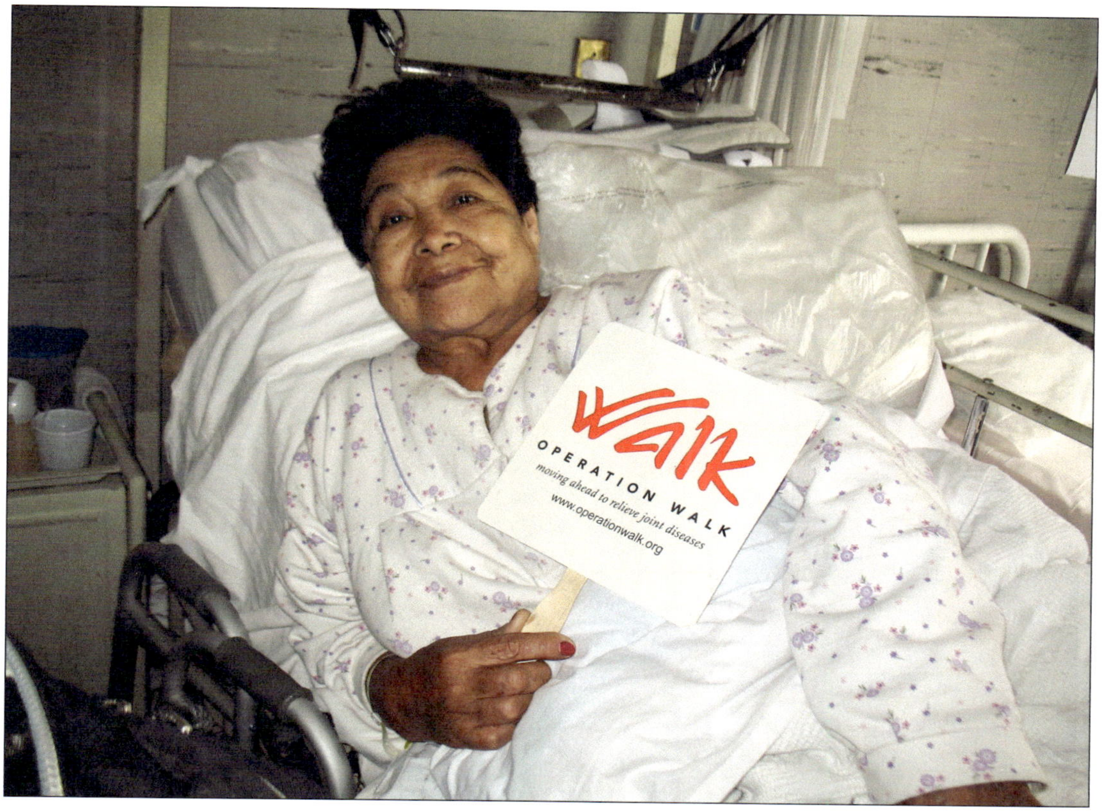

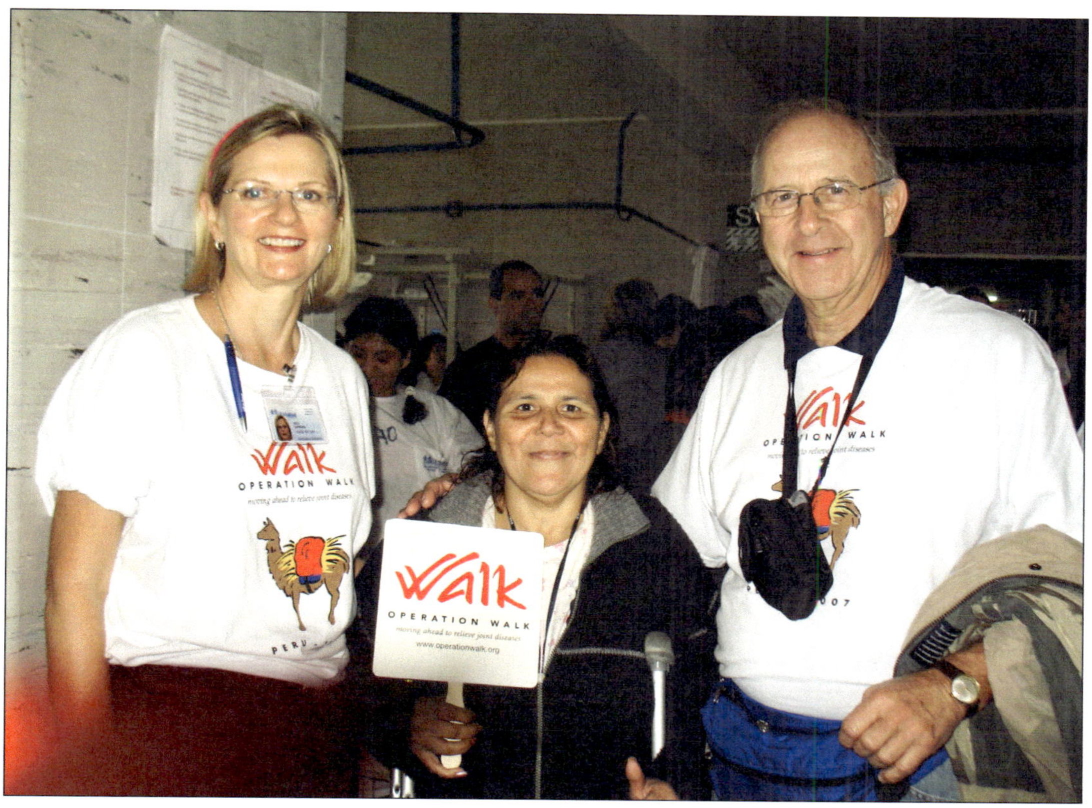

Happy patients

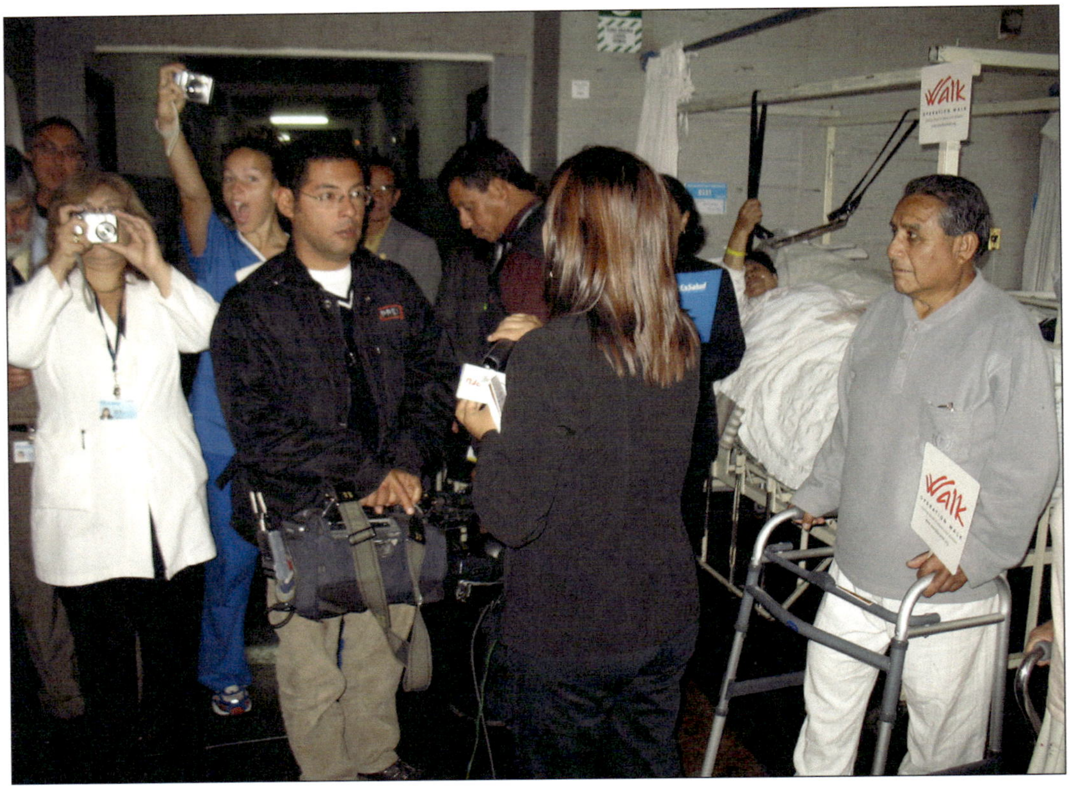

TV crew covering our visit

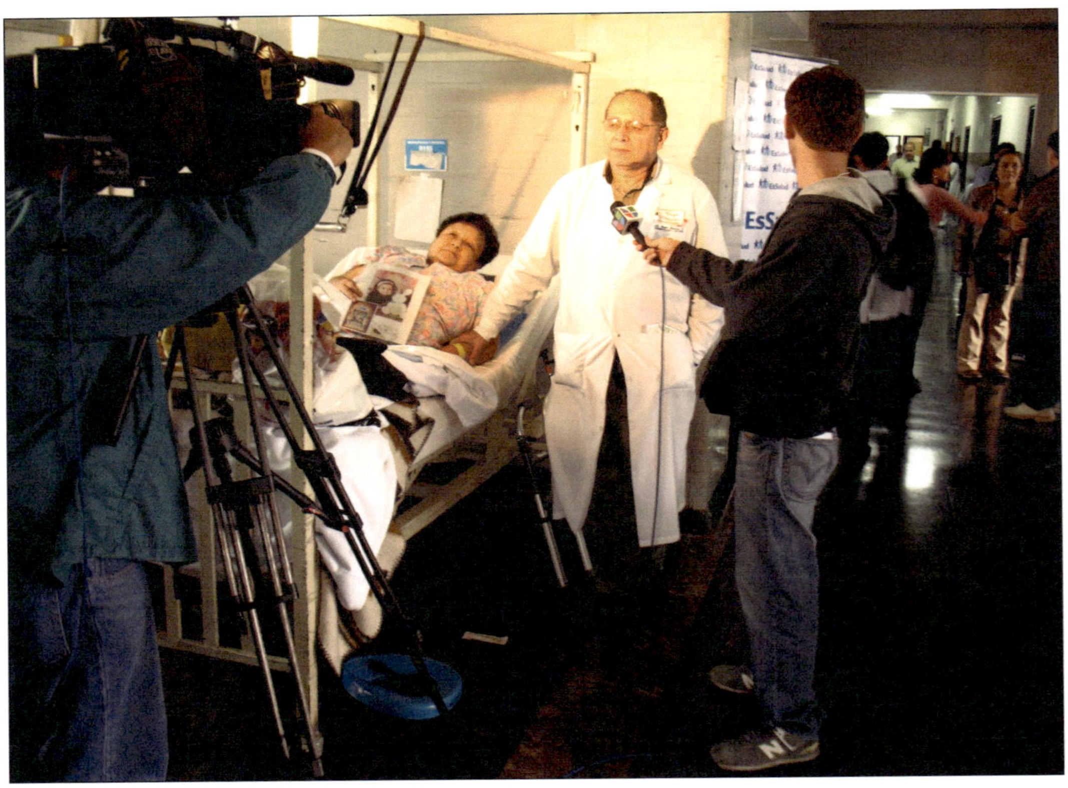

Interviewing Gaston

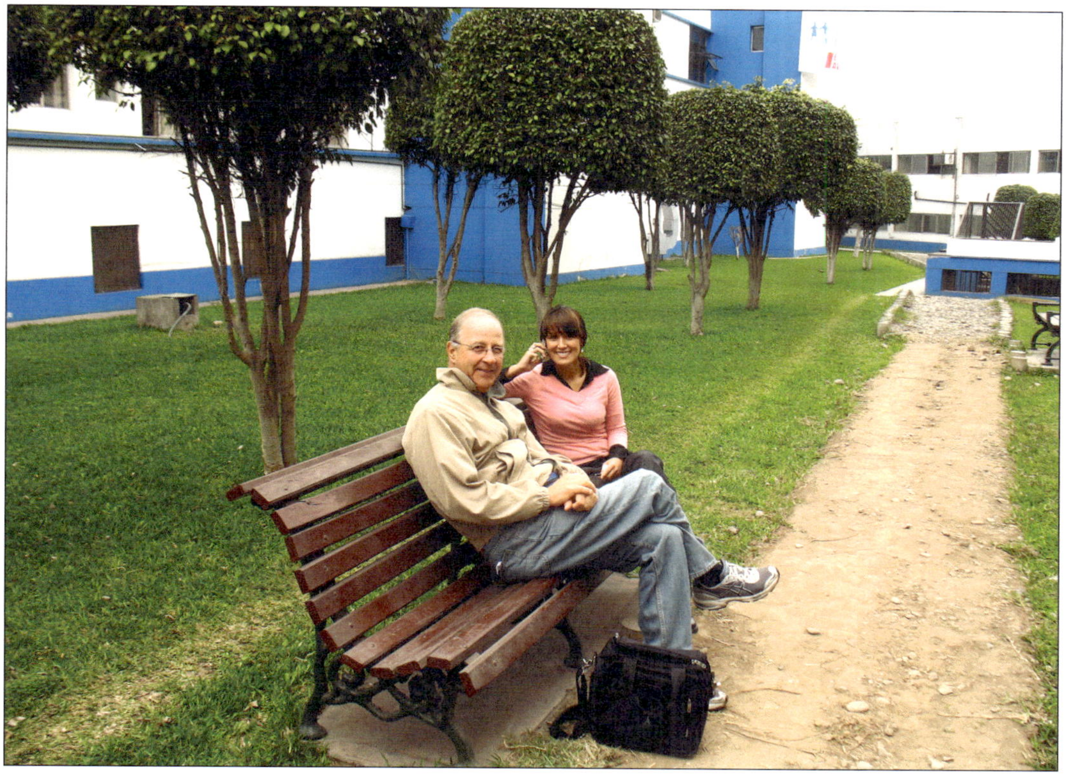

Me being interviewed by local journalist

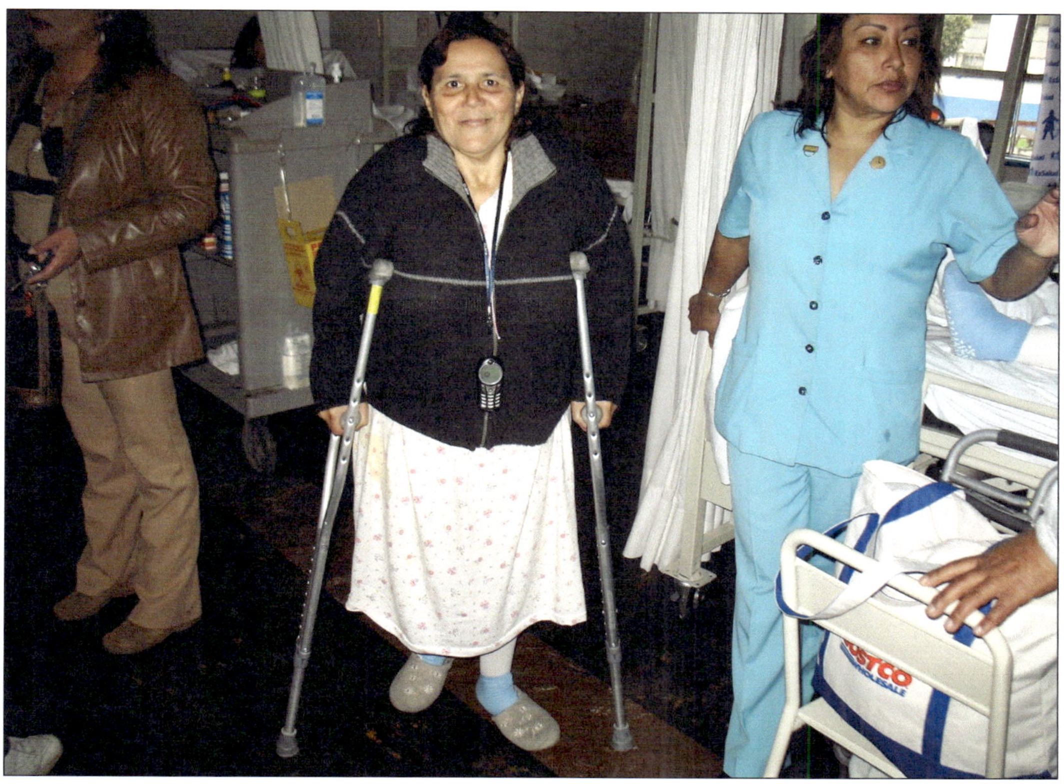

Happy patient

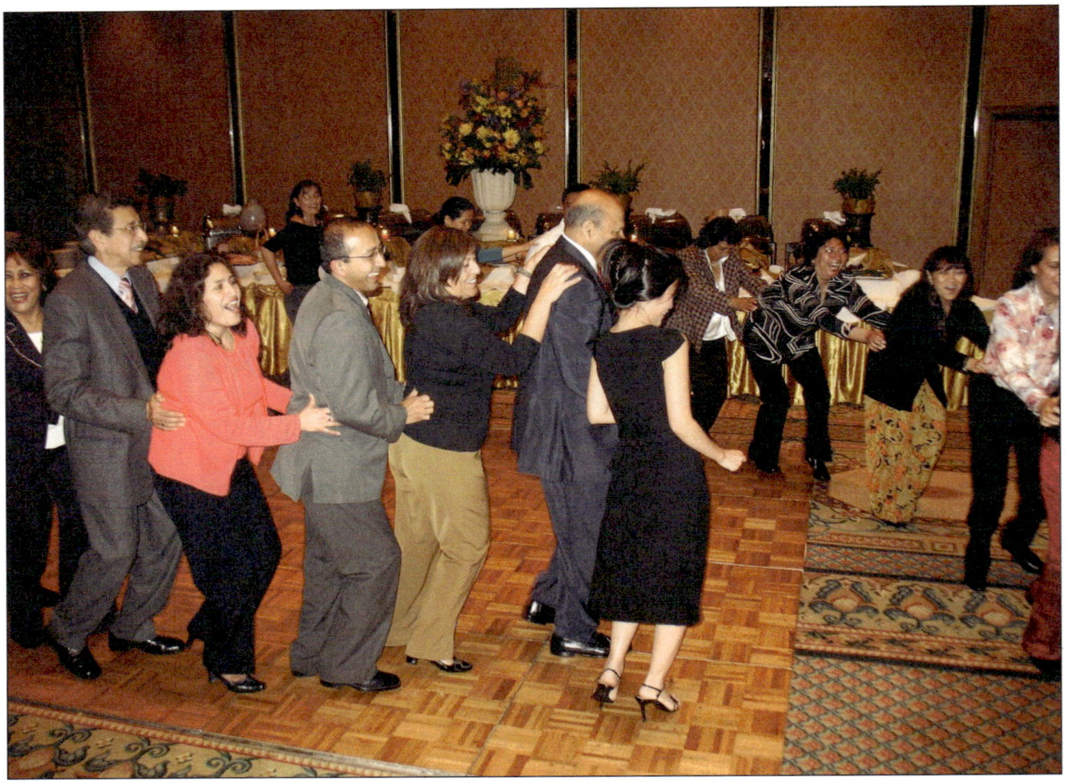

Dinner celebration with hospital personnel

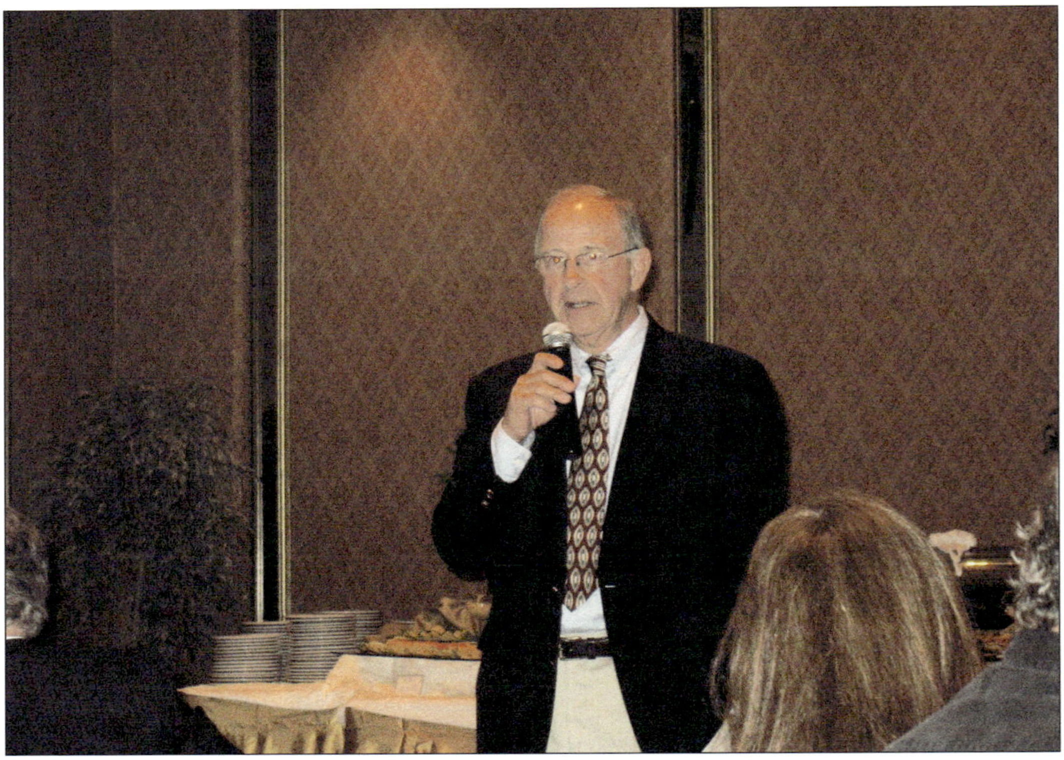

Thanking them for their assistance

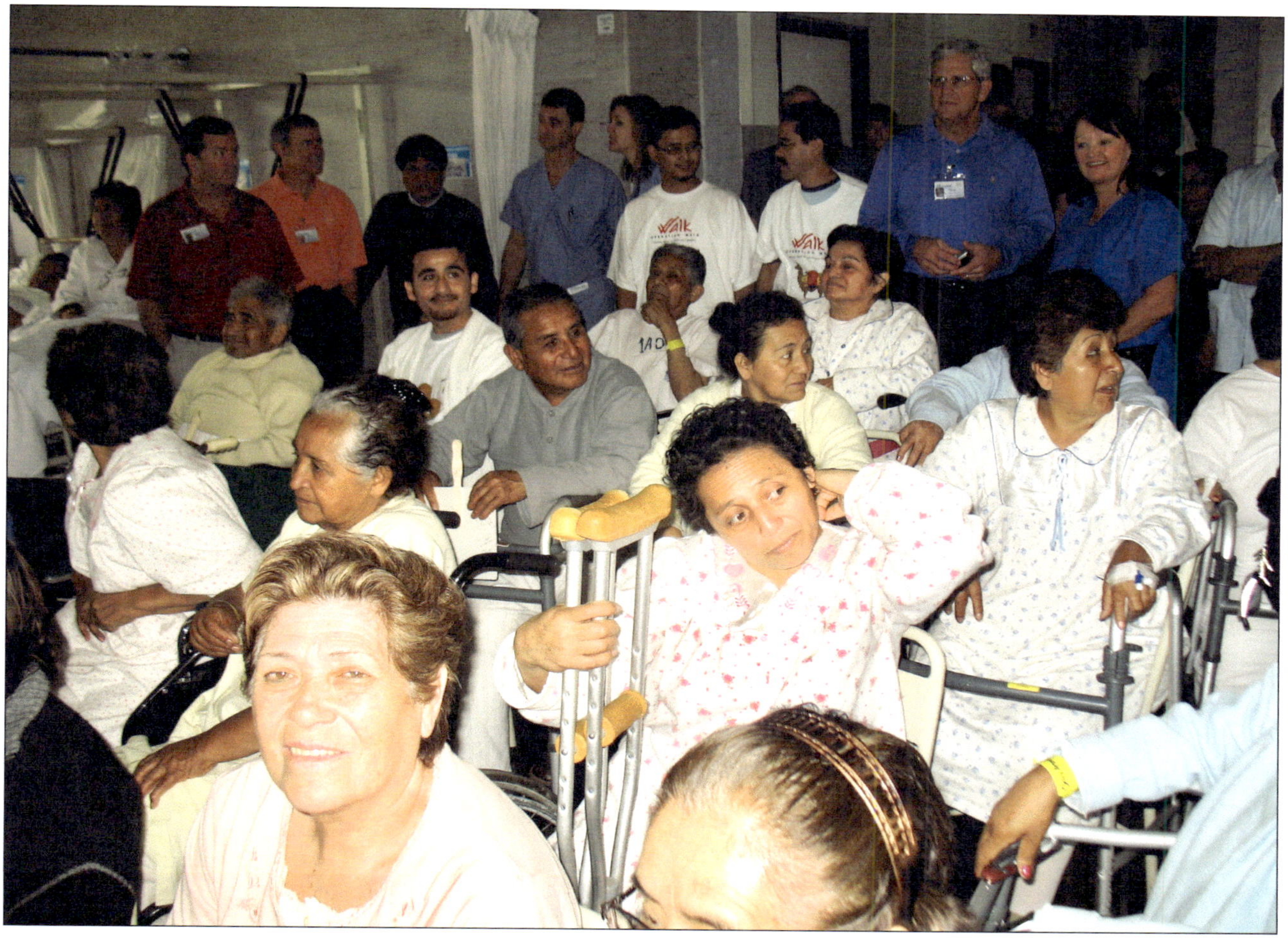

Post-op patients being given final instructions

Cuba

Over the years, we made five additional trips with Operation Walk: twice to Nicaragua, once to China, Nepal, and Cuba, and an aborted trip to La Paz in Baja California, canceled because supplies could not be cleared through customs.

Cuba was our first trip in '96 and was a most interesting experience, being able to witness the country firsthand after reading and hearing so much about the evils of Fidel Castro and communism.

> *Cuba was our first trip in '96 and was a most interesting experience ...*

We worked in a large, state-run tertiary hospital that appeared well equipped and modern. The local orthopedists were very respectful, helpful, and quite interested in learning newer techniques of joint-replacement surgery. Our team of six surgeons rotated between three operating rooms, moderating the surgery in one of the rooms through closed circuit TV broadcast into an adjoining conference room to a group of local physicians.

We were housed in government facilities nearby and were fed and entertained daily by "representatives" of the government, who were with us at all times.

Cuba was striving to become a center of healthcare excellence to the rest of Latin America, hoping to attract wealthy, paying patients by charging a fraction for their care compared to having surgery done in the US. Thus their eagerness to learn the latest and best techniques.

We visited a local research facility that was working on state-of-the-art pharmaceuticals and also toured a local physician clinic, where we were introduced to the Cuban healthcare system.

While their economic system is believed to be a failure, their education and healthcare were impressive. Cuba has one of the highest literacy rates in the world, and everyone has access to healthcare.

Healthcare is delivered by primary-care physicians, who are responsible for a certain number of patients, with whom they are familiar, making sure they have the necessary screening and vaccinations and treating them when they are injured or sick. If the primary-care doctor is unable to handle the situation, the patient is transferred to a regional clinic or hospital; if these facilities are unable to provide the necessary care, they are referred to a tertiary hospital located throughout the island. One glaring inadequacy at the local level, however, was the lack of supplies and medicines.

We implanted fifty joints during our stay. One woman was a 50+ female with severe arthritis in both hips, with such limited mobility that she was unable to sit in a chair. I told her we would do both hips and restore movement in her hips, allowing her to do things she had not done in years. She stated she was too fearful of having both surgeries and would only agree to one. When I told Larry of her decision, he said, "We'll do both hips." Then he walked over to her, took her hand, and, in a forceful, yet caring way, told her we would do both of her hips and that she would do well. In my practice, I never tried to talk patients into an elective procedure. She had her surgery, did well, and was extremely grateful.

One glaring inadequacy at the local level was the lack of supplies and medicines.

Another young girl with severe rheumatoid arthritis of both hips and such limited mobility that toilet care was problematic and she was unable to have sexual relations with her husband. Needless to say, following surgery, there was one happy family.

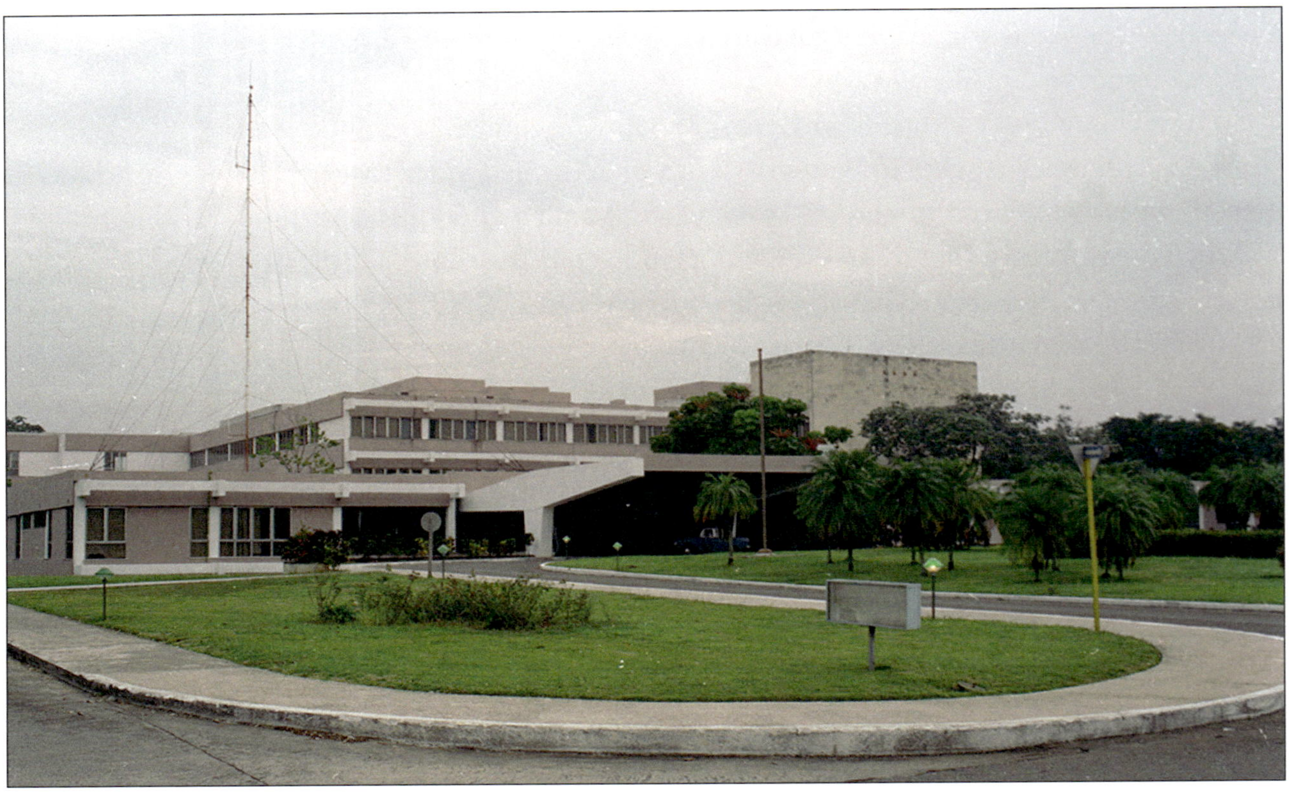

Havana hospital

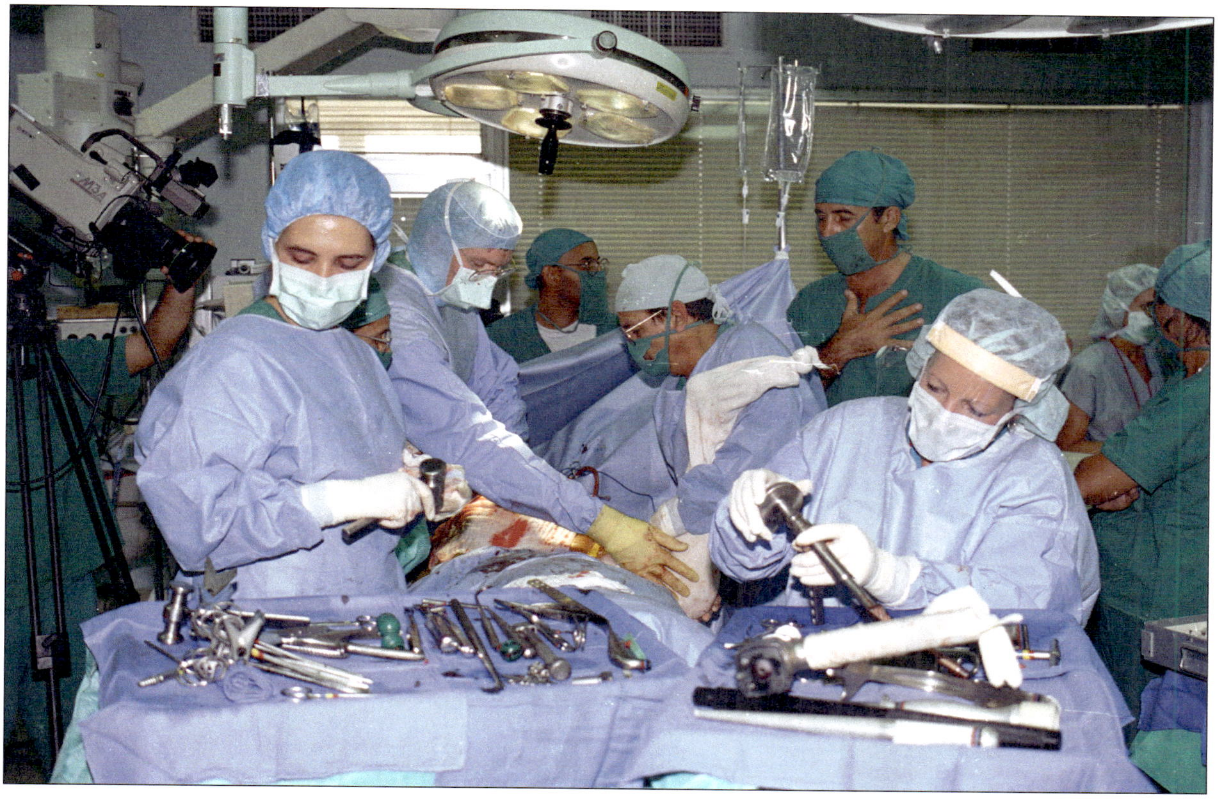

Crowd in Cuba's ORs: Local doctors, closed circuit TV broadcasting surgery to auditorium filled with other local physicians.

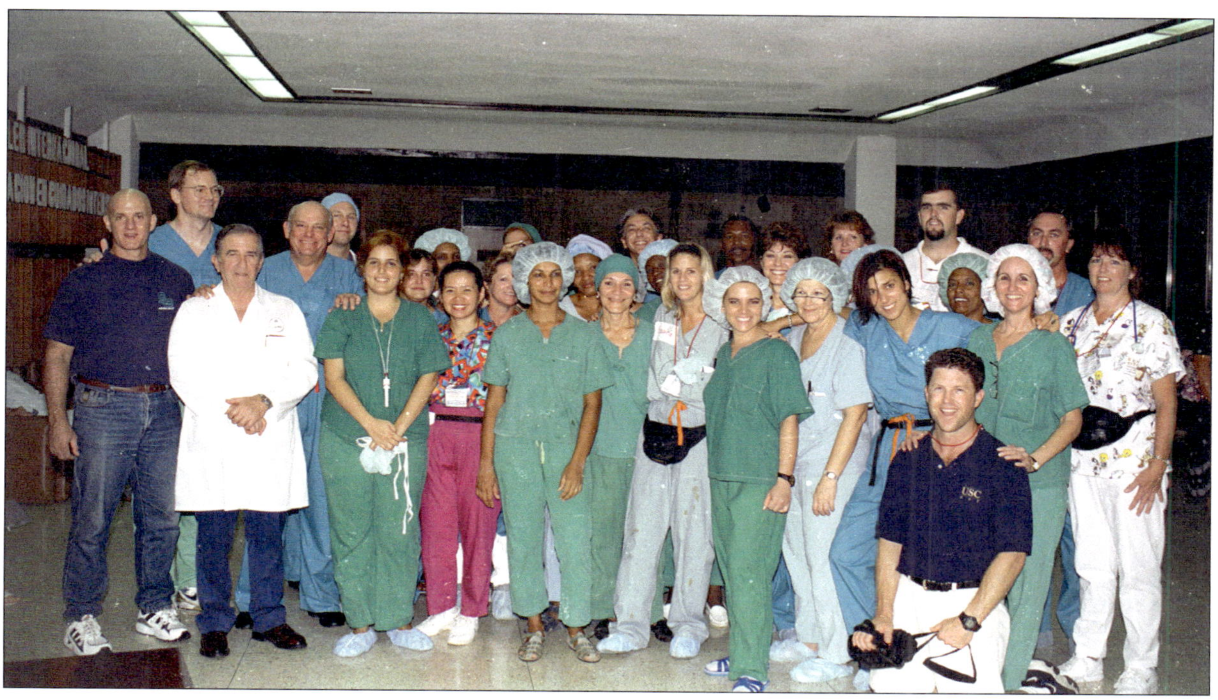

Operation Walk Team

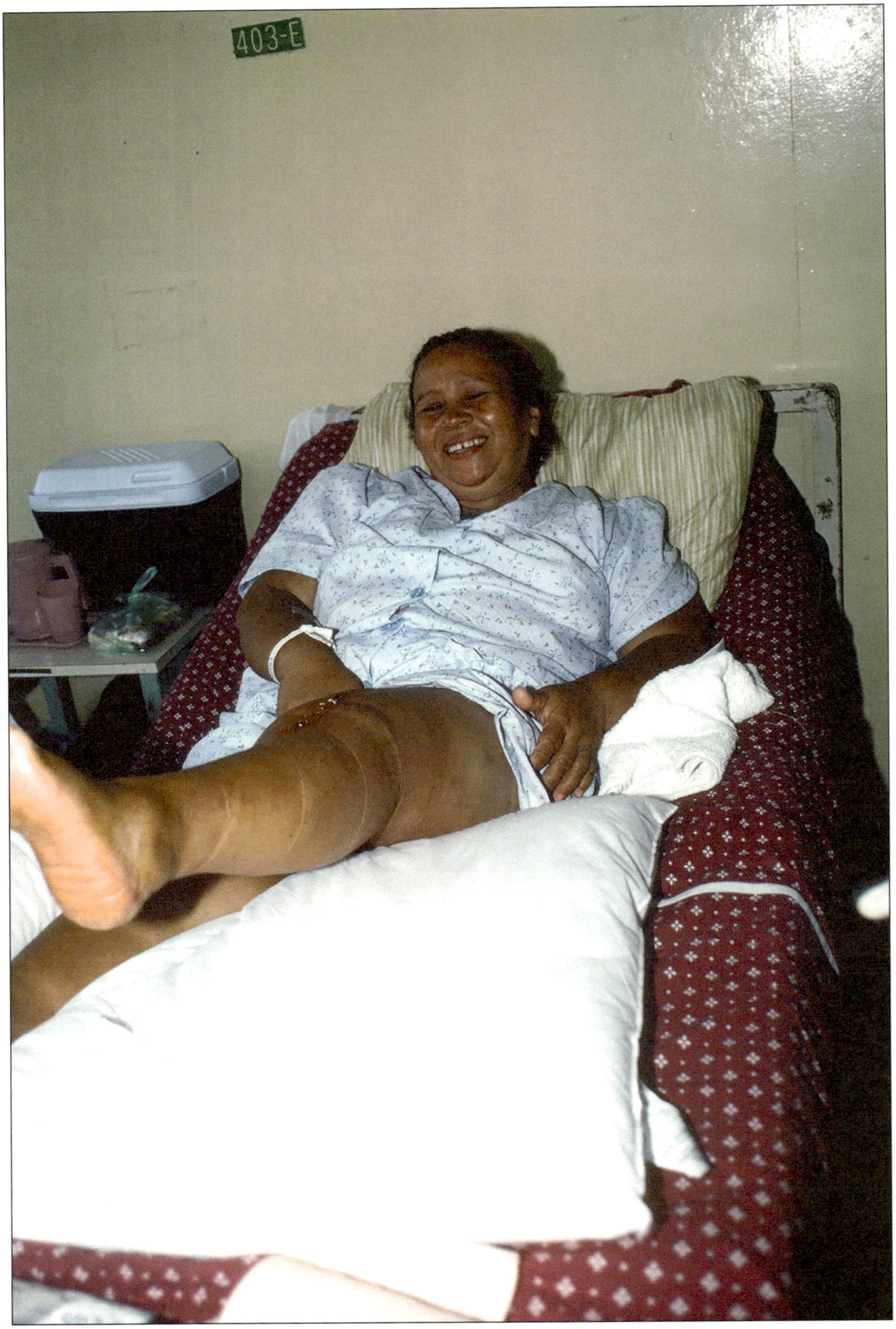

Happy and grateful patients

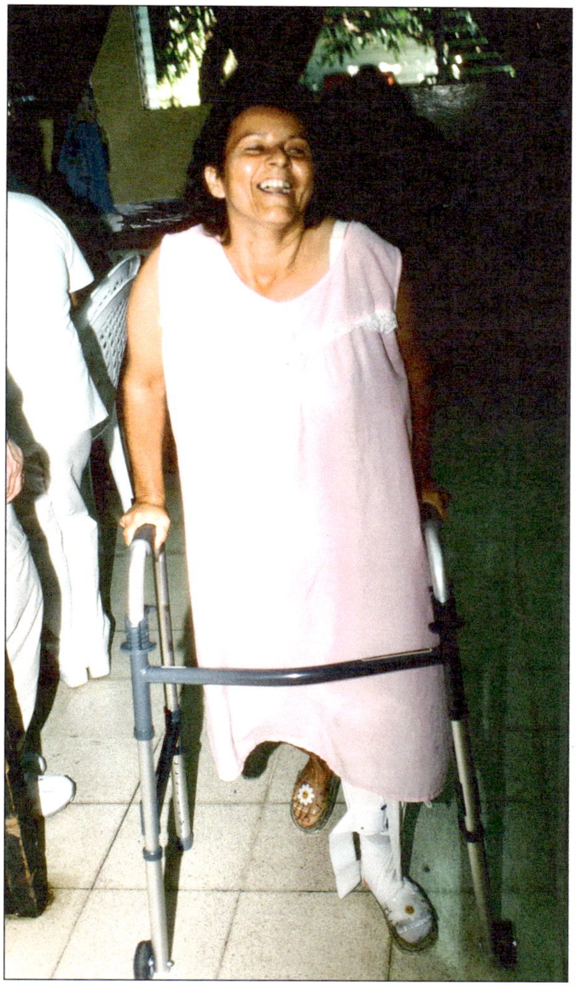

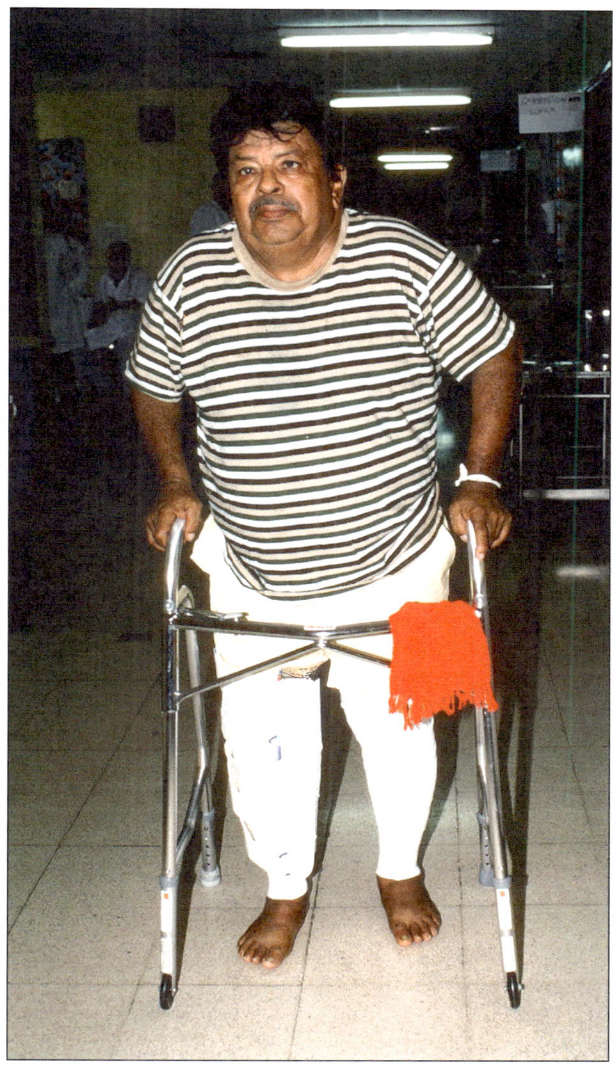

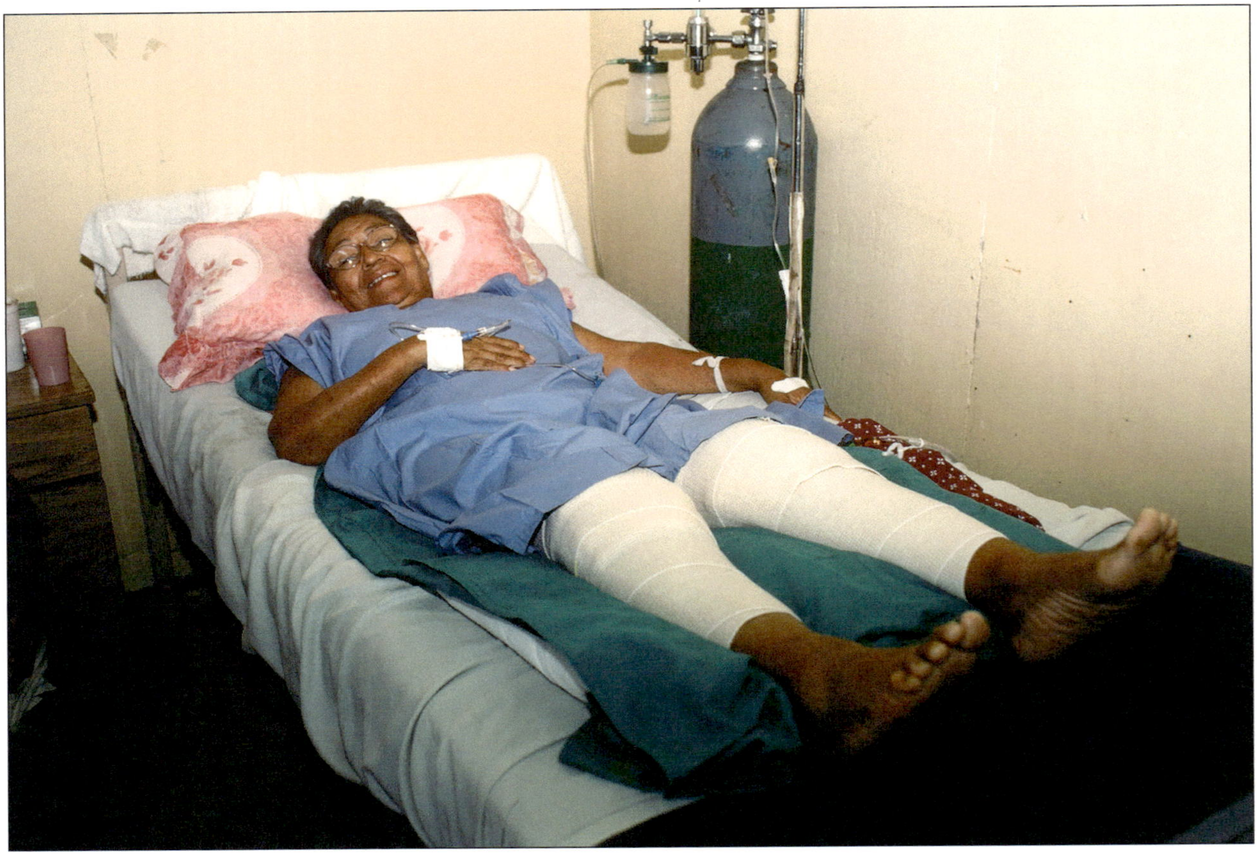

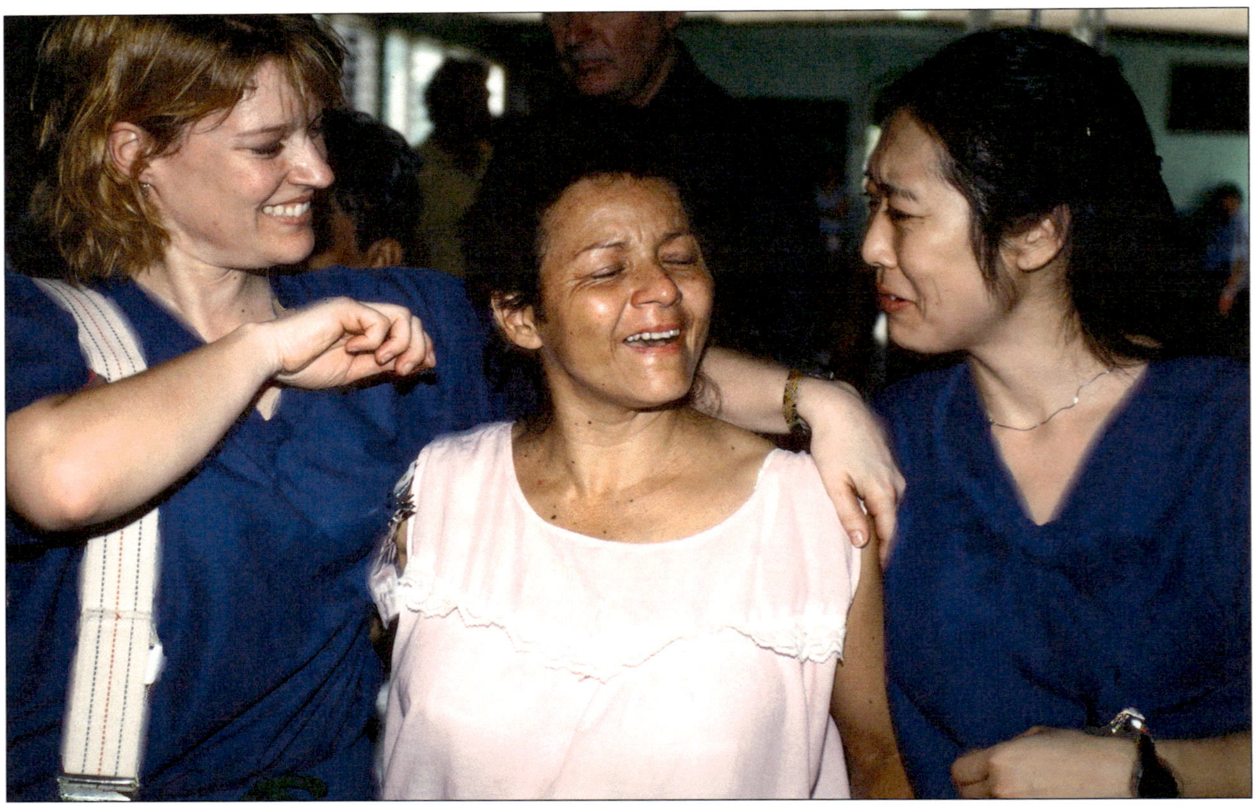

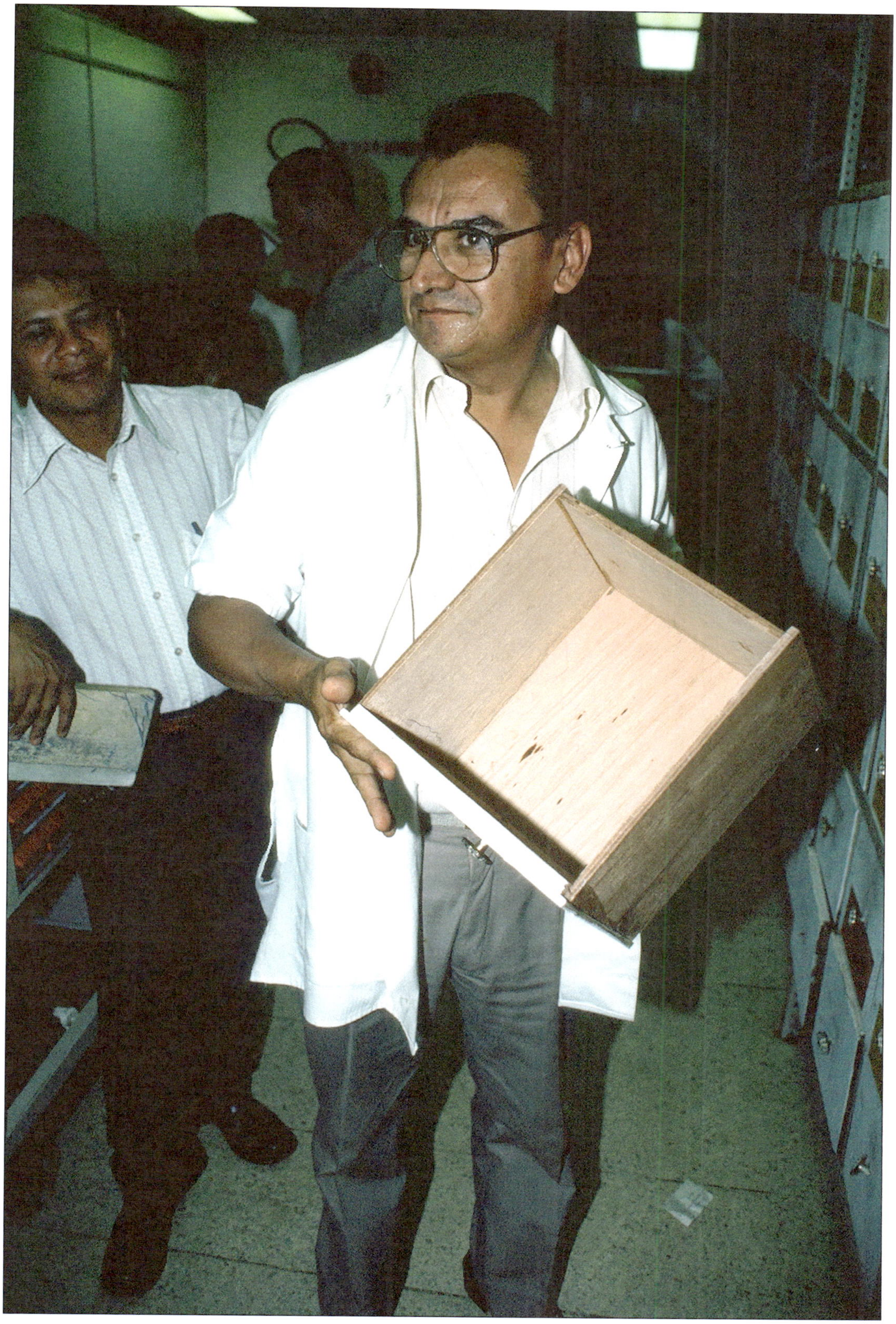

Local doctor displaying empty medicine drawer

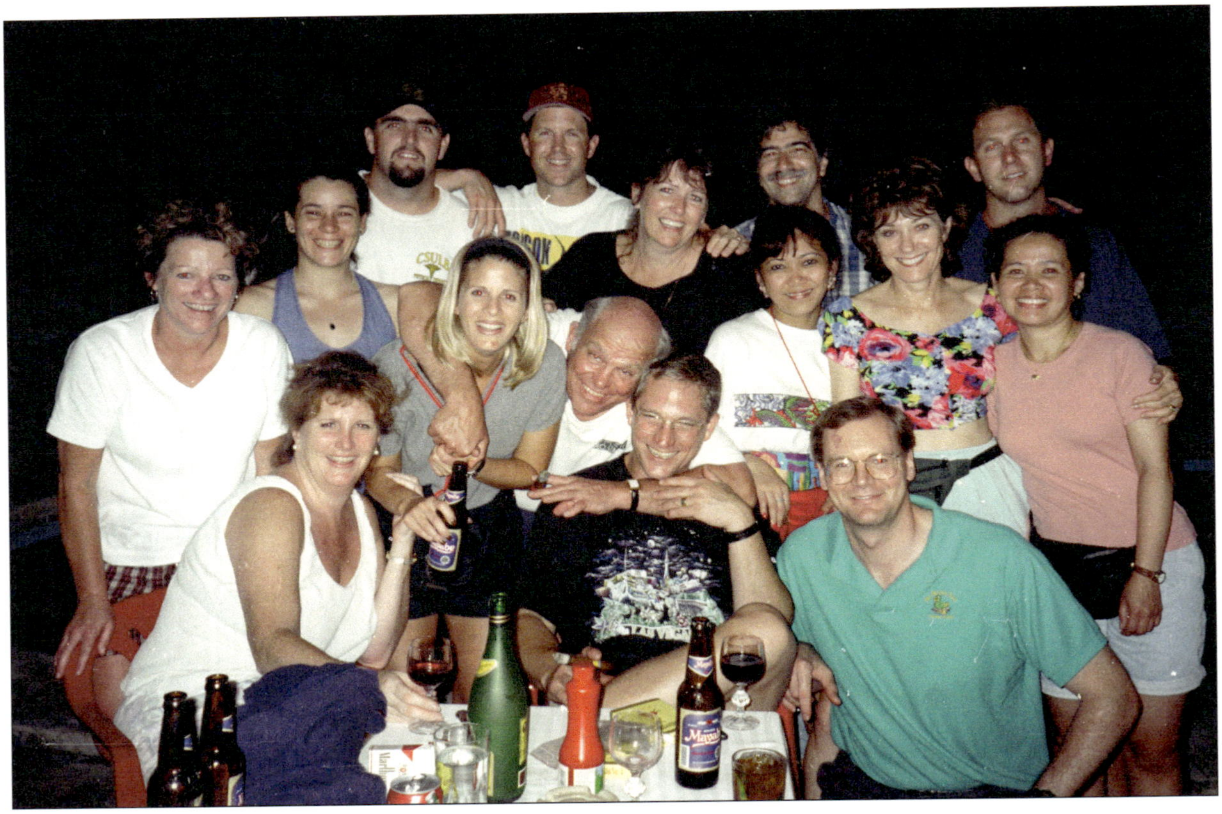

Party Time

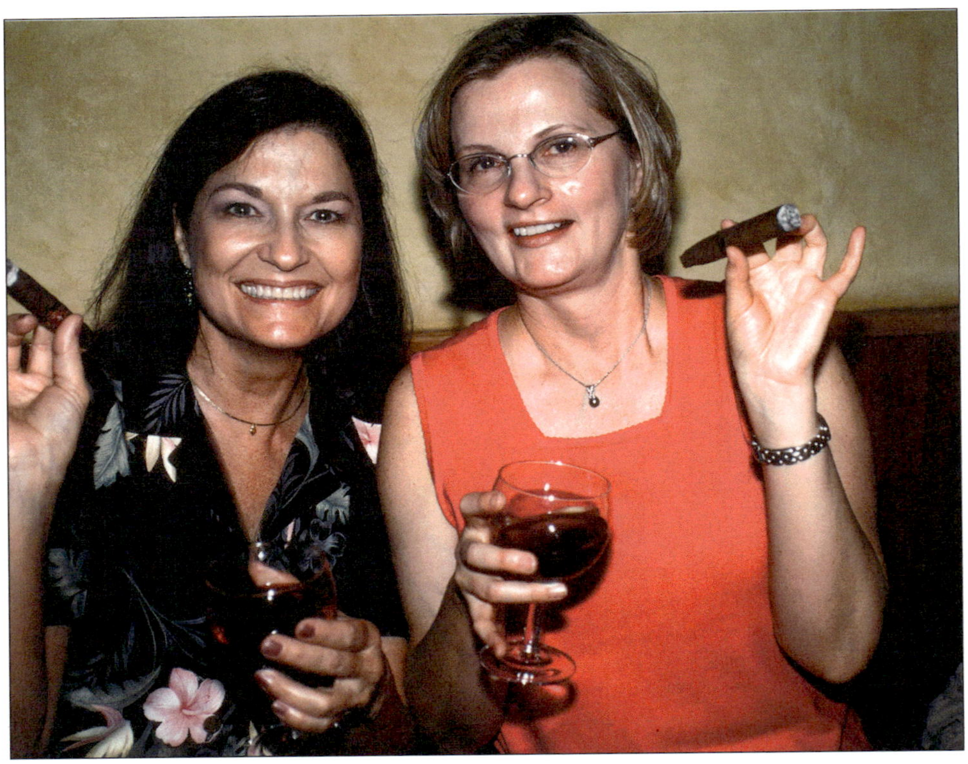

Enjoying a fine Cuban Cigar

China

In 2005 we traveled to Chengdu China with Operation Walk, working in the Sichuan Provincial Peoples Hospital, a facility with 4,300 beds. The hospital was quite modern in appearance, and the personnel were very accommodating in assisting our efforts. Our routine was the same as the other countries we had visited: evaluating patients for a half day, having a pre-op surgical conference, and then begin operating for 3 days implanting some 60 total joints. The final day was used for patient and physician post-op instruction.

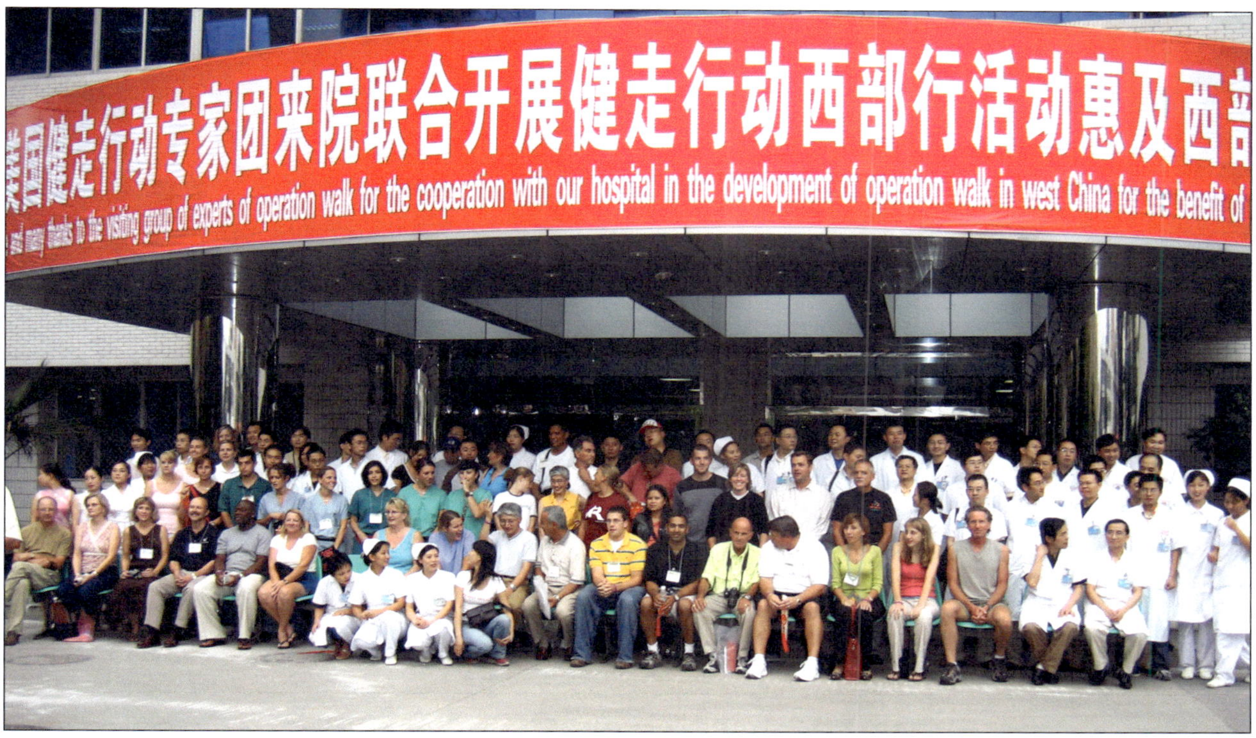

美国健走行动专家团来院联合开展健走行动西部行活动惠及西
and many thanks to the visiting group of experts of operation walk for the cooperation with our hospital in the development of operation walk in west China for the benefit of

Op Walk team and hospital personnel

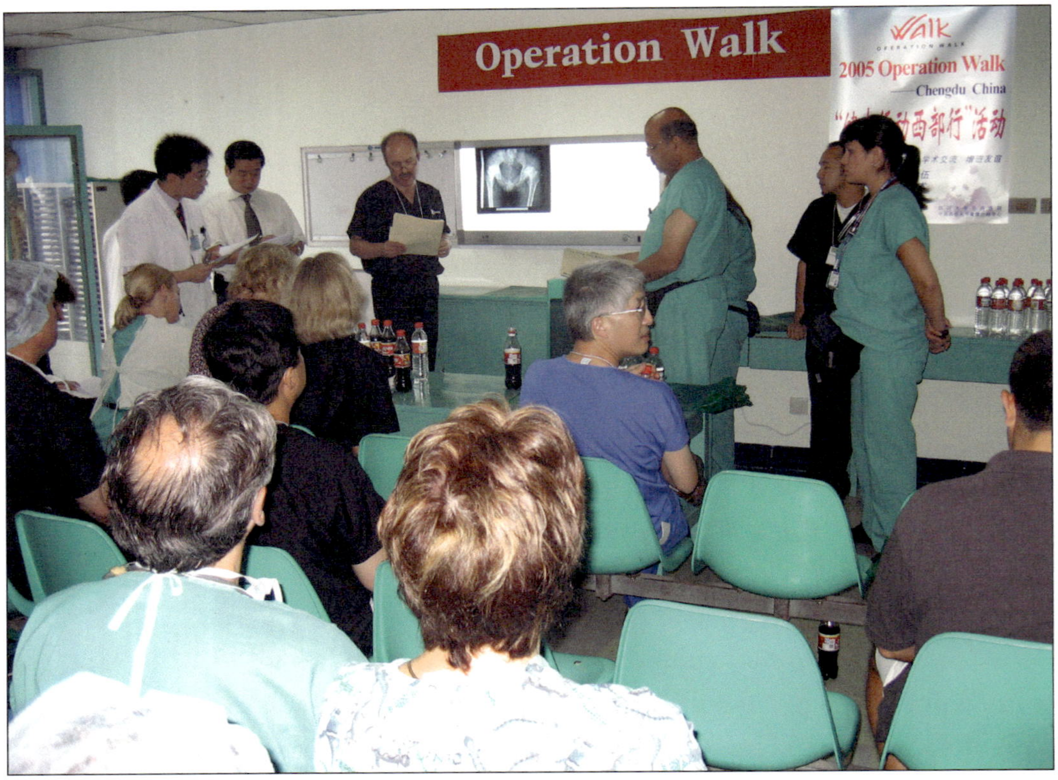

Pre-op conference

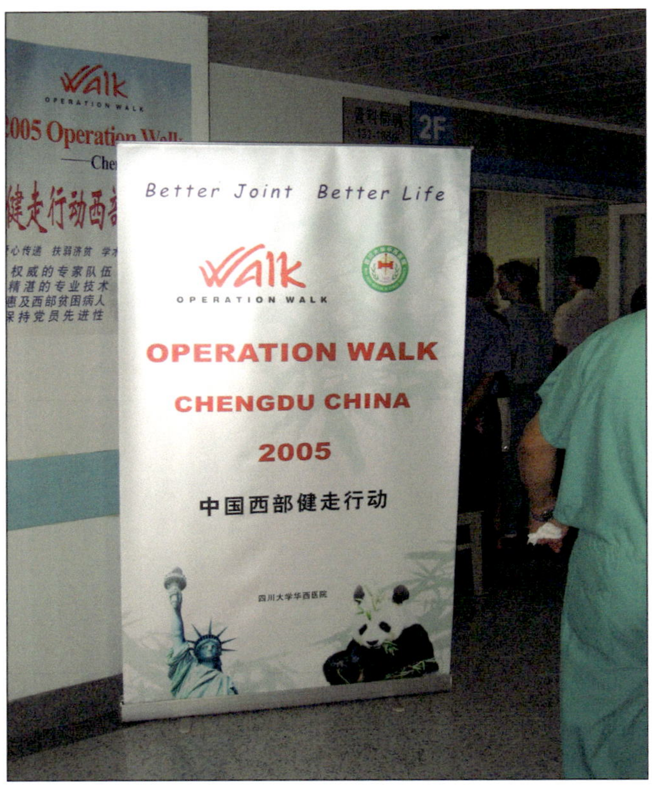

Announcement of our visit

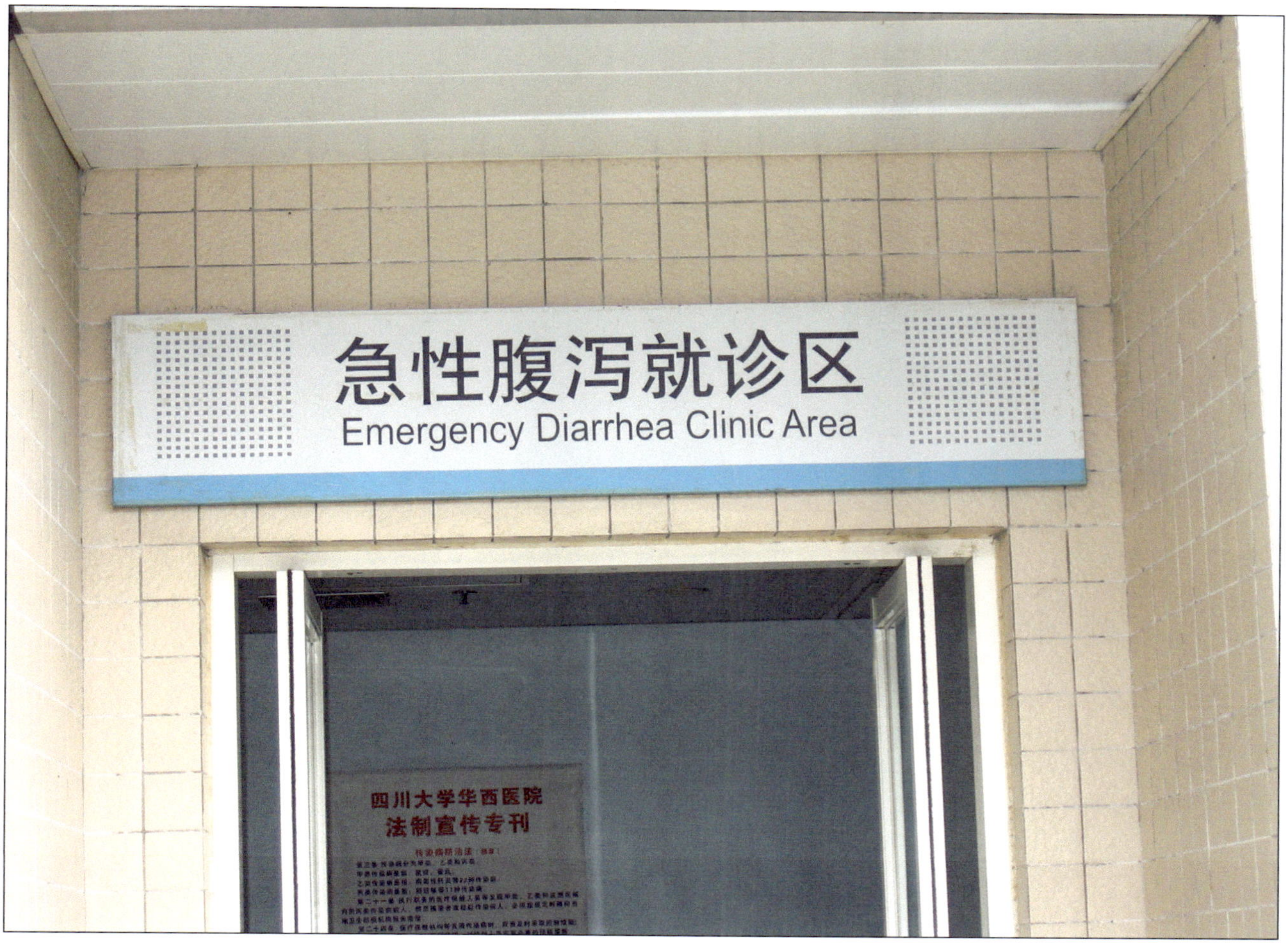

Thankfully, we didn't have to use this facility

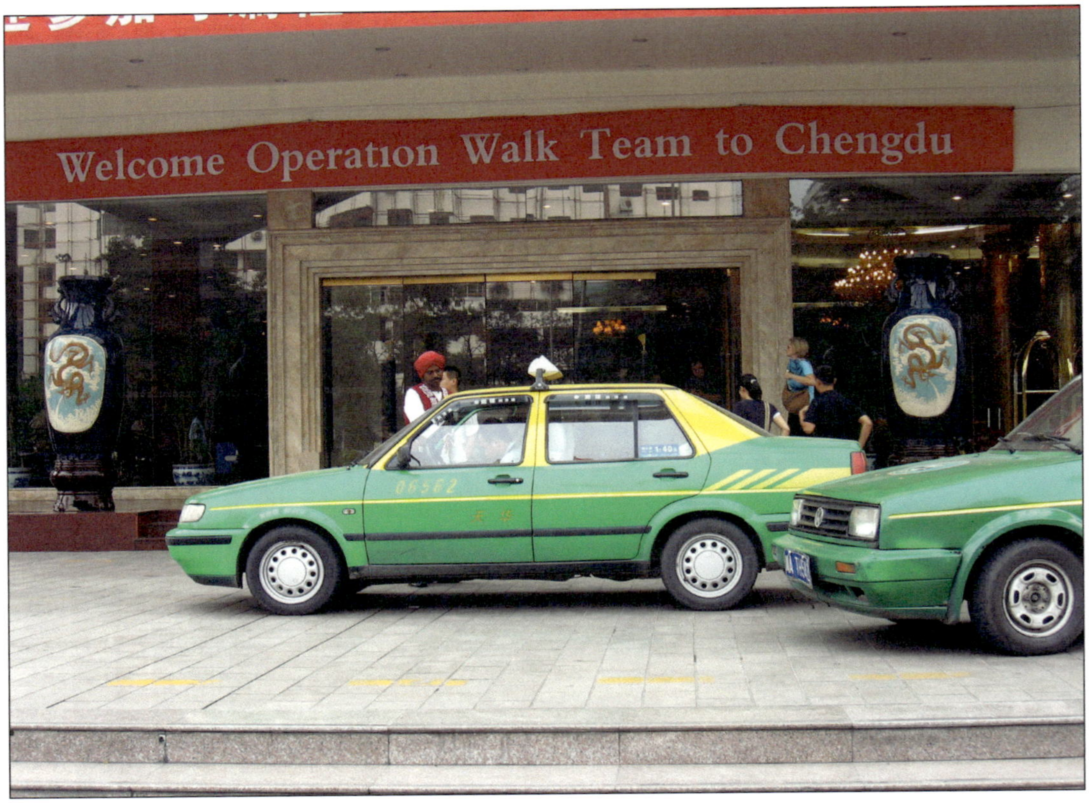

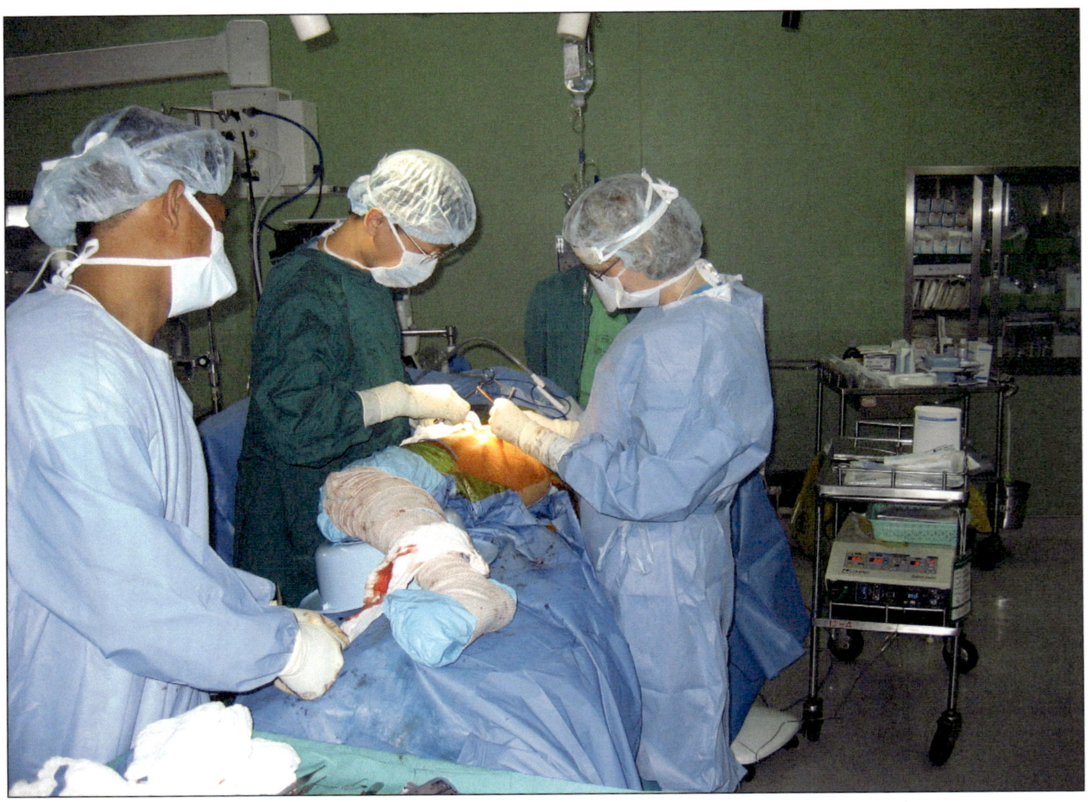

Rita assisting on hip replacement

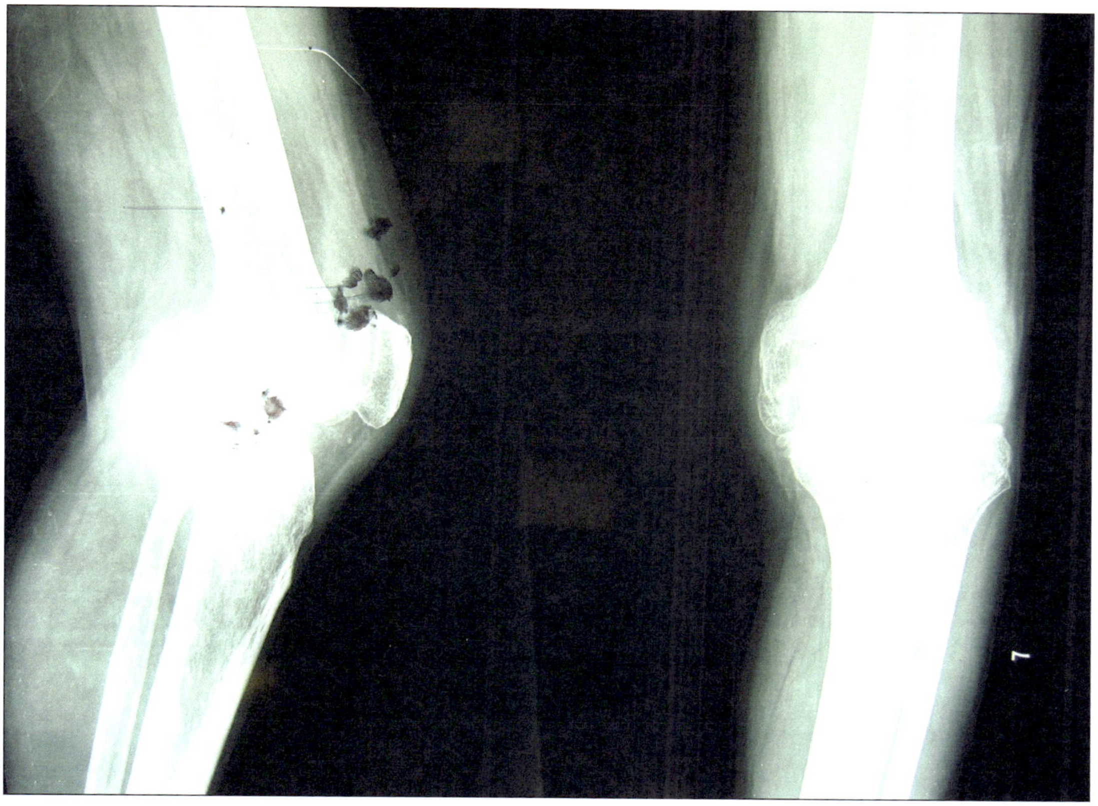

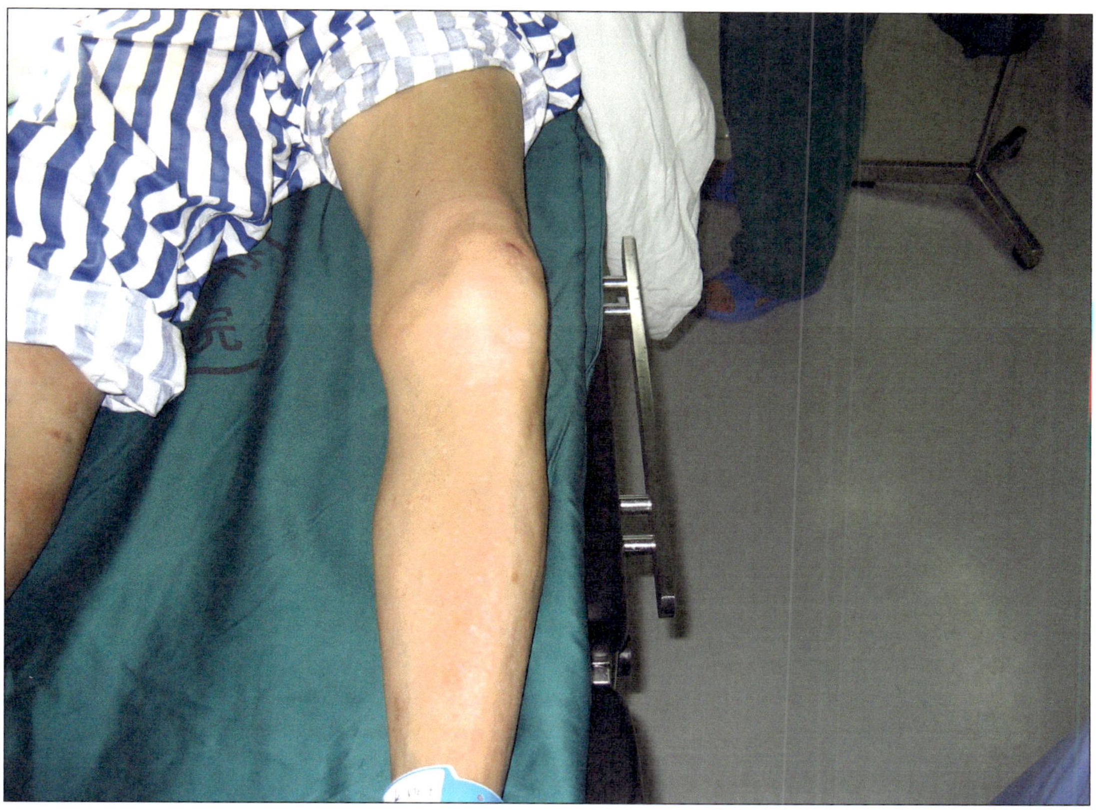

X-ray of arthritic, deformed left knee

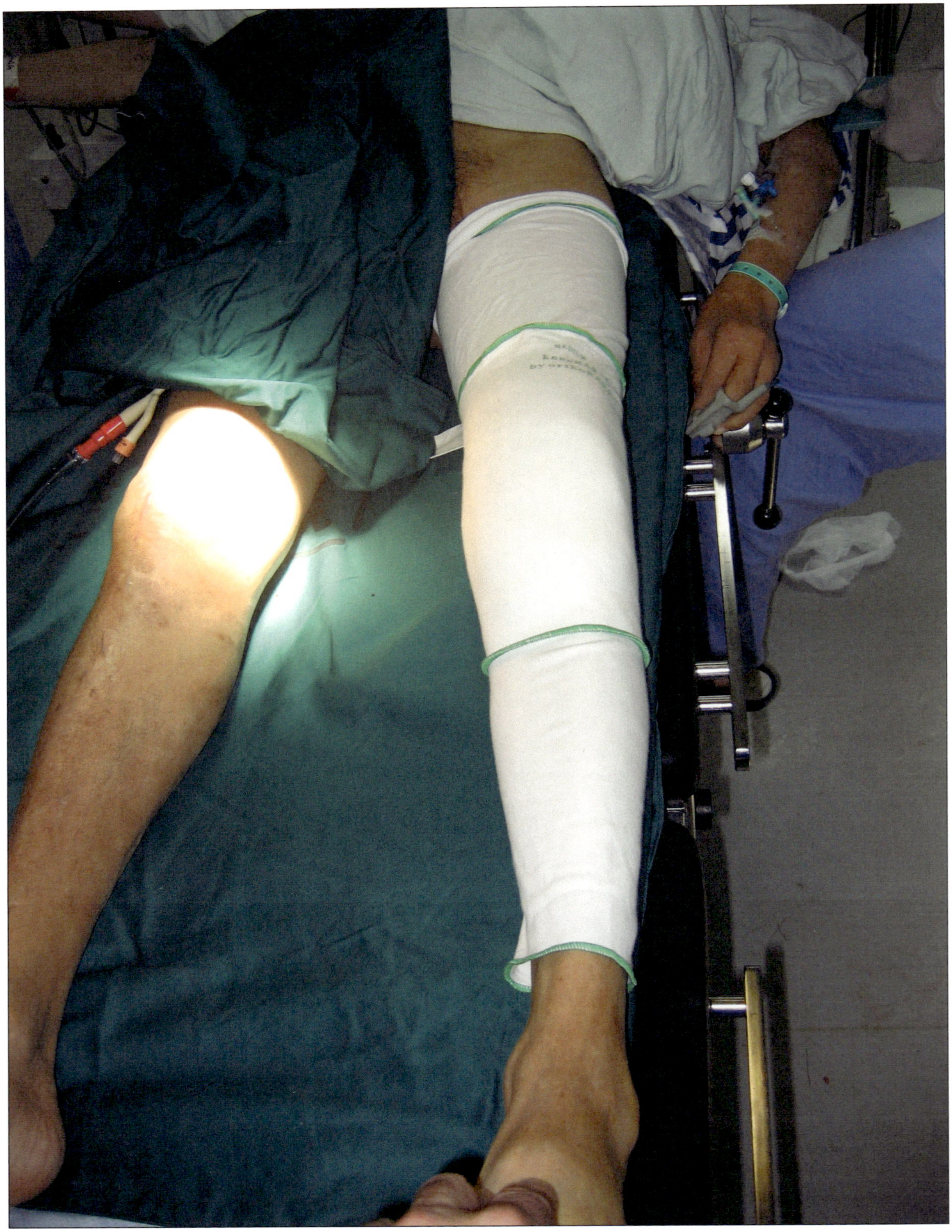

Post-op, knee straightened

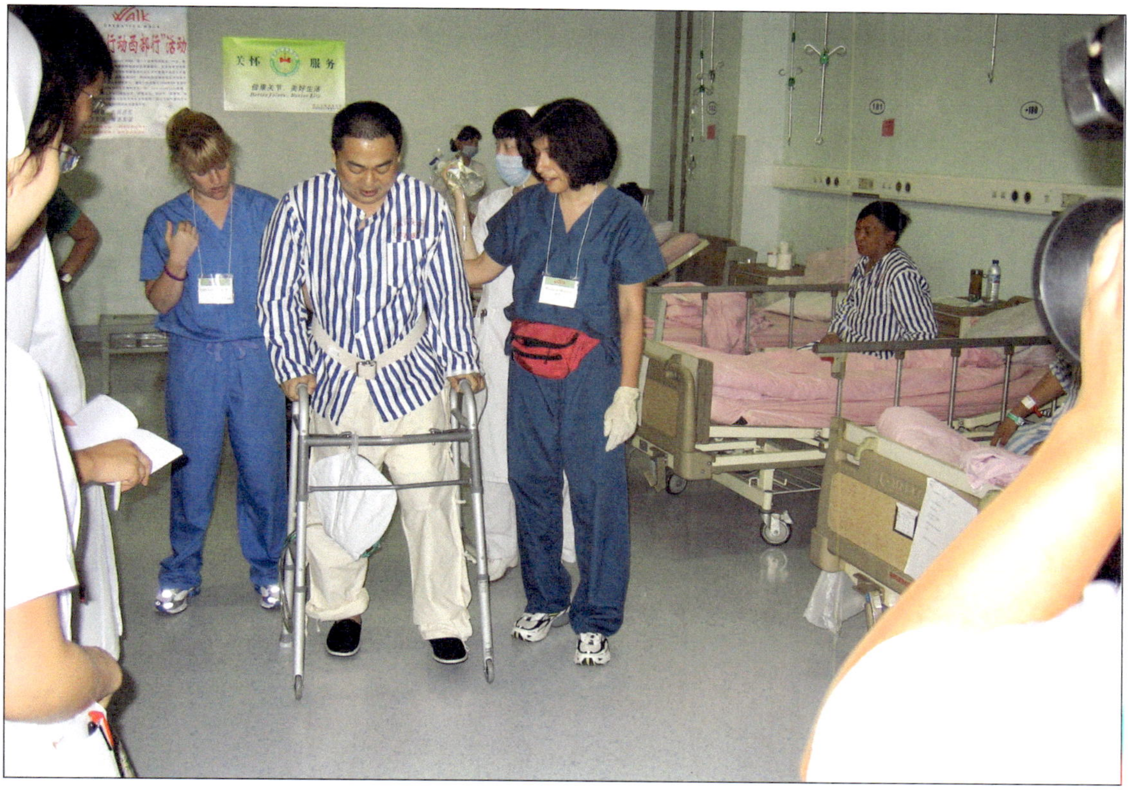
Walk
关怀 服务

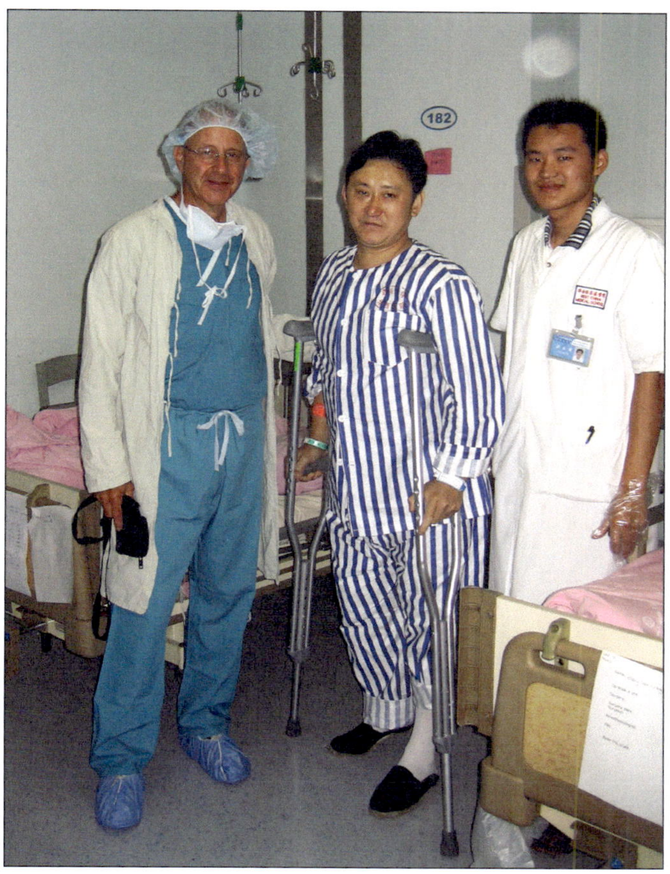
182

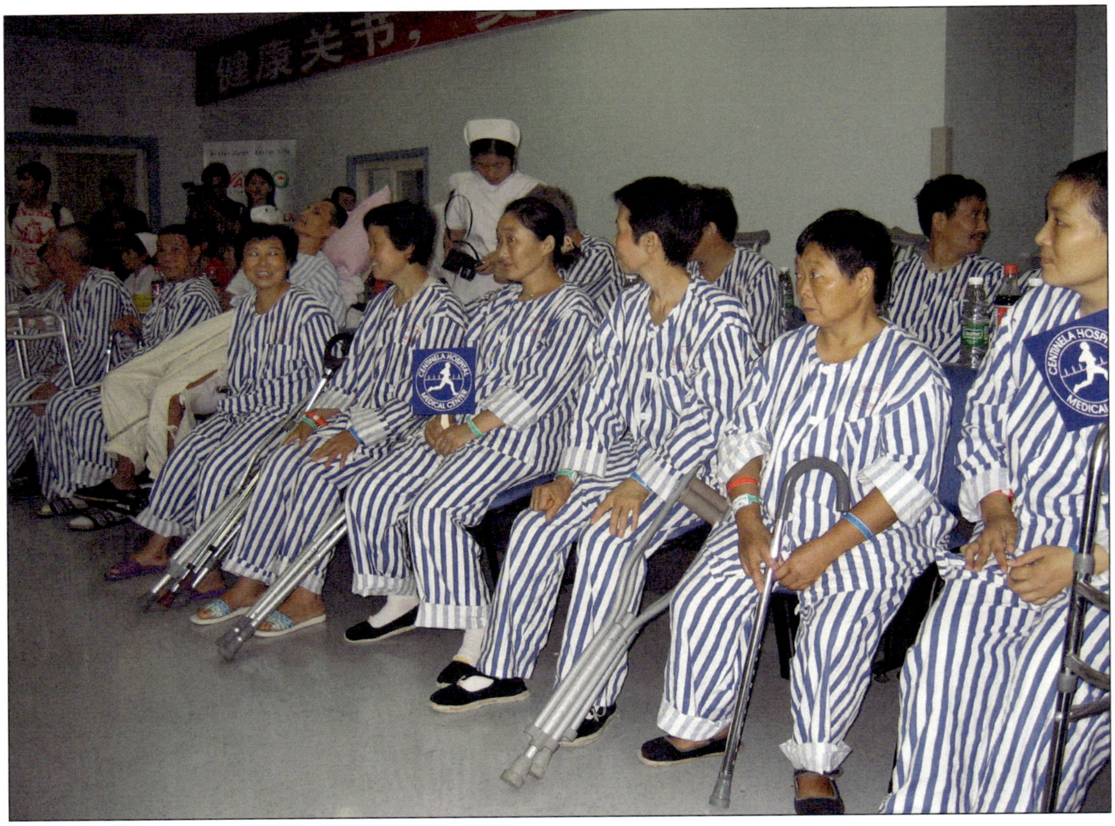

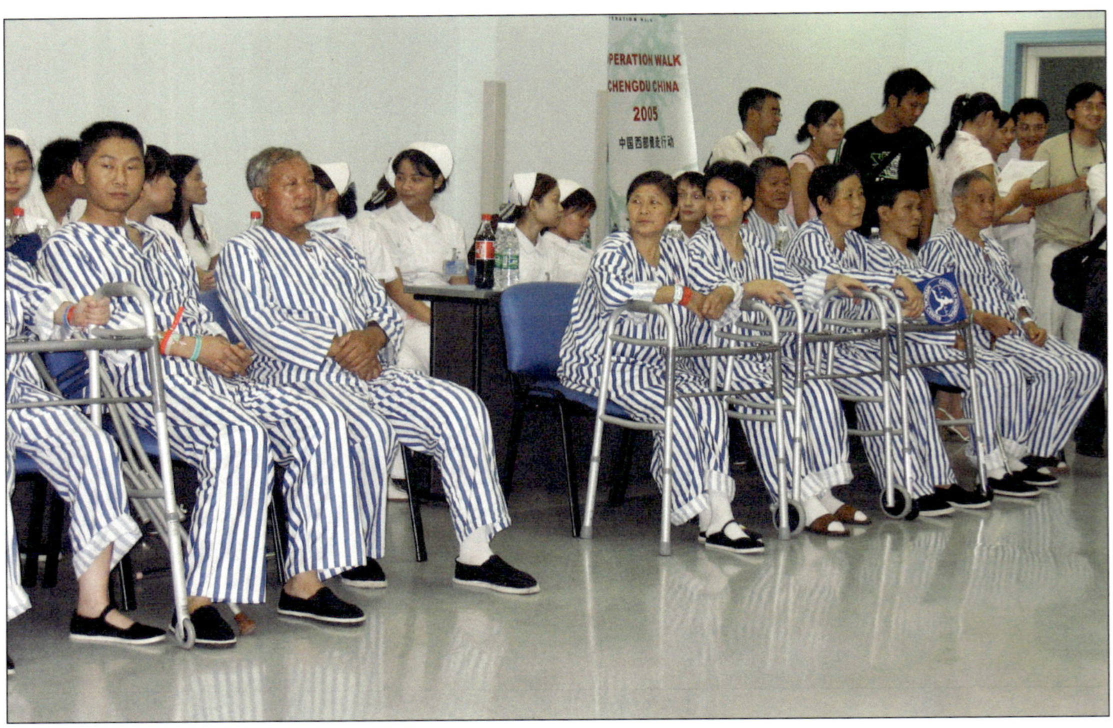

Final-day instructions

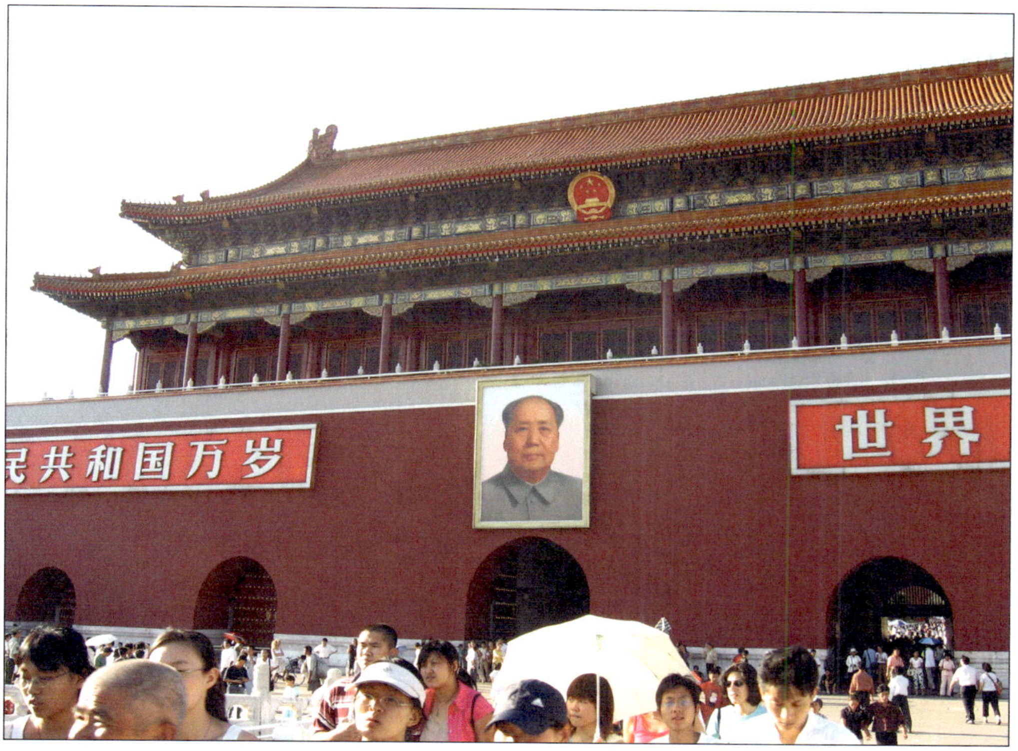

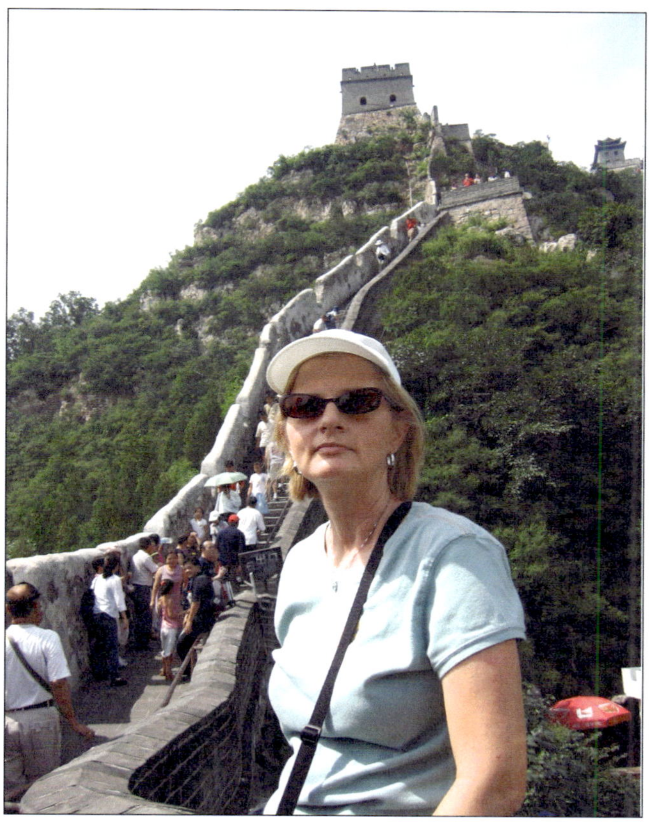

Seeing the sights in China

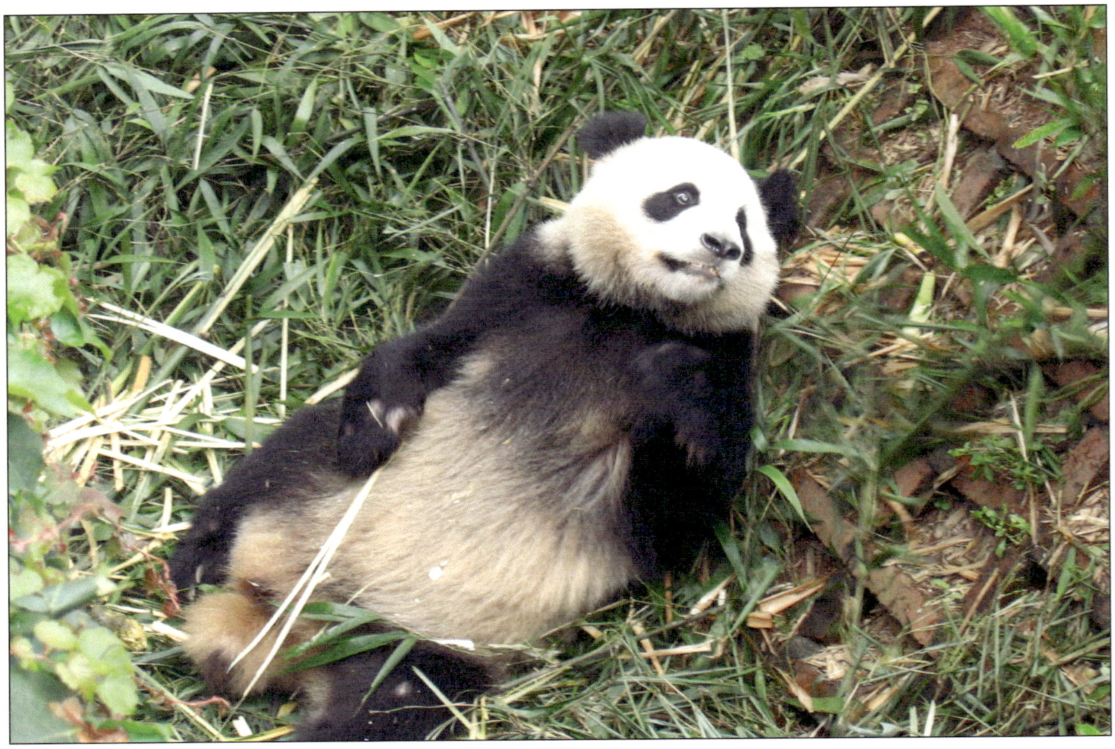

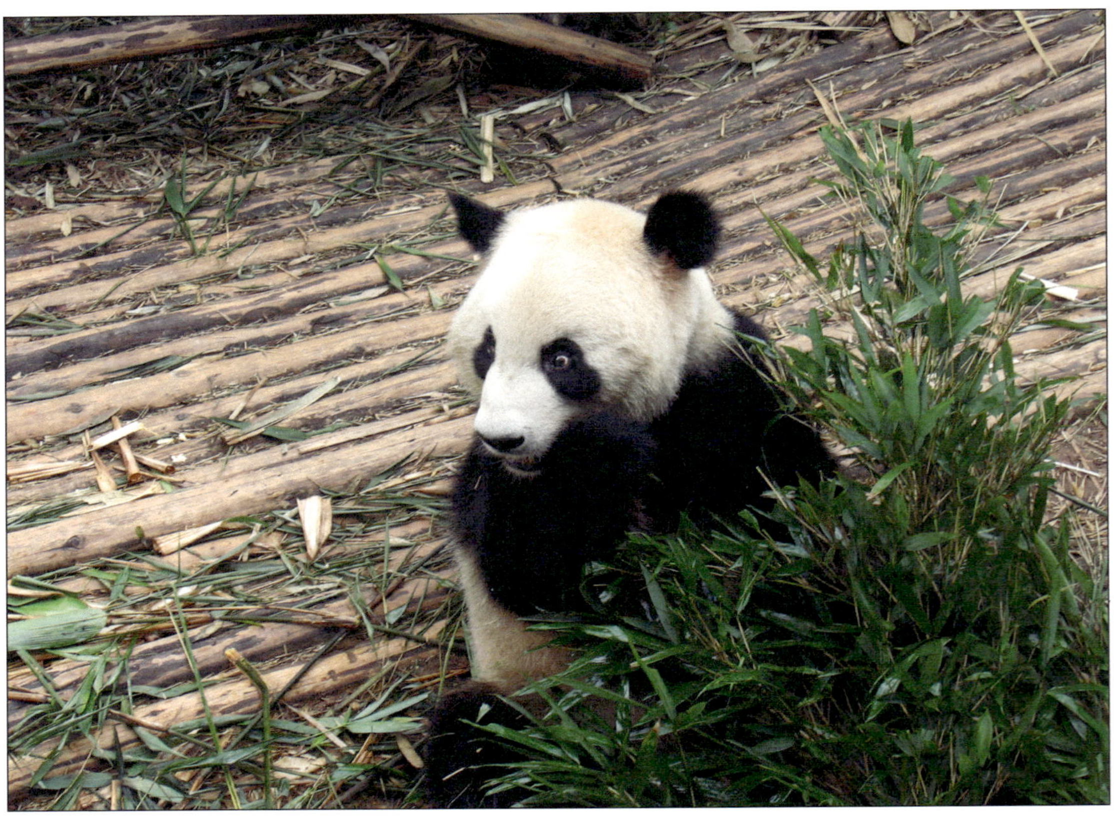

Famous Panda Park in Chengdu

Nicaragua

We journeyed to Nicaragua on three separate occasions — two with Op Walk doing hip and knee replacements and one with the Arizona Medical Team, an organization founded by Cindy McCain, wife of then-Senator John McCain. I traveled to Nicaragua with Cindy on a private jet before the team left to scout out the environment and establish connections with local officials. Returning, with the medical team, we were accompanied by a news crew from one of the local Phoenix TV stations. They recorded our trip daily; sending back images of our activities. At the time, Nicaragua had been ruled by a communist government (Sandinistas) that had recently ended a civil war with anti-Sandinistas forces supported by the US, known as the Iran-Contra Affair. This entailed selling arms to Iran, which was under an embargo and thus illegal, and using the proceeds to fund the Contras, prohibited by Congress. There was still a great deal of dislike and distrust between the pardoned Contra soldiers and the Sandinista sympathizers. Our community, Jinotepe, was in a region of Sandinista supporters. A recent election had ousted the communist leader, Daniel Ortega, and Violeta Chamorro was the sitting president. Her husband was a respected newspaper owner and publisher who'd been assassinated by the Sandinistas for his anti-communist editorial stance in 1978. We went to dinner one evening with a former Contra soldier who had been educated in the US until he was 18 and then returned home to join in the struggle. He was a well-known personality, and due to the residual animosity between two groups, he was always accompanied by a bodyguard. During the meal, there was a power outage, and my

Returning, with the medical team, we were accompanied by a news crew from one of the local Phoenix TV stations.

first thought was that this was an assassination attempt on our guest, and I was expecting gunfire at any moment. Fortunately, the lights were restored quickly, and we all resumed breathing. He told us how the Contra soldiers who had disarmed were assured they would be welcomed and reintegrated with Nicaraguan society. Unfortunately, this turned out not to be true, and, later that evening, he took us to a house that served as a dormitory for 8–12 former fighters, keeping them sequestered and protected from Sandinista sympathizers who had openly killed other returning soldiers.

Fortunately, the lights were restored quickly, and we all resumed breathing.

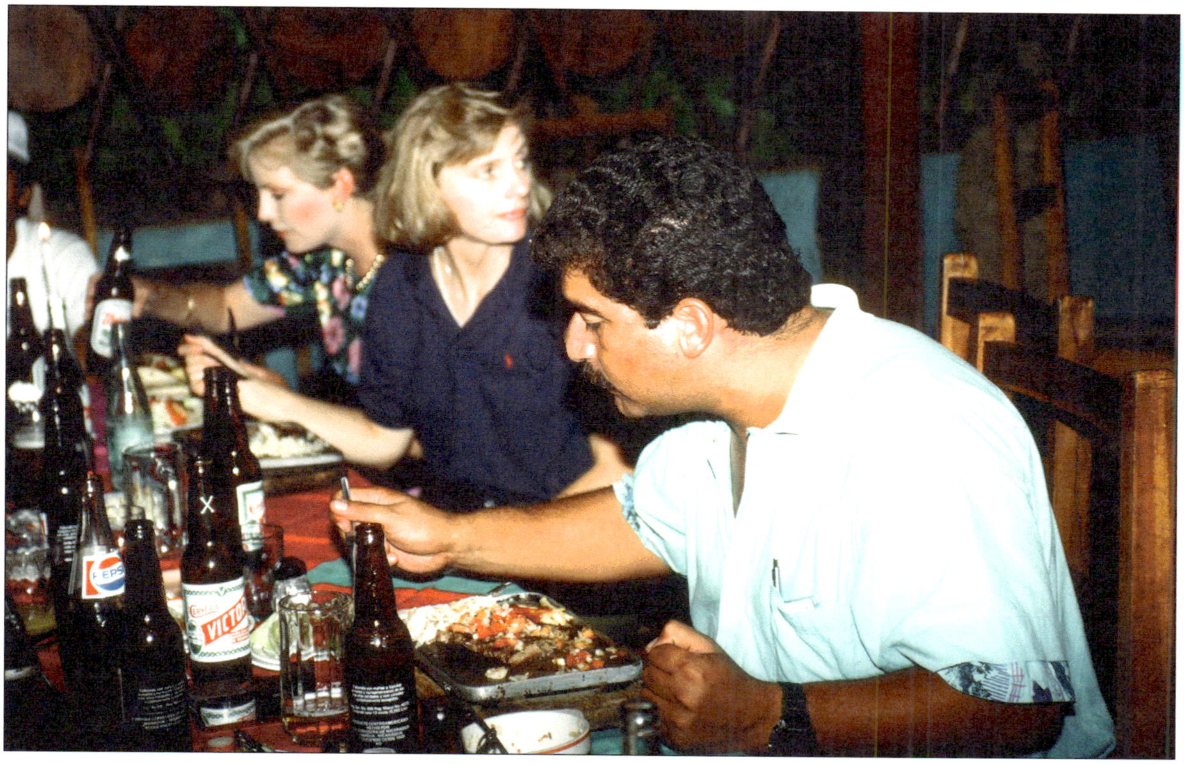

At dinner with former Contra soldier

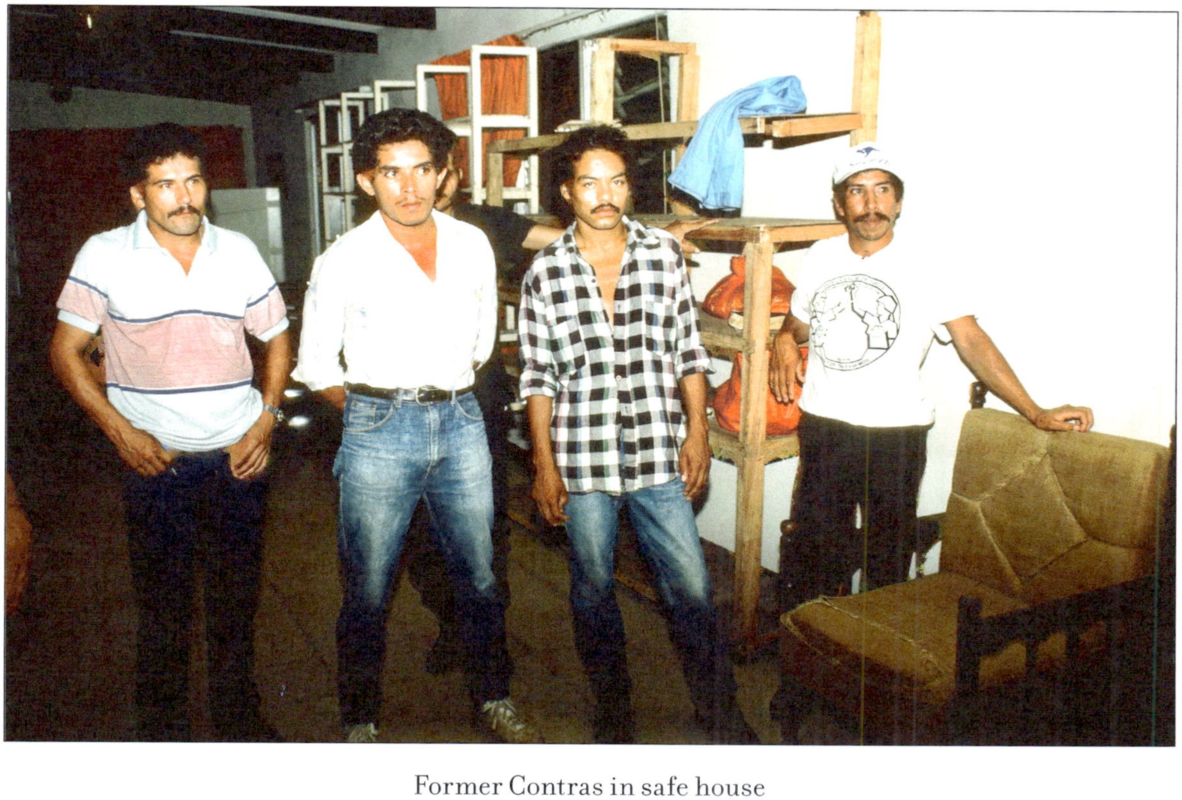

Former Contras in safe house

One of the residents was a young man who had been shot in the lower leg and had never had appropriate treatment, leaving an area of absent bone about half way between his ankle and knee. This left his foot and lower leg to flail about whenever he moved. He had also lost motor control to his foot, rendering that region a useless appendage. He was too fearful to seek treatment at one of the local hospitals, so we took him back to Jinotepe, where I amputated the lower part of his leg the following day. It was hoped he would eventually receive a prosthetic limb, but at least he was free of of the useless, flailing lower leg.

Unfortunately, the Sandinista-sympathizing nurses refused him pain meds during the night, and he suffered horribly. We quickly rectified the situation the following day.

He had also lost motor control to his foot rendering that region a useless appendage.

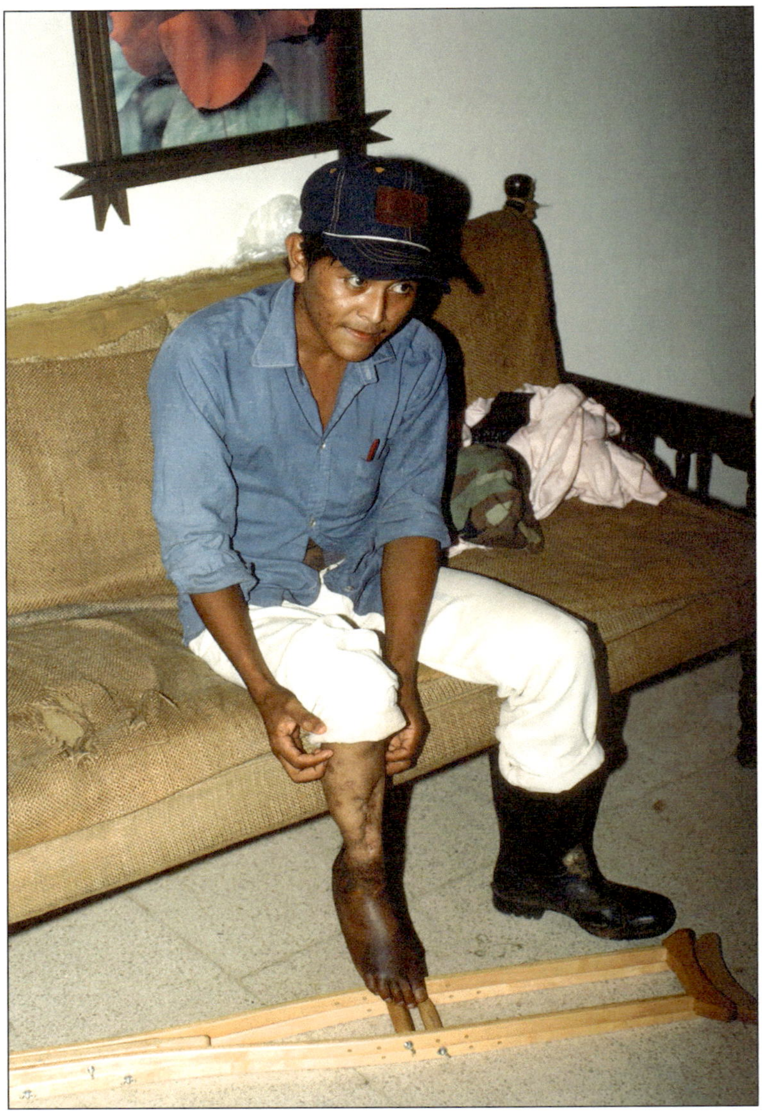

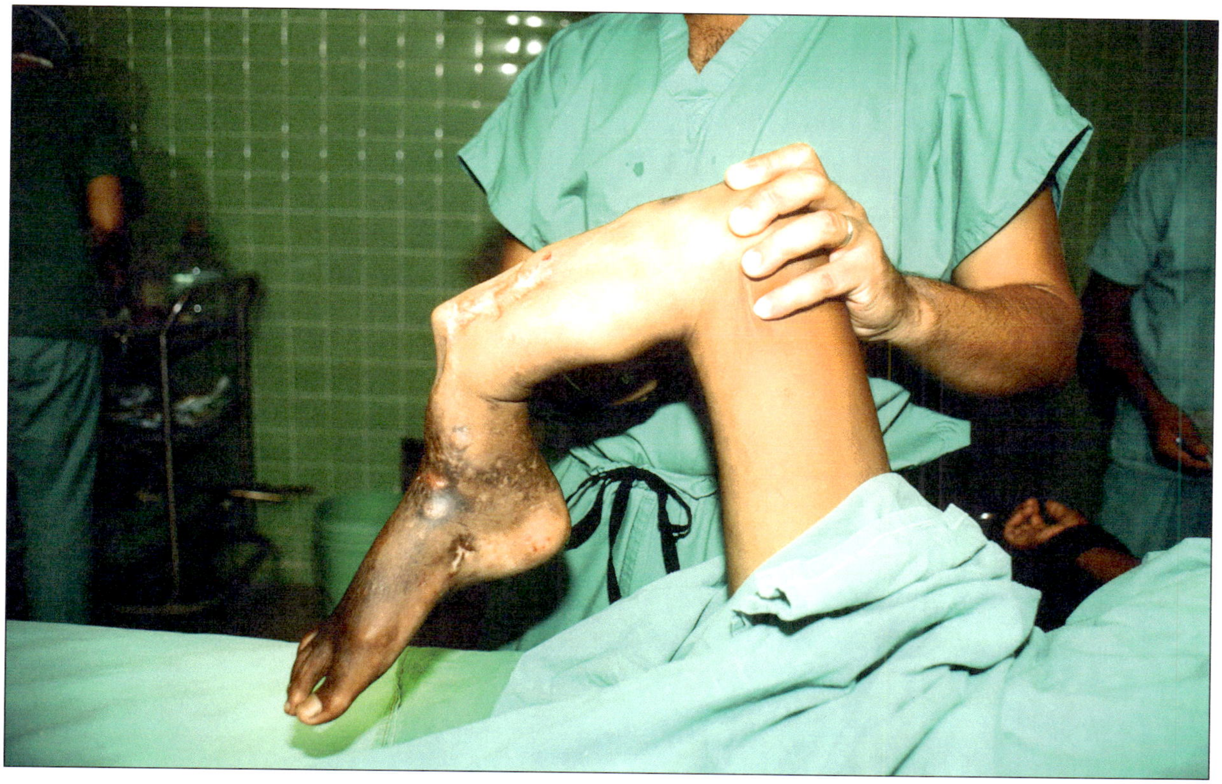

Illustrating useless lower leg and foot

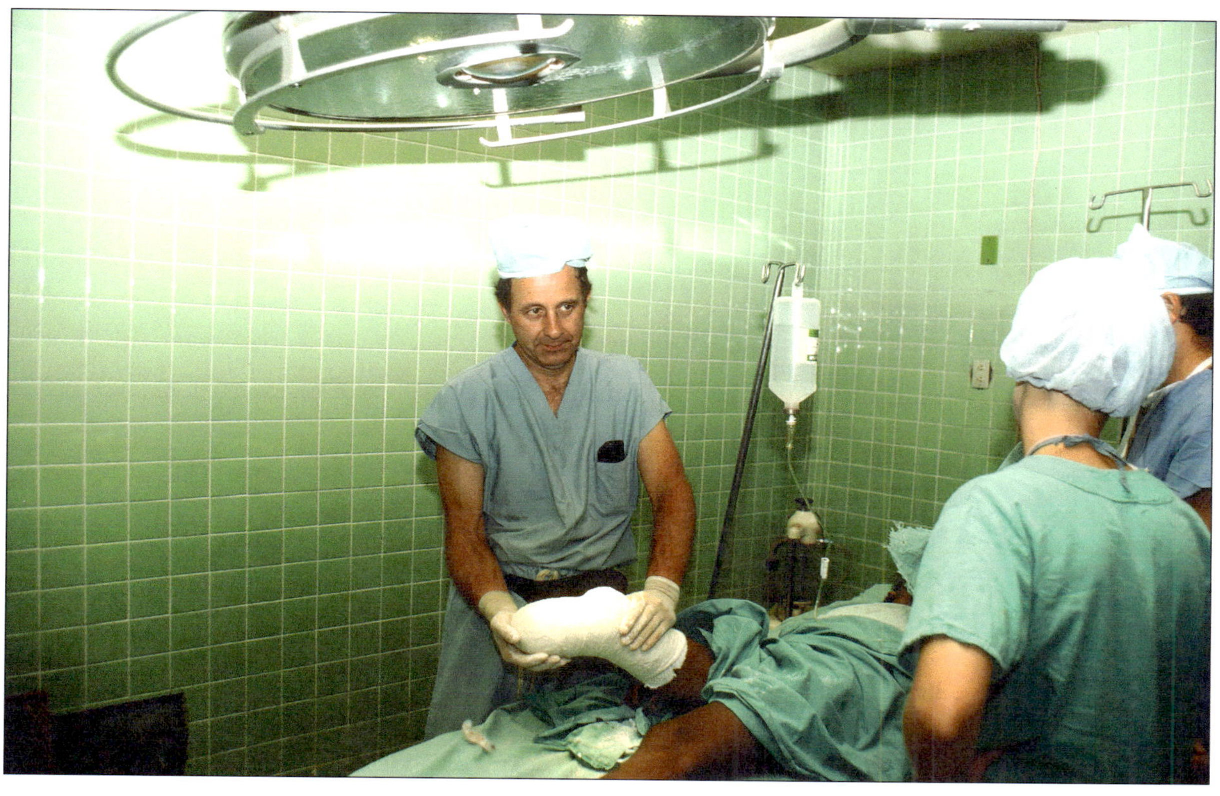

After amputation

With Cindy as our leader, we were able to have a face-to-face meeting with President Chamorro. She was a very charismatic woman and very popular with the people. In her office, she had a large picture of her husband and the bullet-ridden automobile in which he was assassinated.

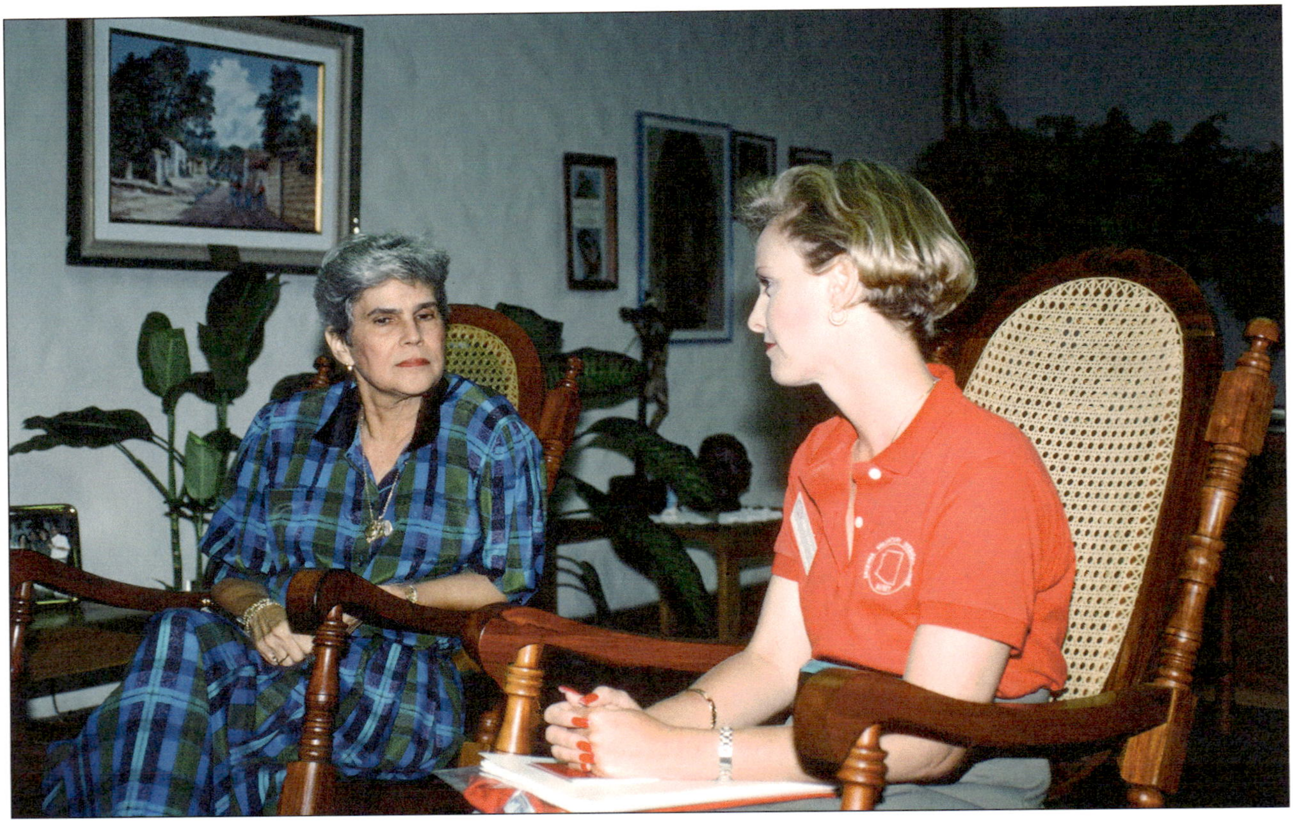

President Chamorro and Cindy McCain

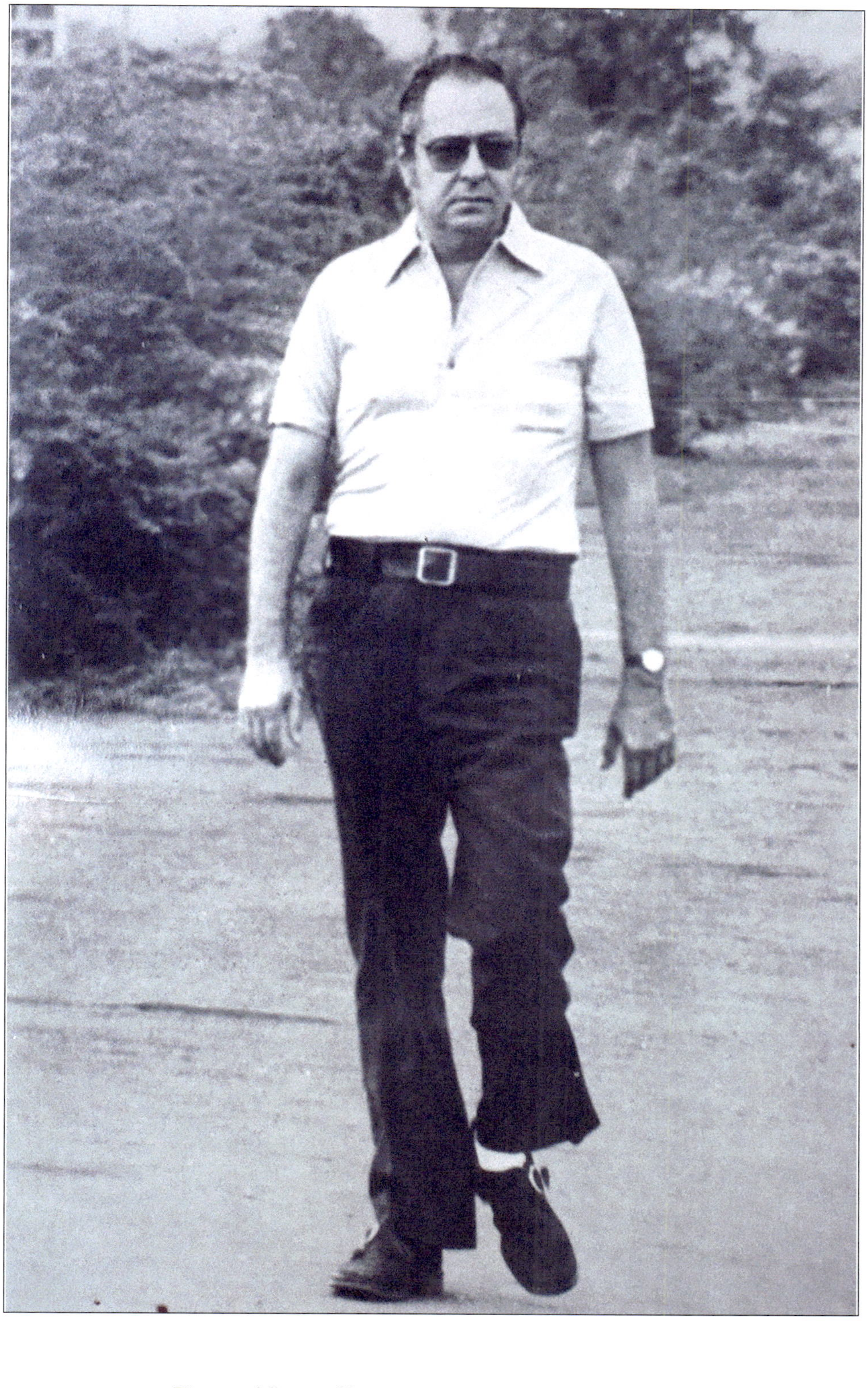

Photo of Señor Chamorro on the President's wall

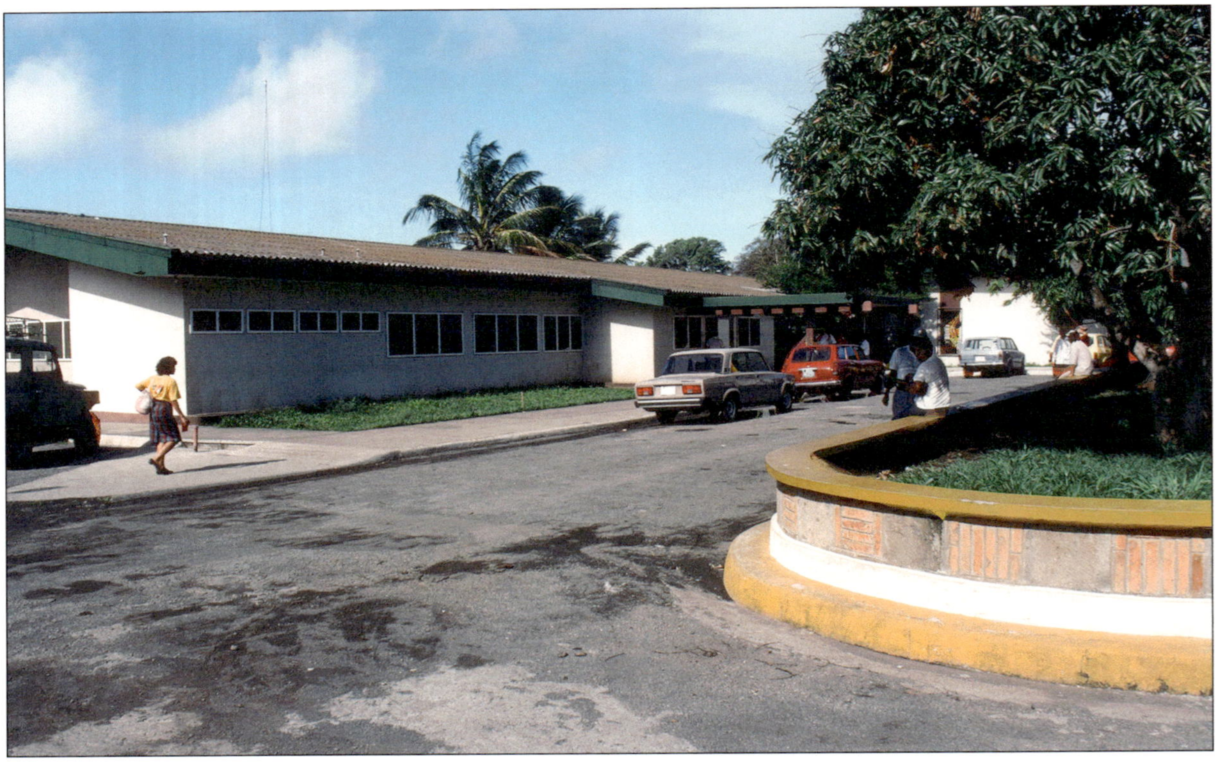

Jinotepe Hospital

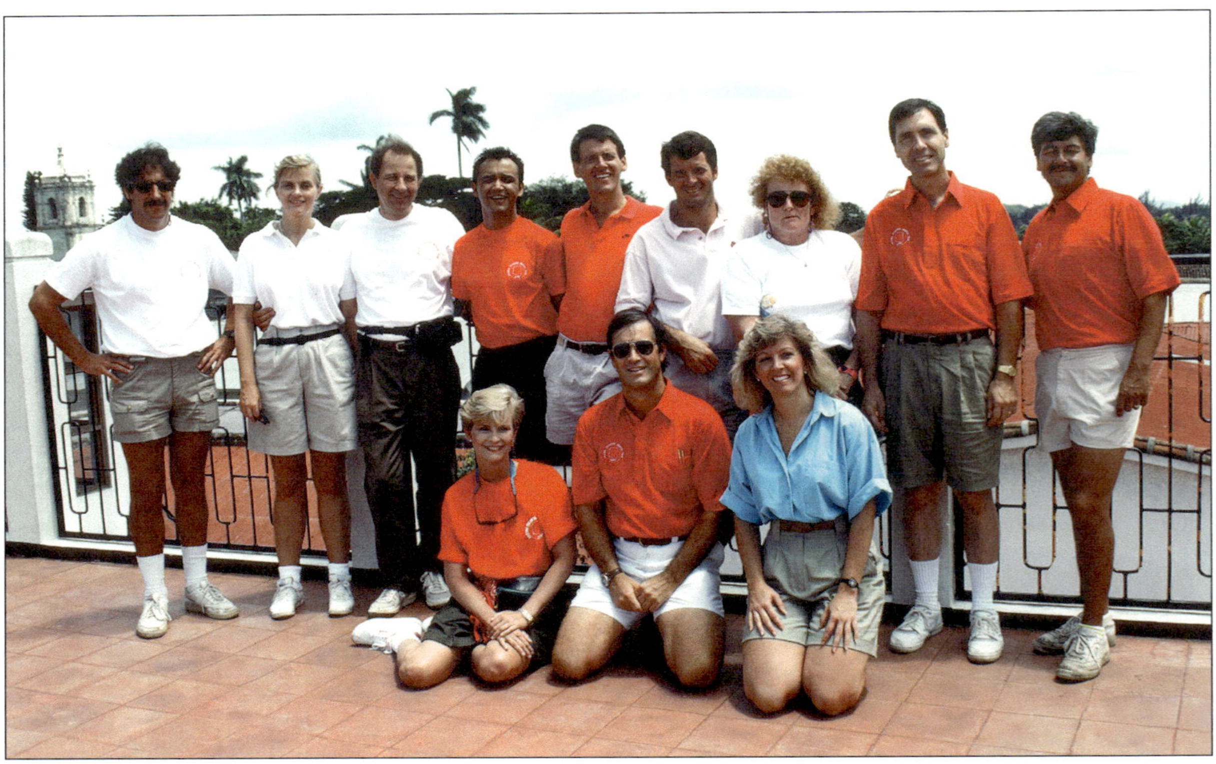

Medical team and Channel 3 reporter bottom right, Cindy on bottom left.

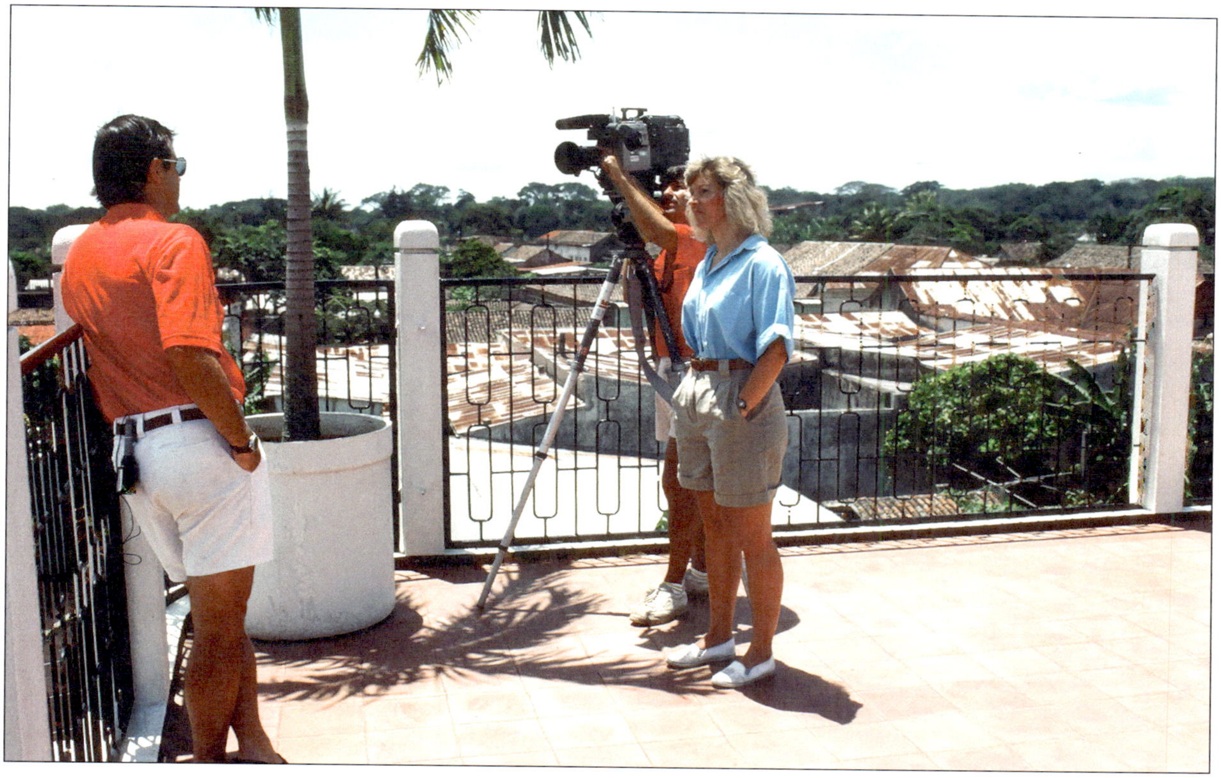

Cater Lee of Channel 3 interviewing one of the doctors

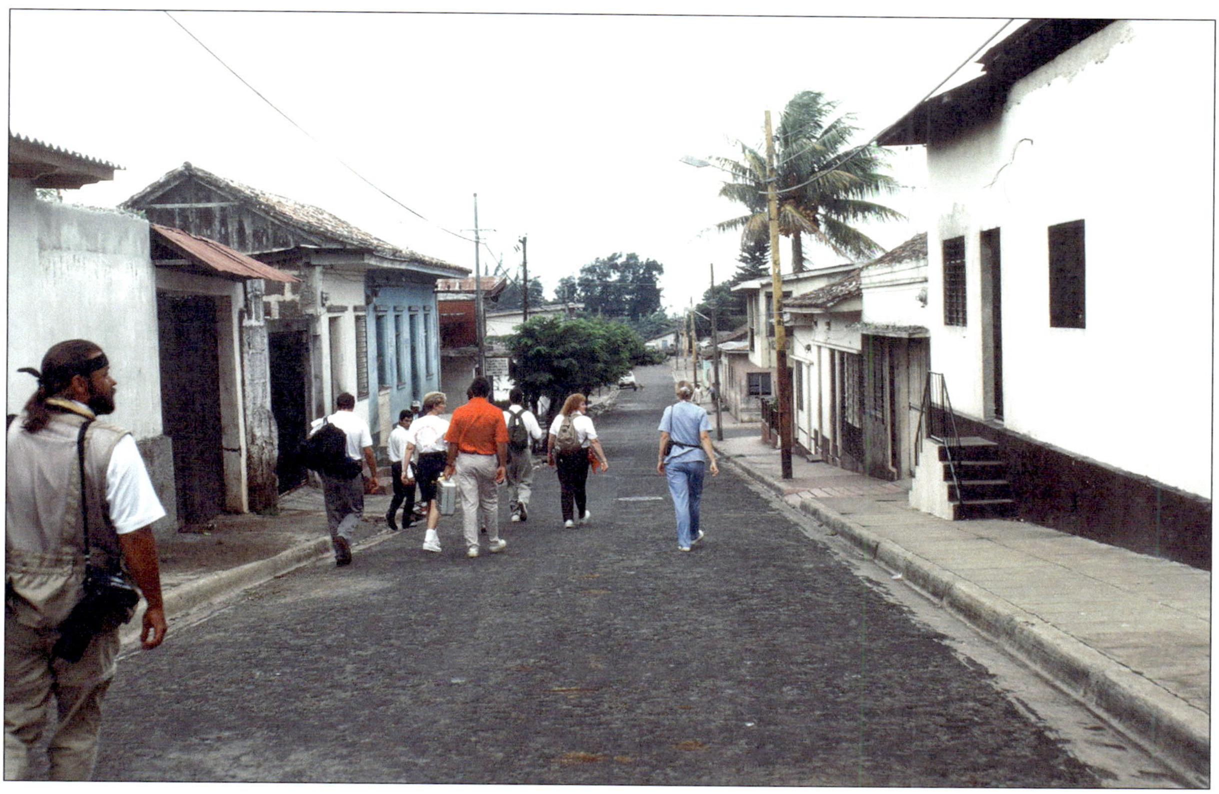

Morning walk to the hospital

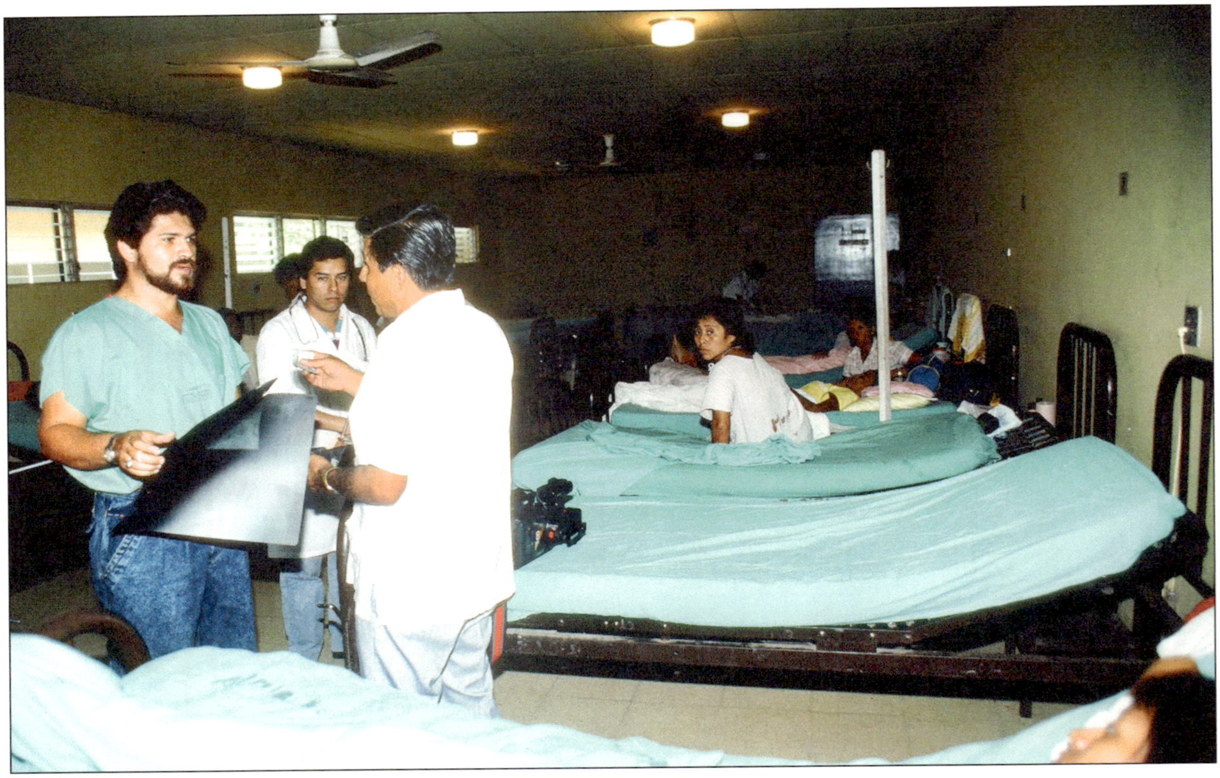

Making rounds with local orthopedist

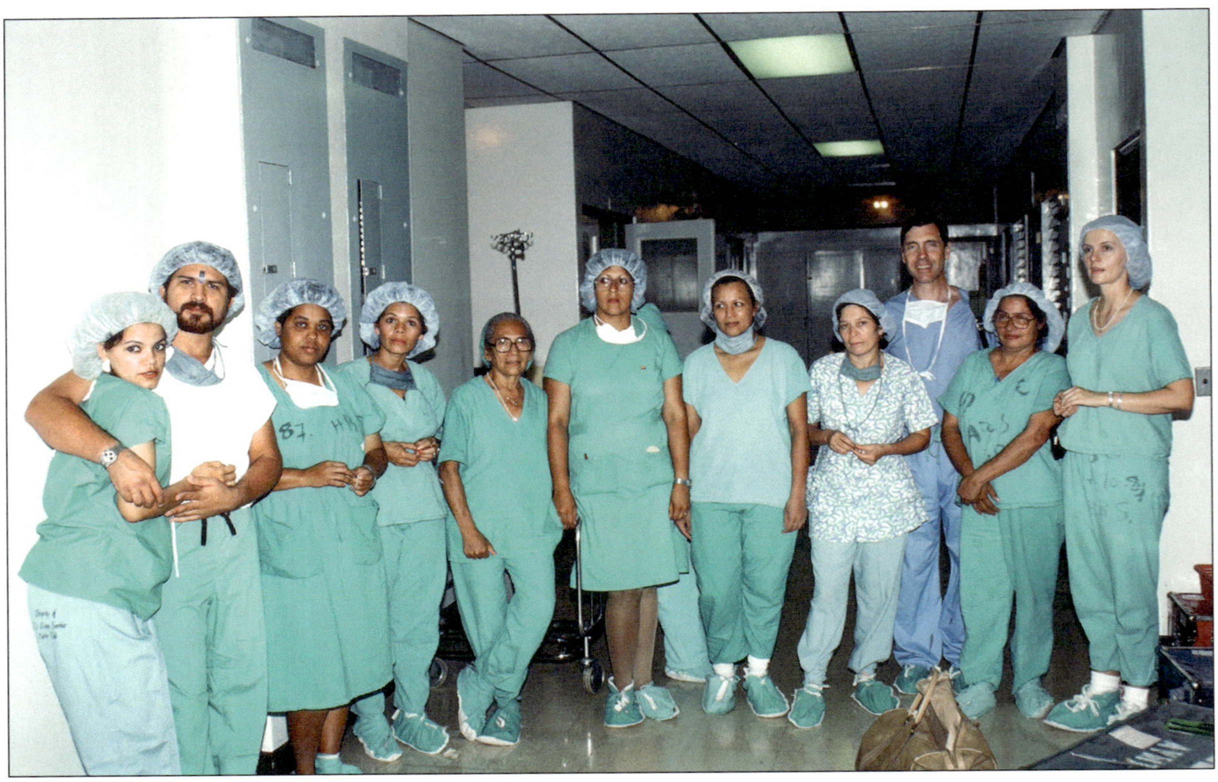

Local operating-room personnel and Rita

During this trip, we traveled to Managua, 40 miles to the north, to visit one of the large community hospitals. There we encountered a triage area, where children suffering from severe diarrhea and subsequent dehydration (a common condition in Third World countries due to water contamination) were on gurneys plugged into IVs for rehydration. We also saw children suffering from sequelae of measles due to a lack of vaccinations. One child had a seizure just as we approached.

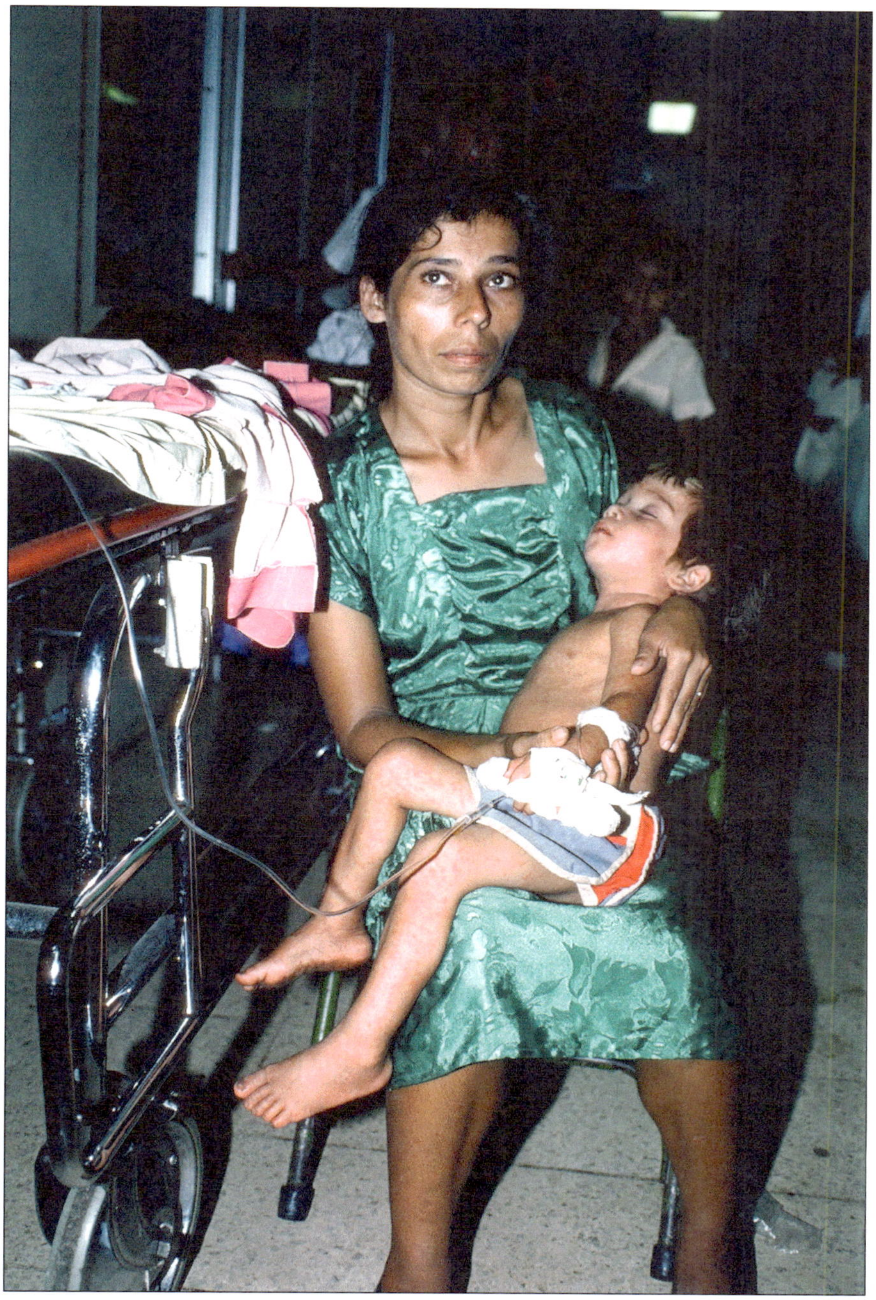

Child receiving IV therapy for dehydration secondary to diarrhea

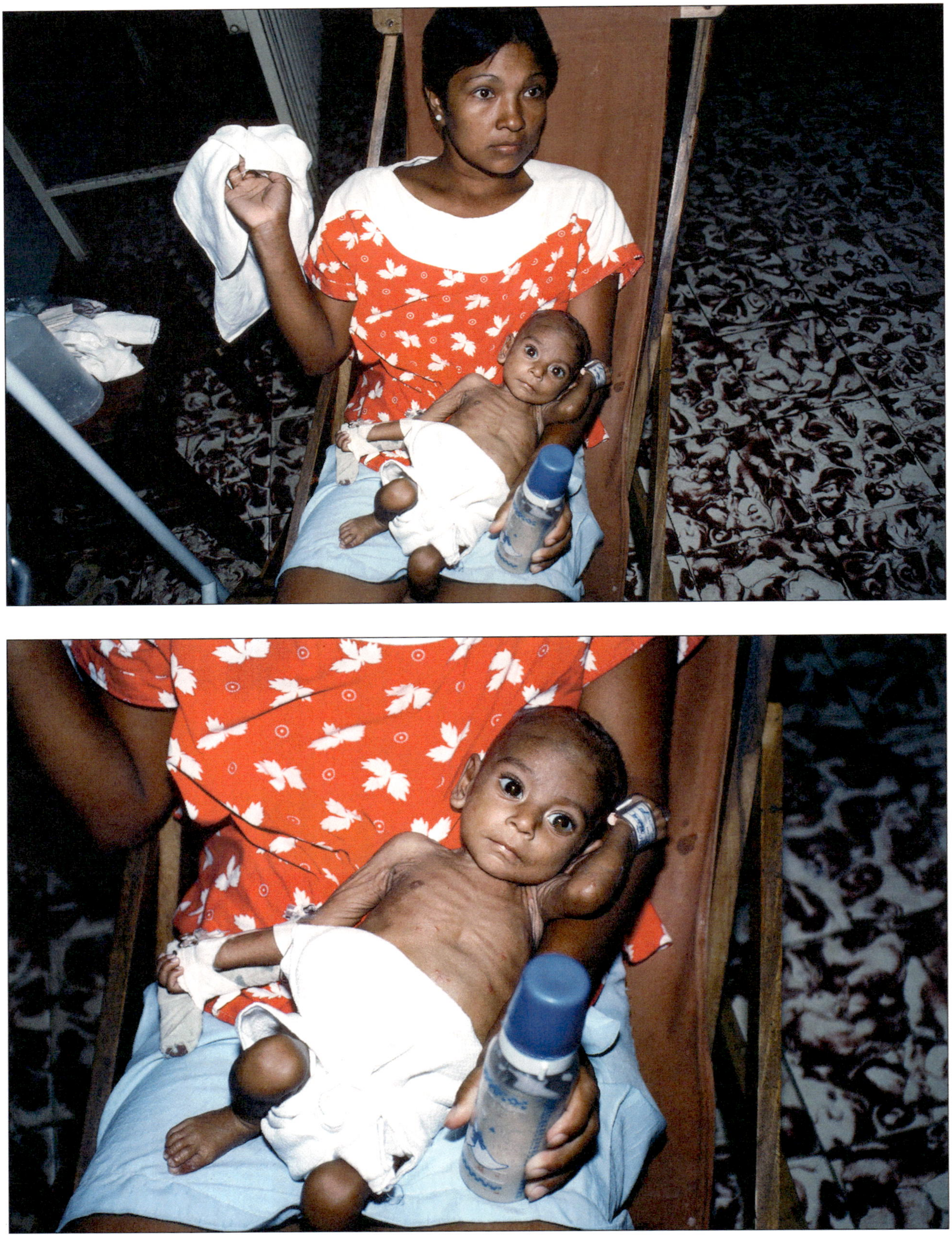

Malnutrition

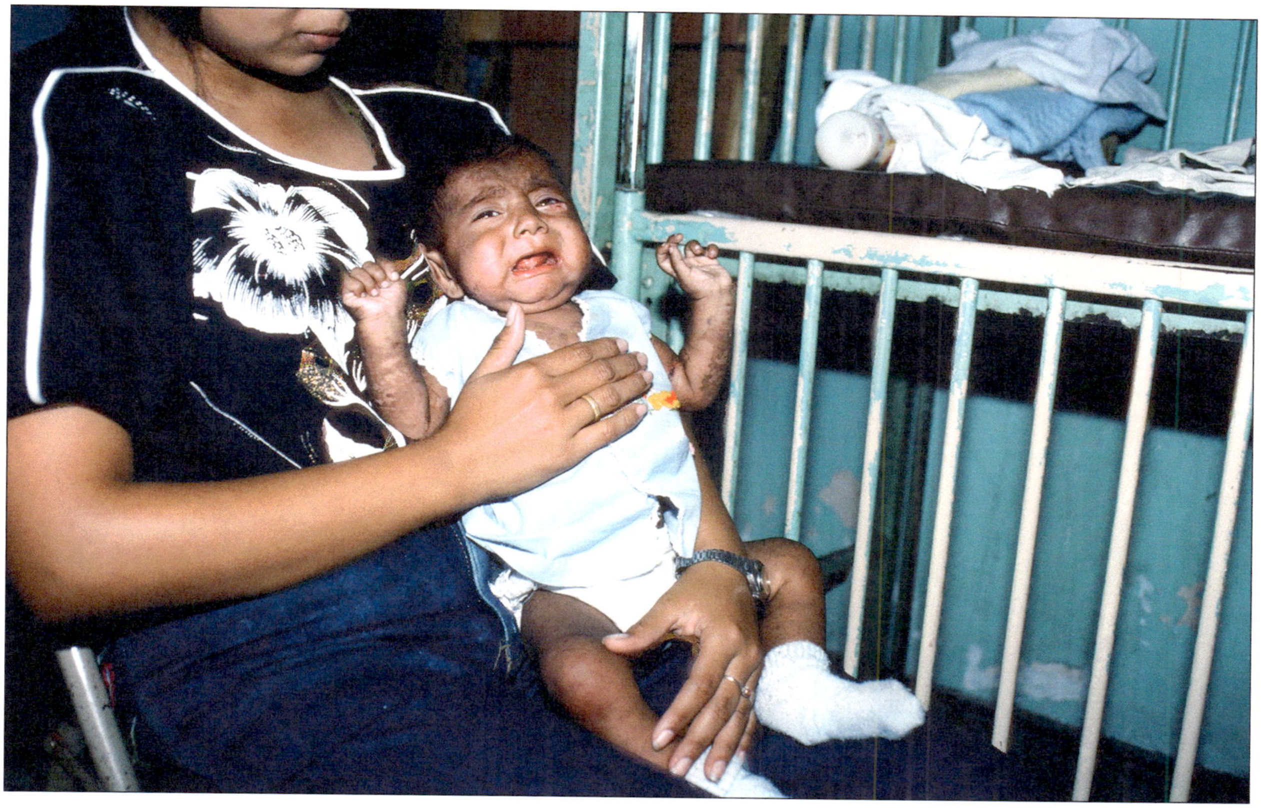

Child with infectious disease had seizure just after this photo

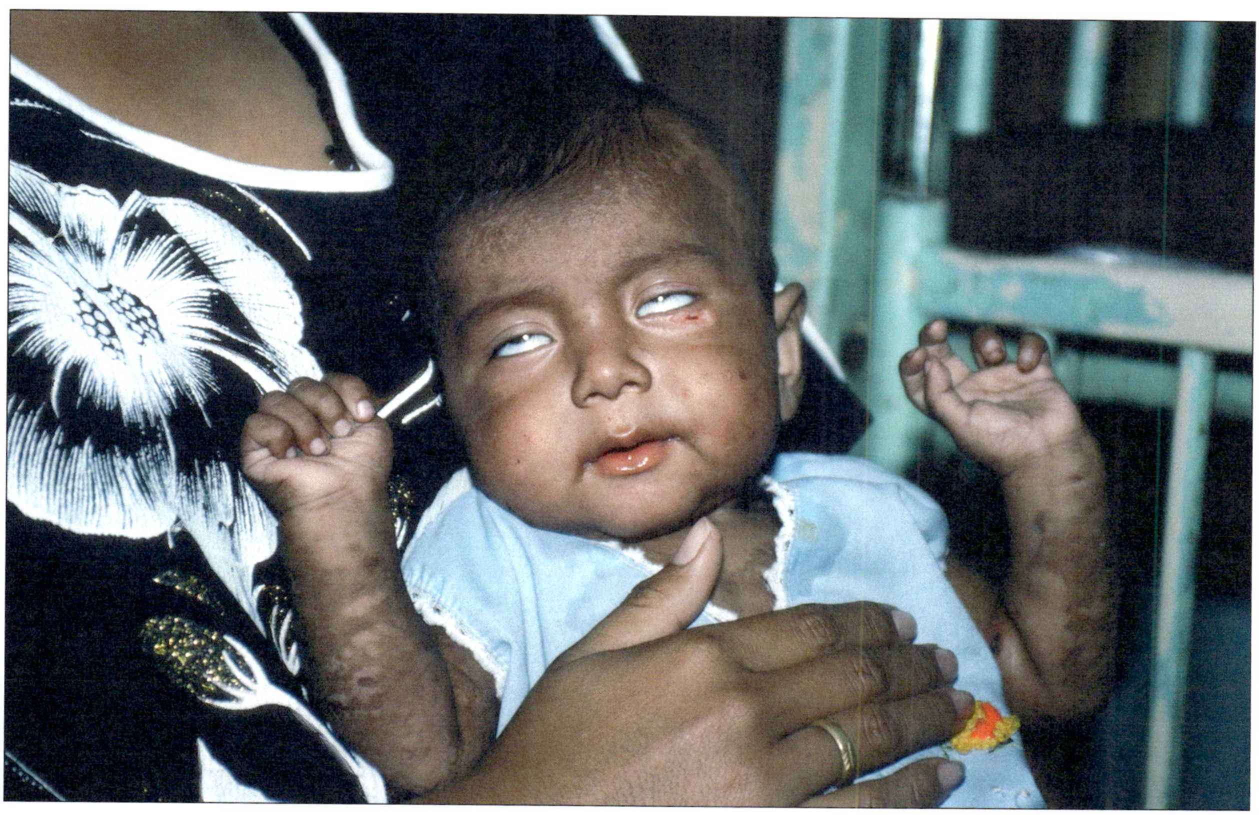

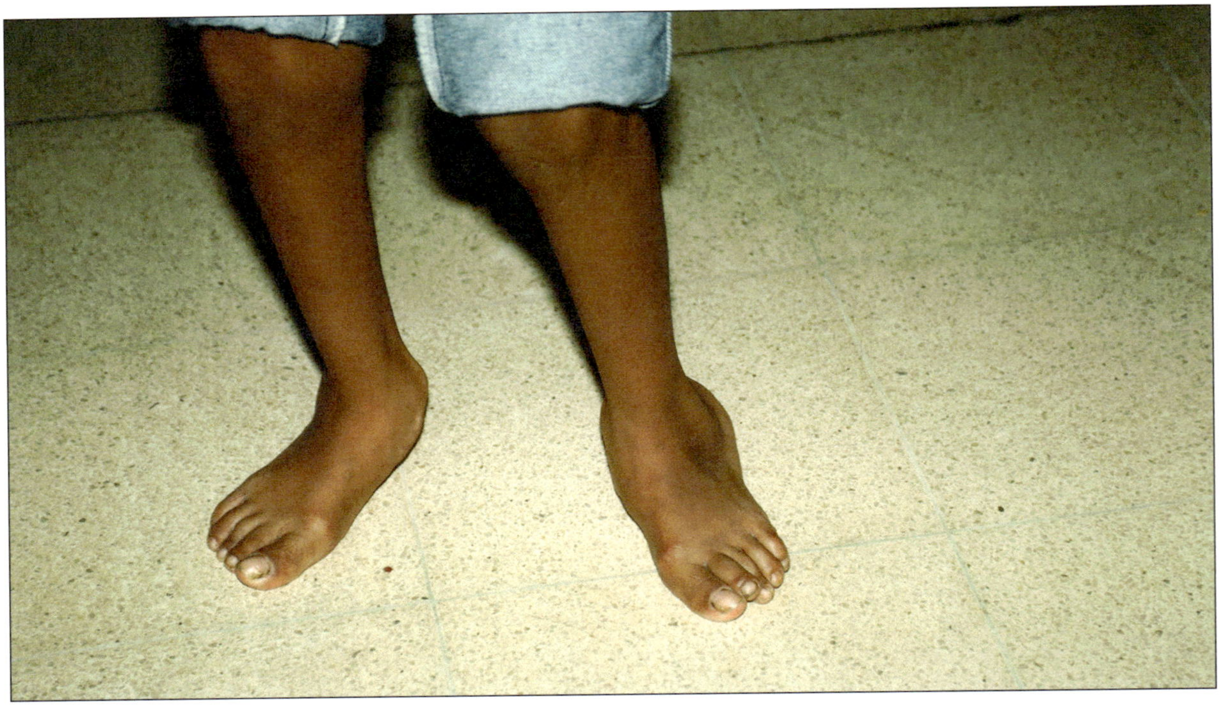

Young boy with foot deformity

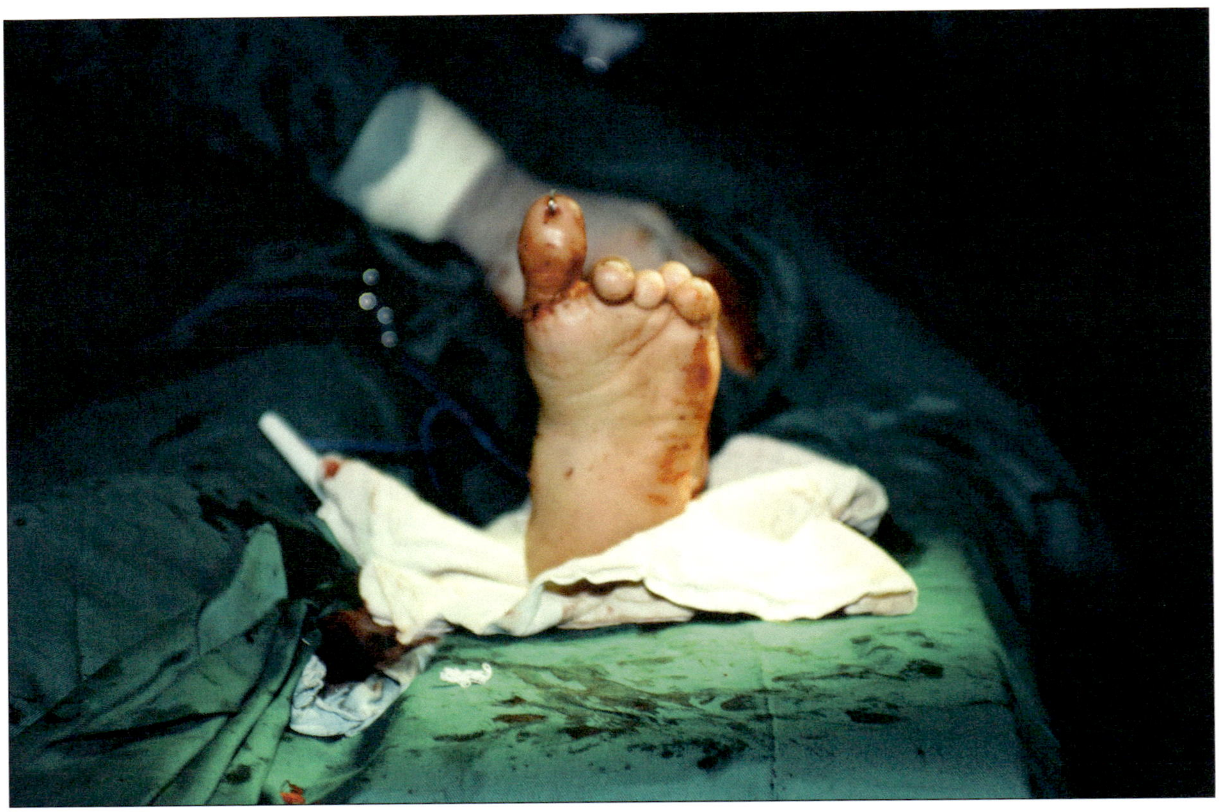

After surgical correction

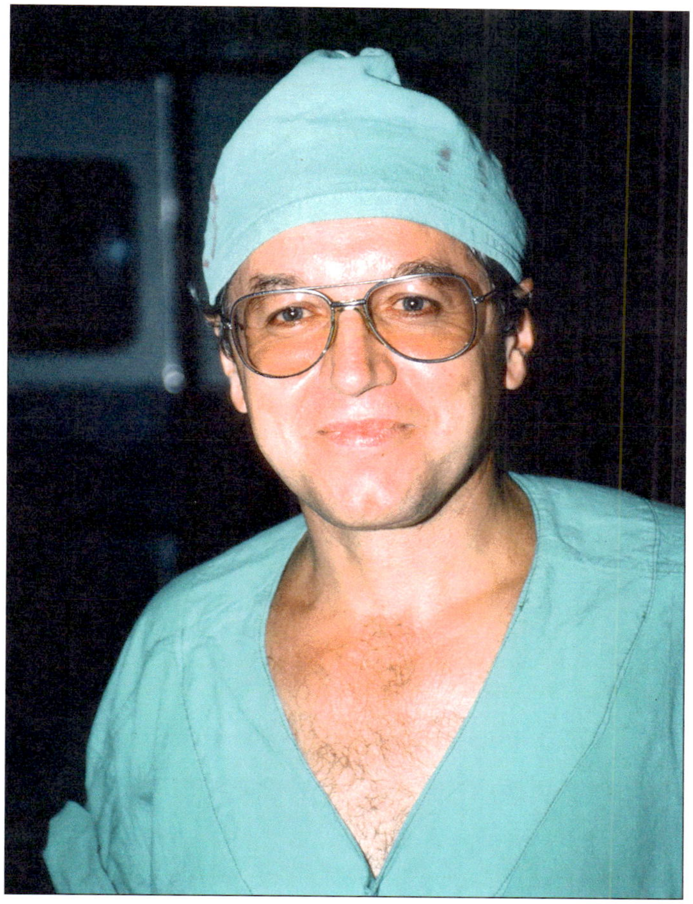

Russian anesthesiologist working in Managua hospital

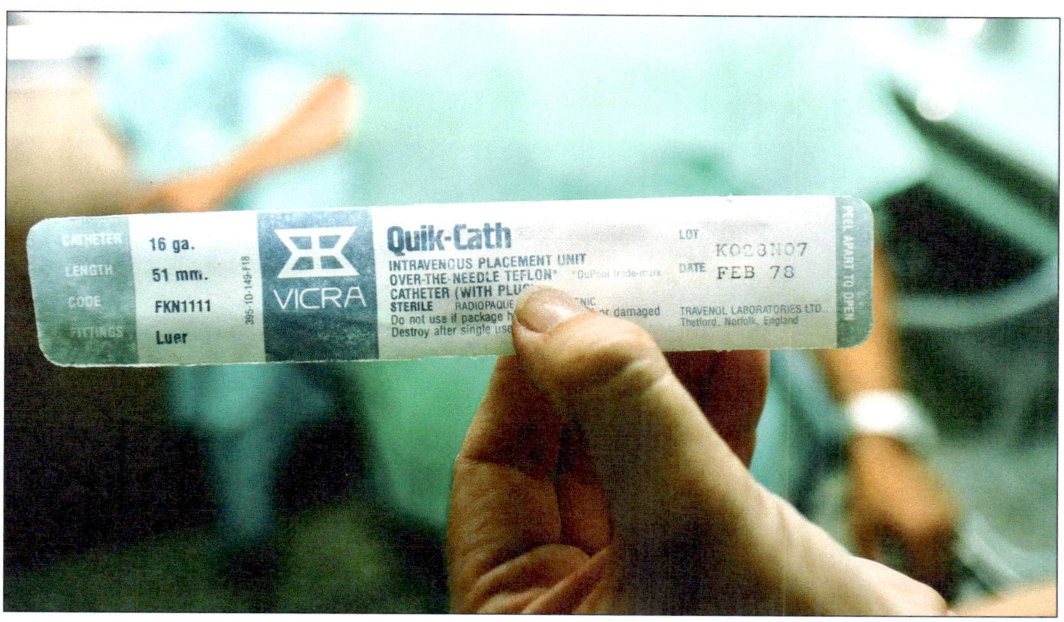

IV needle package he was using with expiration date of Feb 1978

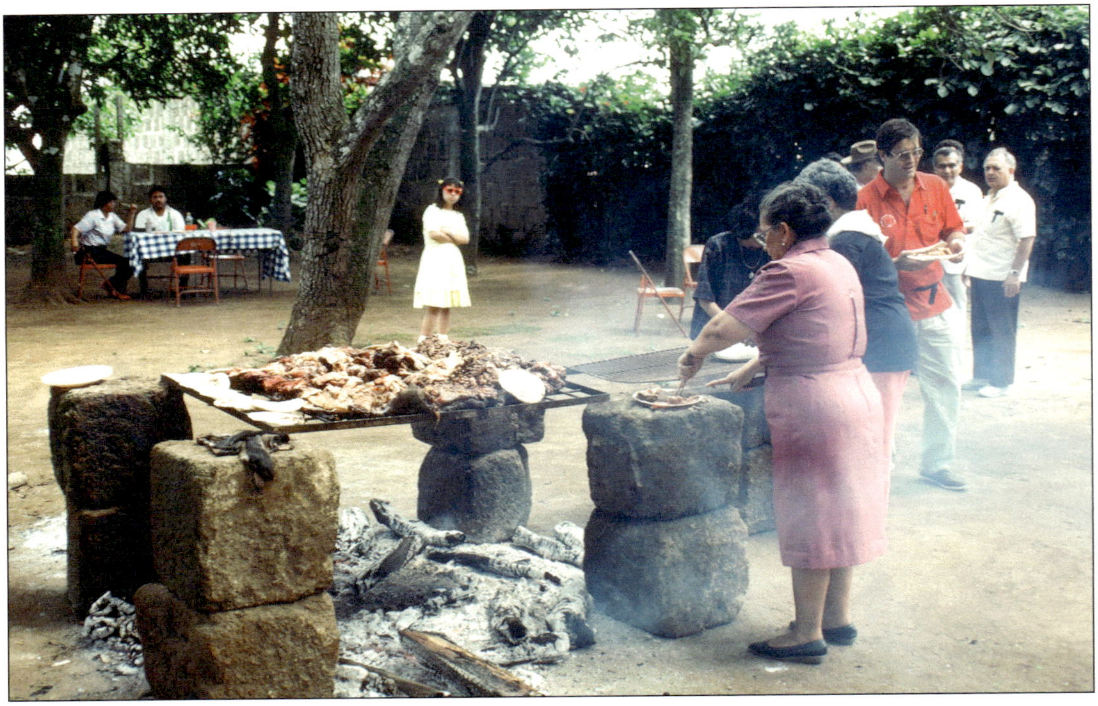

Barbecue for us hosted by local family

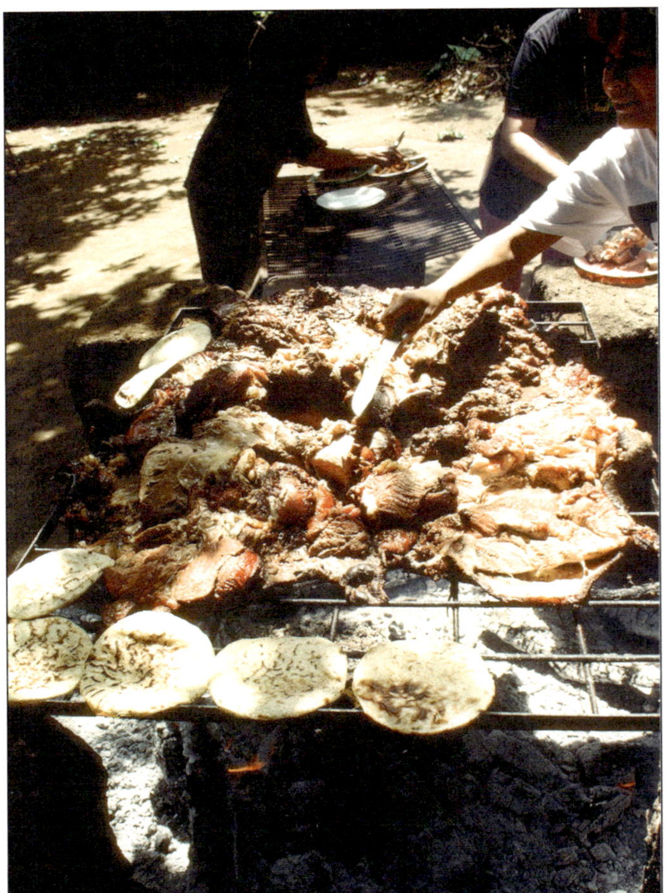

An unfortunate and tragic event happened during this trip when a young baby died during surgery. I was operating on a child with a dislocated hip, and anesthesia was being administered by a Nicaraguan anesthesiologist. During the procedure, he left the room to use the bathroom and asked one of the aides to watch the anesthesia machine during his absence. I was nearing the end of the procedure when he announced he could not hear a heartbeat. I closed the wound rapidly, and we administered CPR on the child manually for six hours before we gave up. The child was from a village outside of Jinotepe, and the mother was the only parent at the hospital. By the time we terminated the resuscitation, it was nighttime, and we had to drive the mother and baby back to their village. Unfortunately, it was a local holiday, and excessive drinking was commonplace for these occasions. Also, due to the recent war, guns were prevalent amongst the general population, and the local doctor was concerned that the father would be intoxicated and have a gun, which could lead to a very volatile encounter once he was informed of his daughter's death. Fortunately, our fears were misplaced, but it created some anxious moments as we met with the father.

An unfortunate and tragic event happened during this trip when a young baby died during surgery.

We made two additional trips to Nicaragua with Operation Walk, working in the Roberto Calderon Hospital doing 100 hip and knee replacements and enriching the lives of patients who would not have had access to these procedures otherwise.

Haiti

My last trip was to Haiti in 2010, two months following a catastrophic earthquake of 7.0 magnitude and more than 52 aftershocks of 4.5 or greater. The death toll was between 100,000 and 160,000. An estimated 250,000 residences and 30,000 commercial buildings were destroyed. Thousands of survivors suffered lacerations, contusions, fractures, dislocations, amputations, and other manifestations of traumatic injuries. I travelled with Bob Porter, a fellow orthopedist and friend from medical school and internship. Bob was from Des Moines and had been Larry Dorr's roommate in college and medical school. The Orthopedic Academy was coordinating efforts with various relief organizations and orthopedic volunteers. We were notified on a Wednesday that a charter flight was leaving Miami for Haiti on Saturday, and we were invited to participate. We met in Miami Friday evening, with an anticipated departure of noon the following day. Upon arrival to Miami, however, we were informed the departure time had been pushed back to 5 p.m. We showed up at 3 p.m. for our departure but did not depart until 7:30! We landed in a rainstorm, and the terminal was closed, so we waited on the tarmac another hour while all the luggage was unloaded. We were then transferred by a bus, badly in need of repair, with other volunteers, arriving at our destination around 11:30 that night. We were housed in tents on the grounds of an abandoned home. It served as an outpatient clinic from Monday to Saturday. Volunteer nurses, PAs, and physicians set up cots or mats inside and saw patients from 8 am to 6 p.m. These volunteers stayed from one to three weeks and were from all over the US and a few from Canada.

My last trip was to Haiti in 2010, two months following a catastrophic earthquake of 7.0 magnitude and more than 52 aftershocks of 4.5 or greater.

The following day, we assessed the facility and discovered it was an outpatient clinic treating patients for all types of general medical disorders, something that we, as surgeons, had little interest in or expertise with, and thus set out on our own to find a hospital that could utilize our services. An early lesson was that there was no informed central location coordinating the supplies and personnel who intermittently streamed onto the island, but we ended up working at the Seventh Day Adventist Hospital, which was just up the street from where we were residing. Since we arrived some six weeks after the quake, the work remaining was a bit different than that required right after the event.

Most of the amputations and acute-fracture repair had been completed in the initial few weeks. Upon our arrival, most surgical treatment involved repair of delayed or malunited fractures, rehabilitation of the injured, and occasionally redoing previous surgeries. Our first few days involved making rounds on all post-operative patients who were still residing in tents on the hospital grounds. This was necessary, as the hospital did not have enough beds to accommodate the large number of surgical cases, and many of these individuals had no other place to go, as their homes had been destroyed. The surgeons in the hospital did not have time to evaluate the large number of patients housed on the outside. Some patients remained outside due to fear of aftershocks and fear that the hospital would collapse, resulting in devastating injuries from which they were now recuperating. The grounds were filled with fifty to sixty patients and their families living in tents, sometimes two families to a tent. We evaluated all of the patients, examining their wounds, changing dressings, ordering X-rays, and prescribing their future treatments, especially the timing of weight bearing for fractures of the lower extremity.

Most of the amputations and acute-fracture repair had been completed in the initial few weeks.

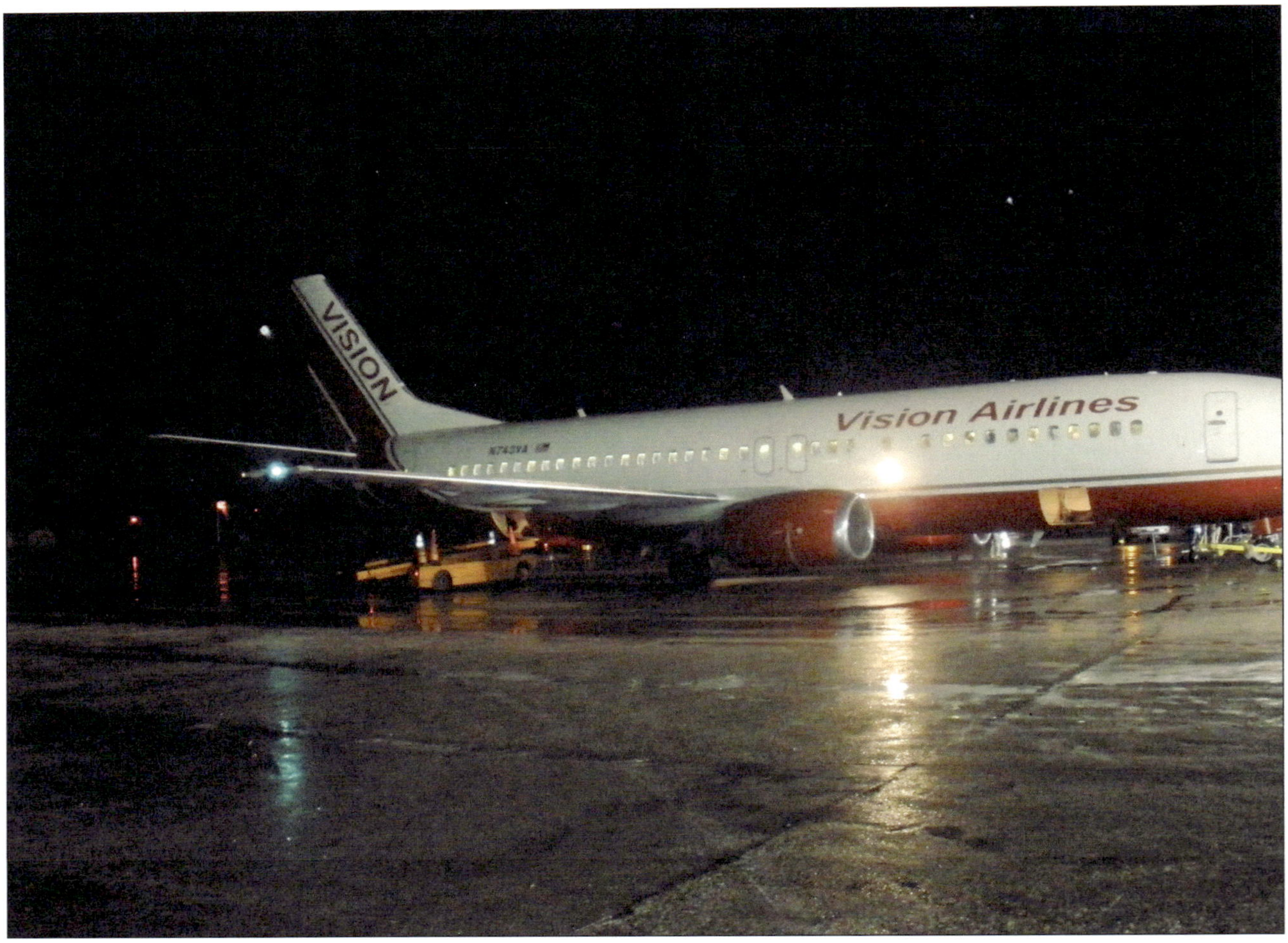

Charter from Miami

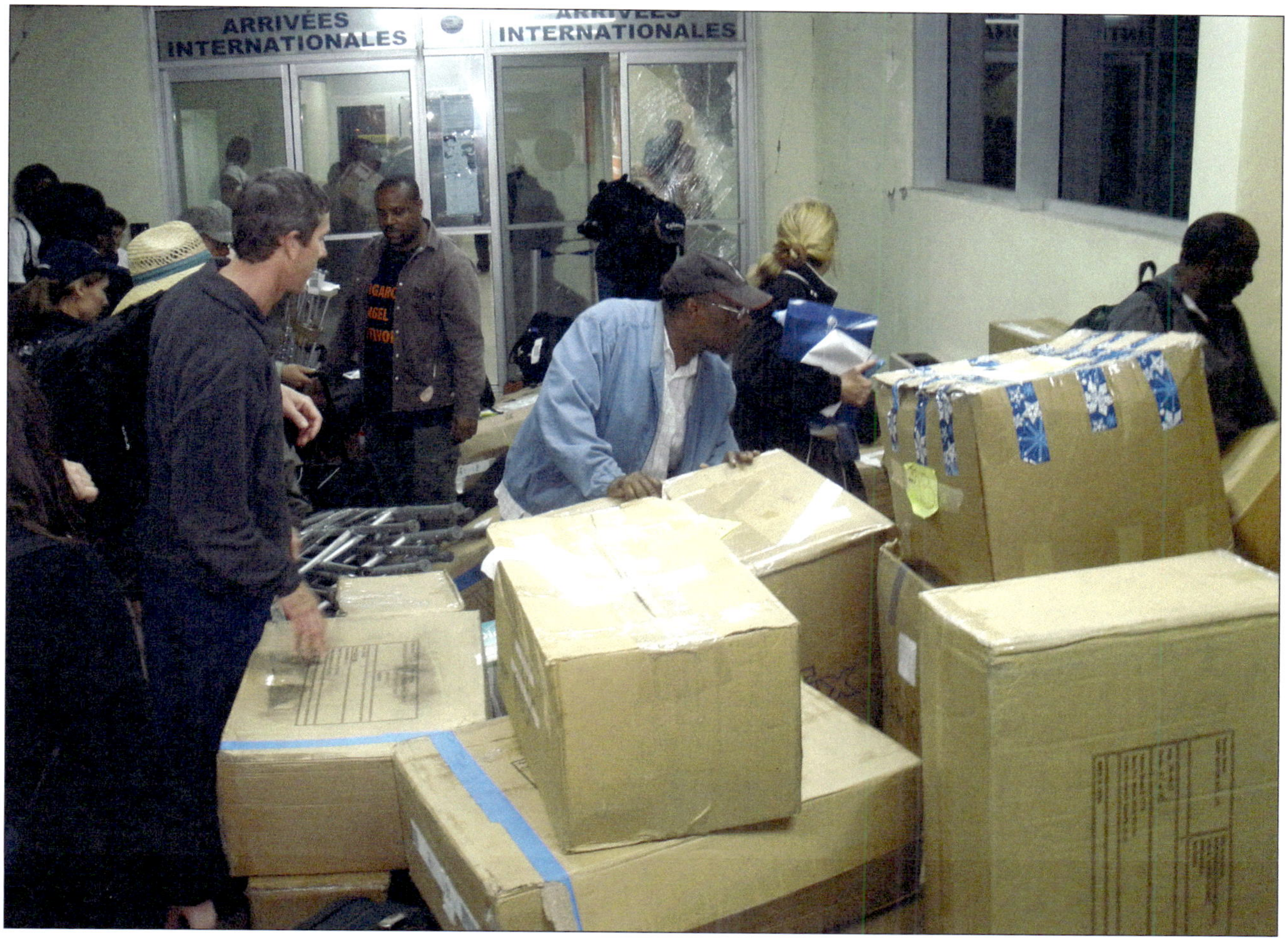

Unloaded supplies at airport

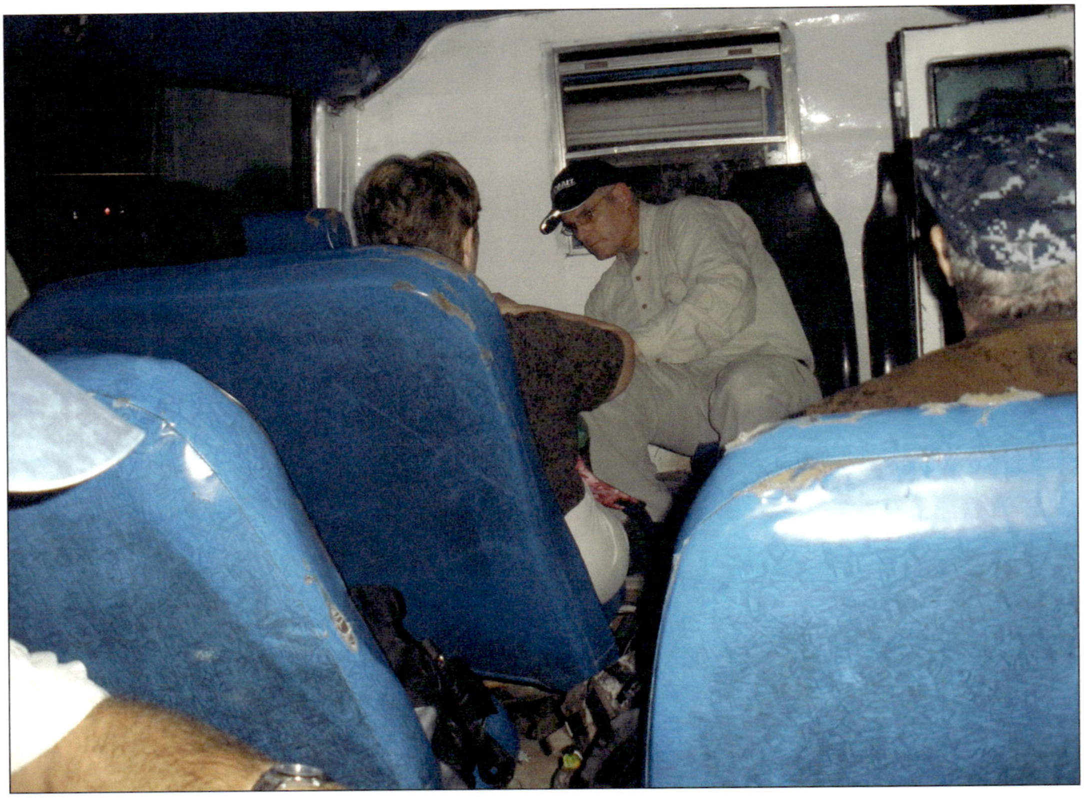

Inside bus from airport

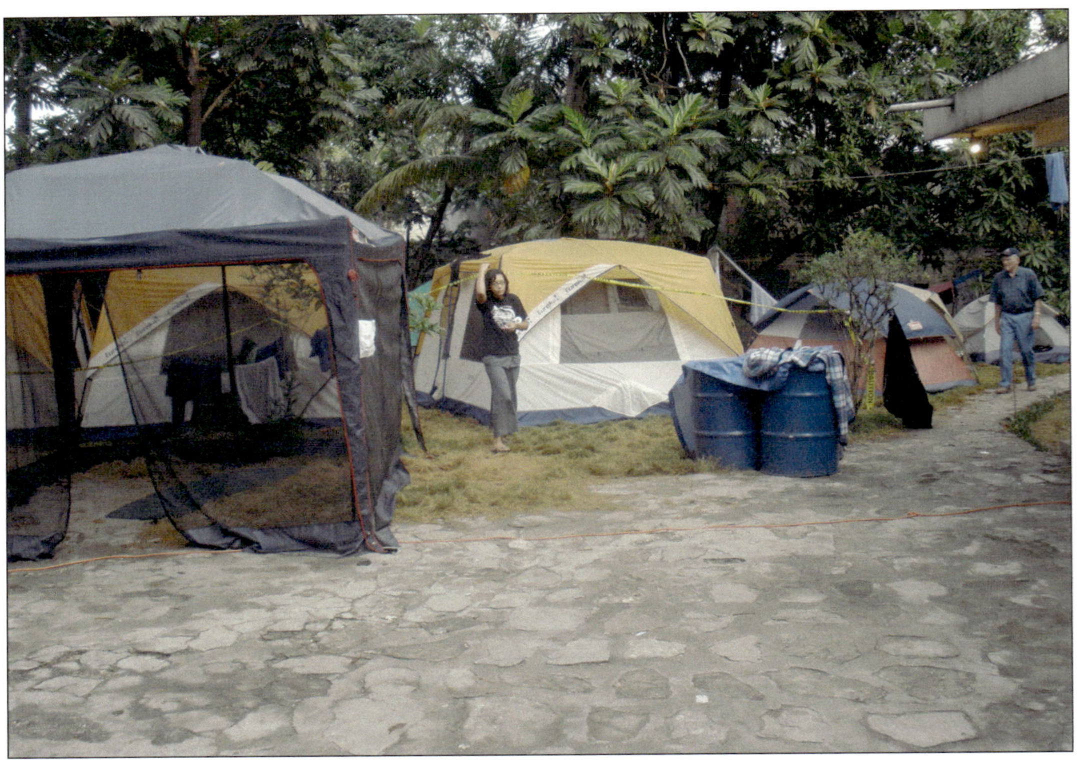

Our quarters

Destroyed remnants of earthquake

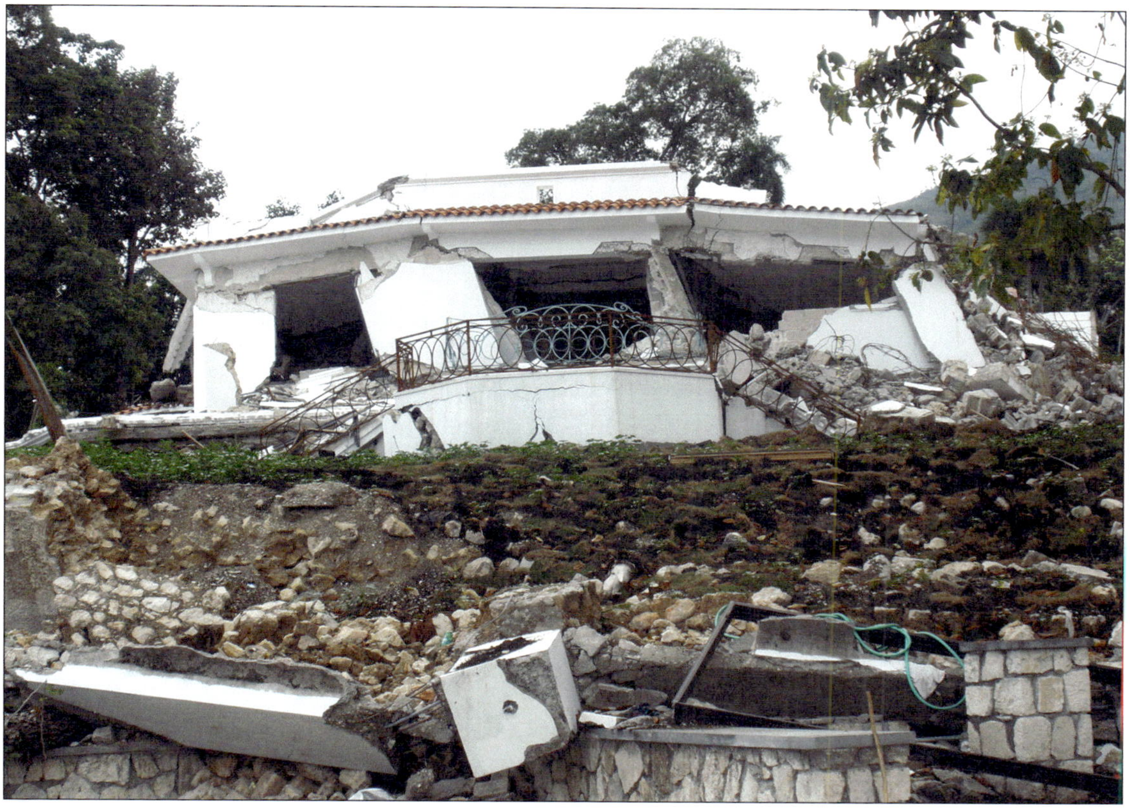

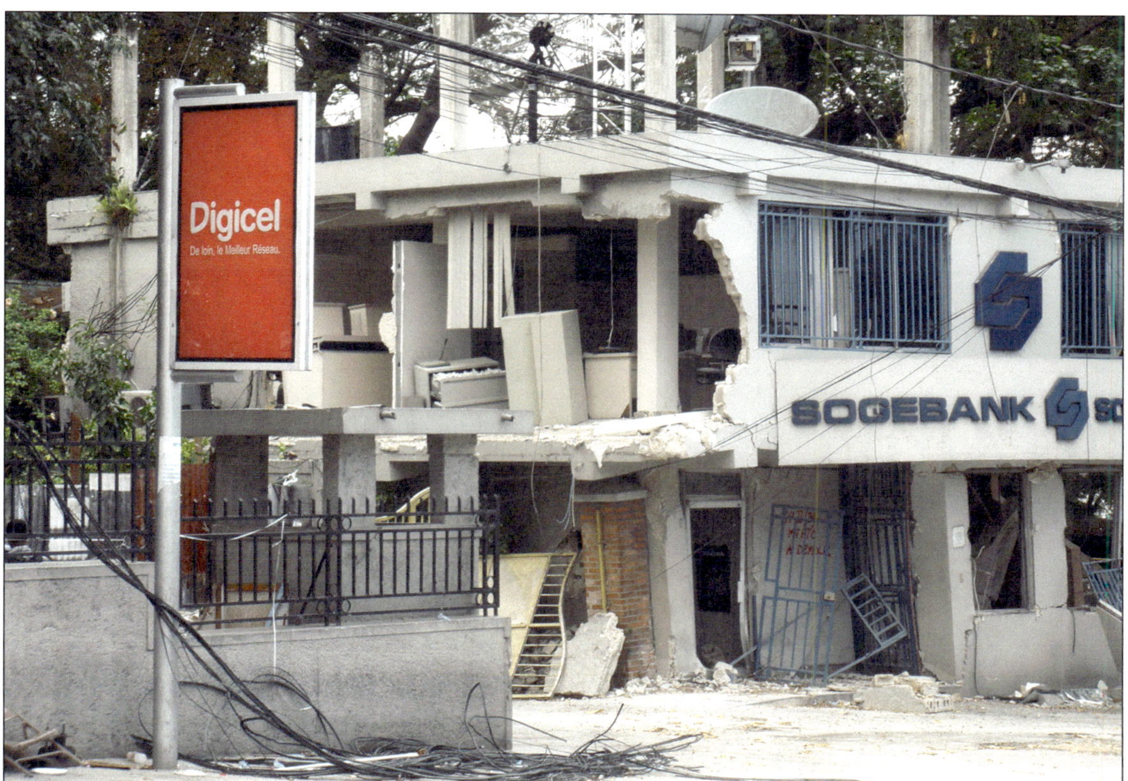

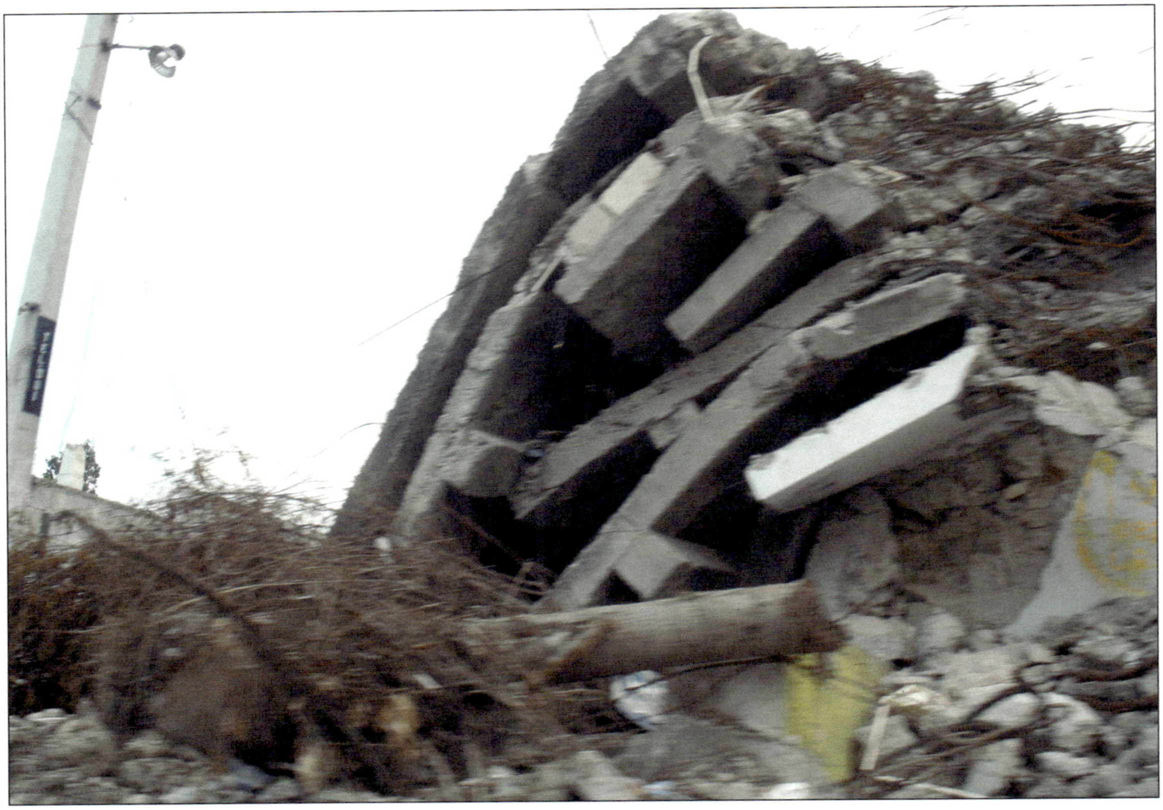

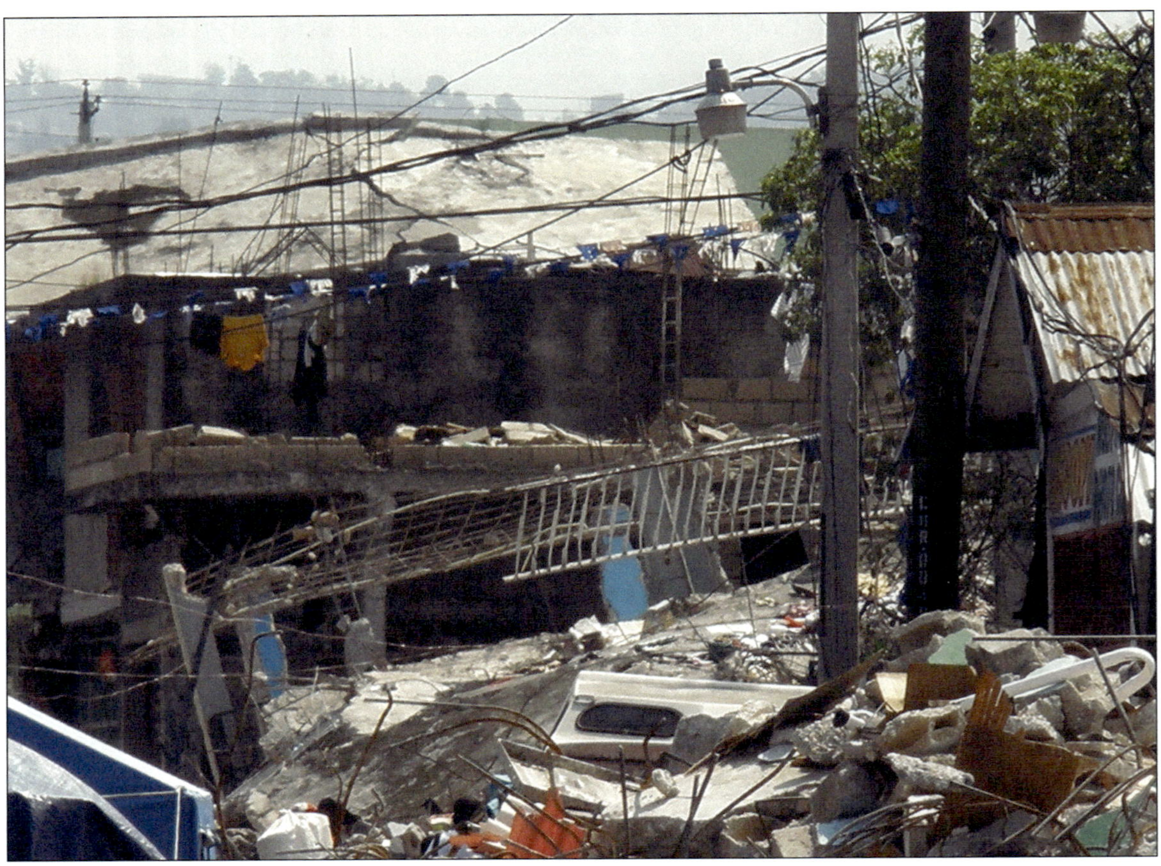

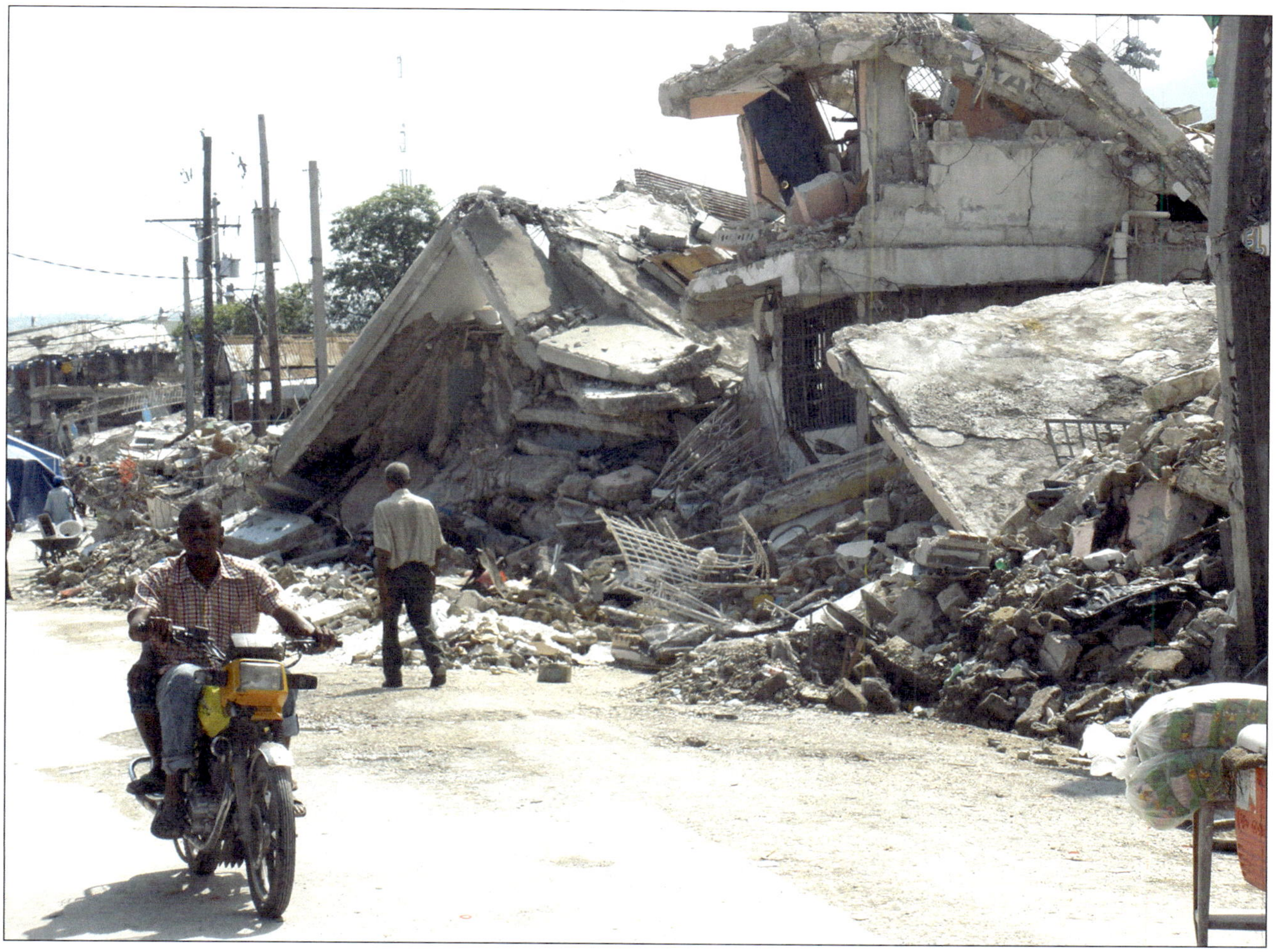

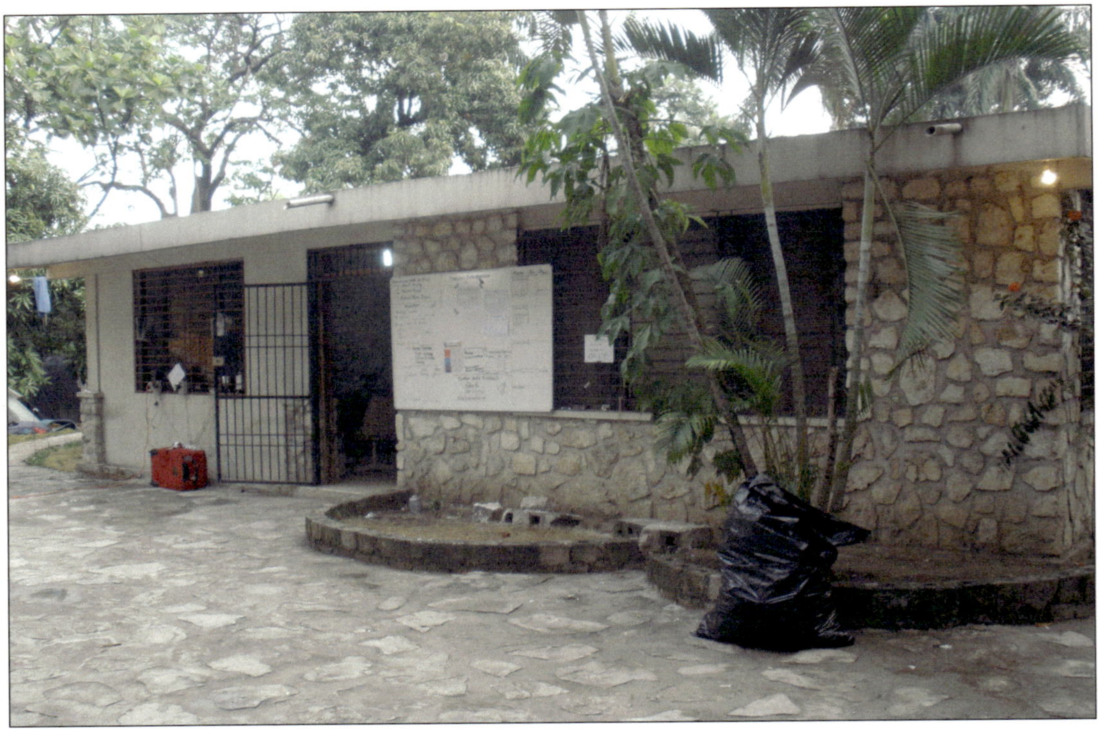

House that was outpatient clinic

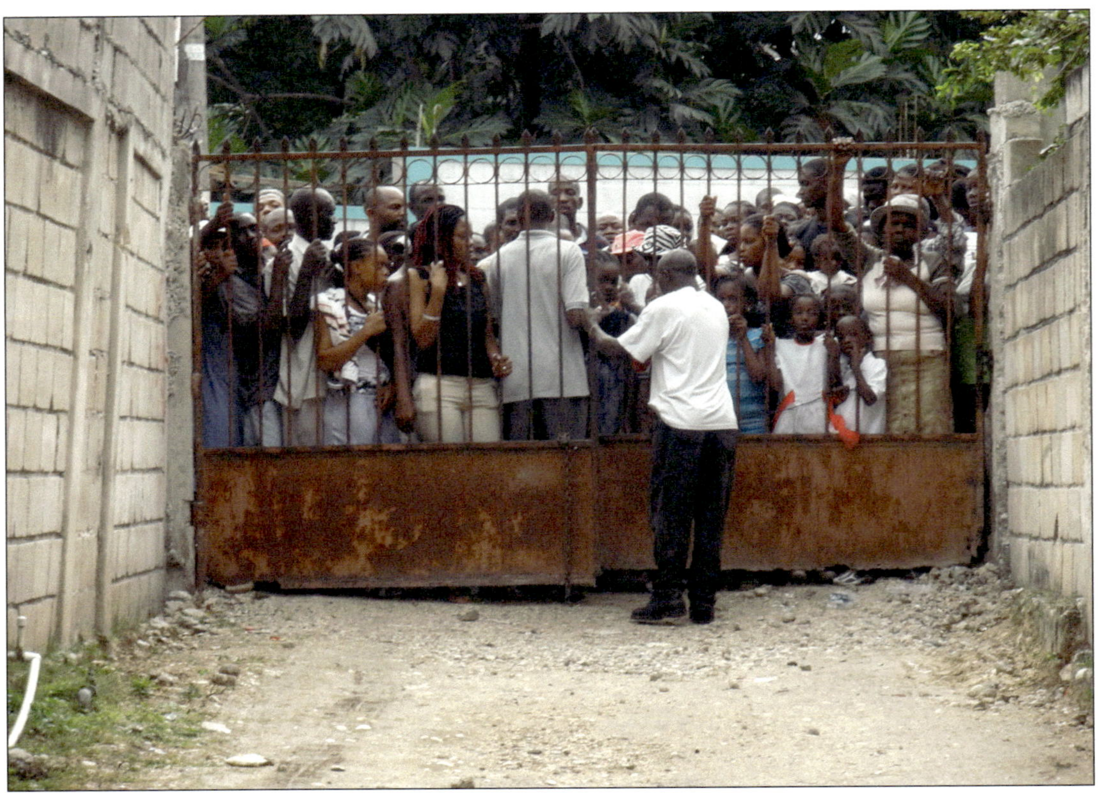

Guard opening gate at 8 a.m.

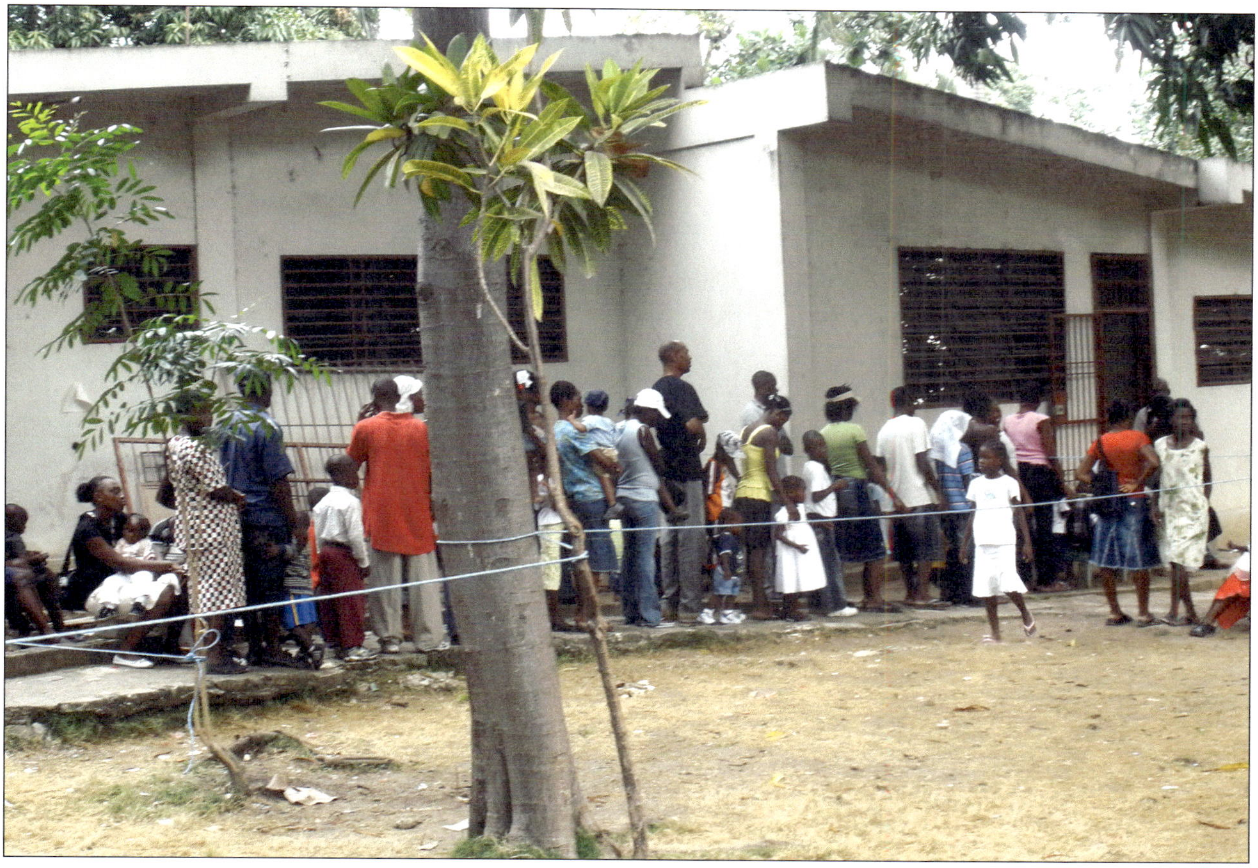

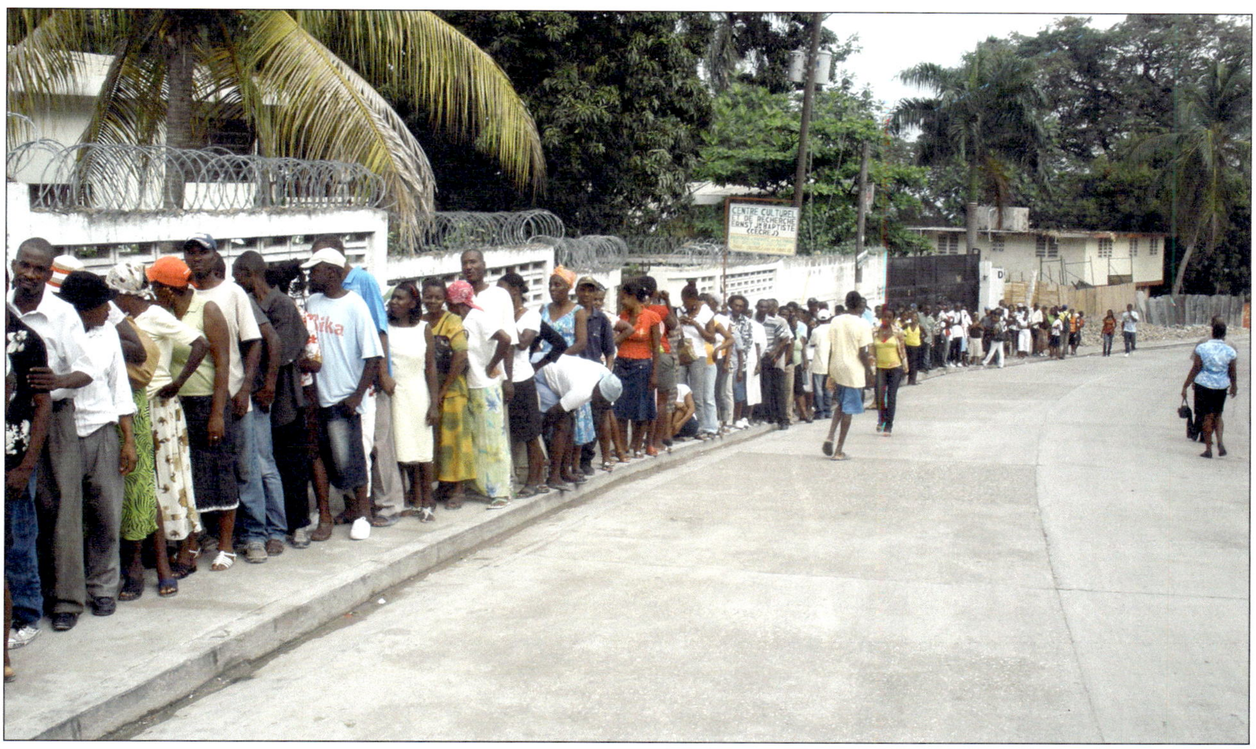

Patients waiting to be seen at clinic

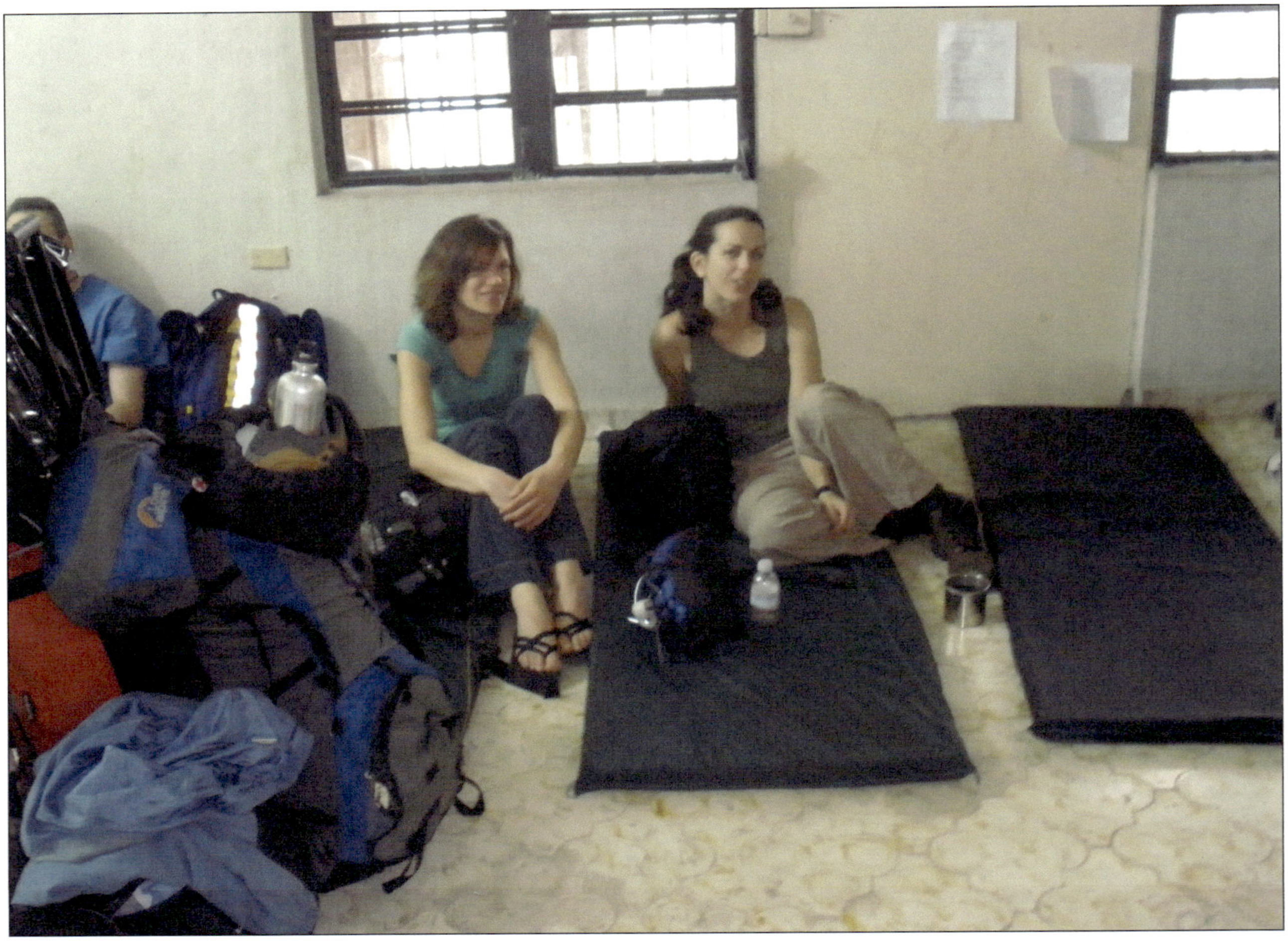

Two nurses and their exam tables

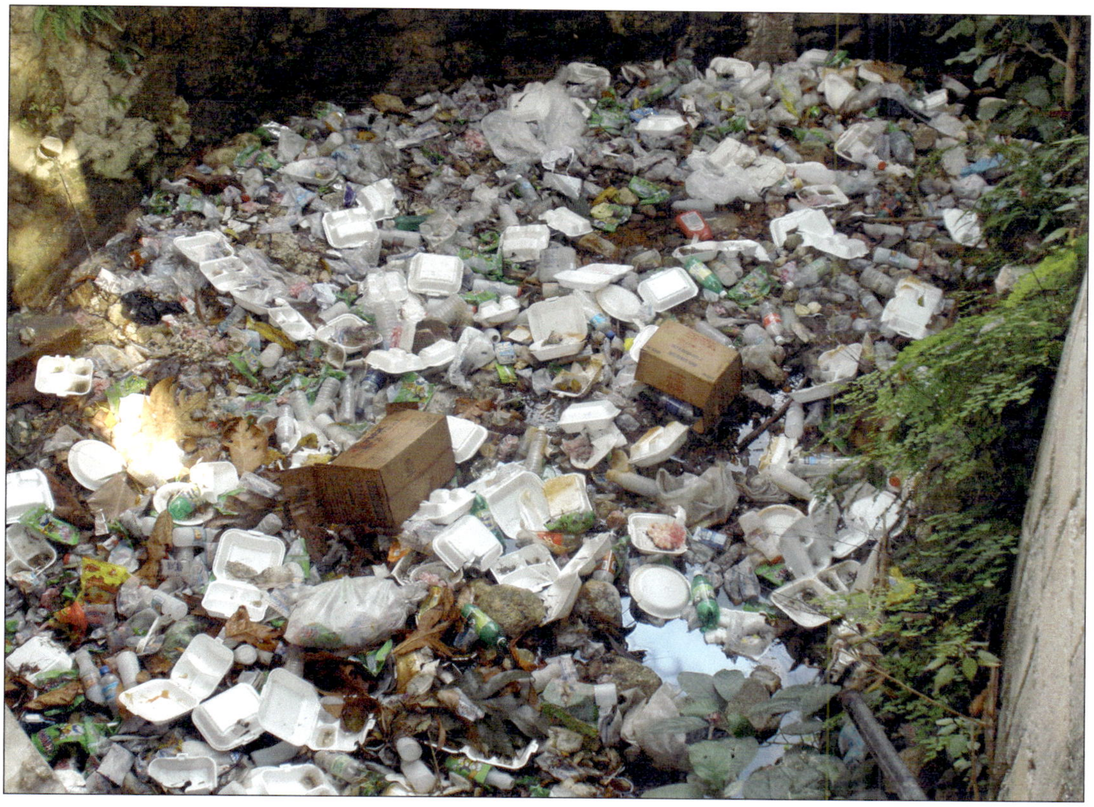

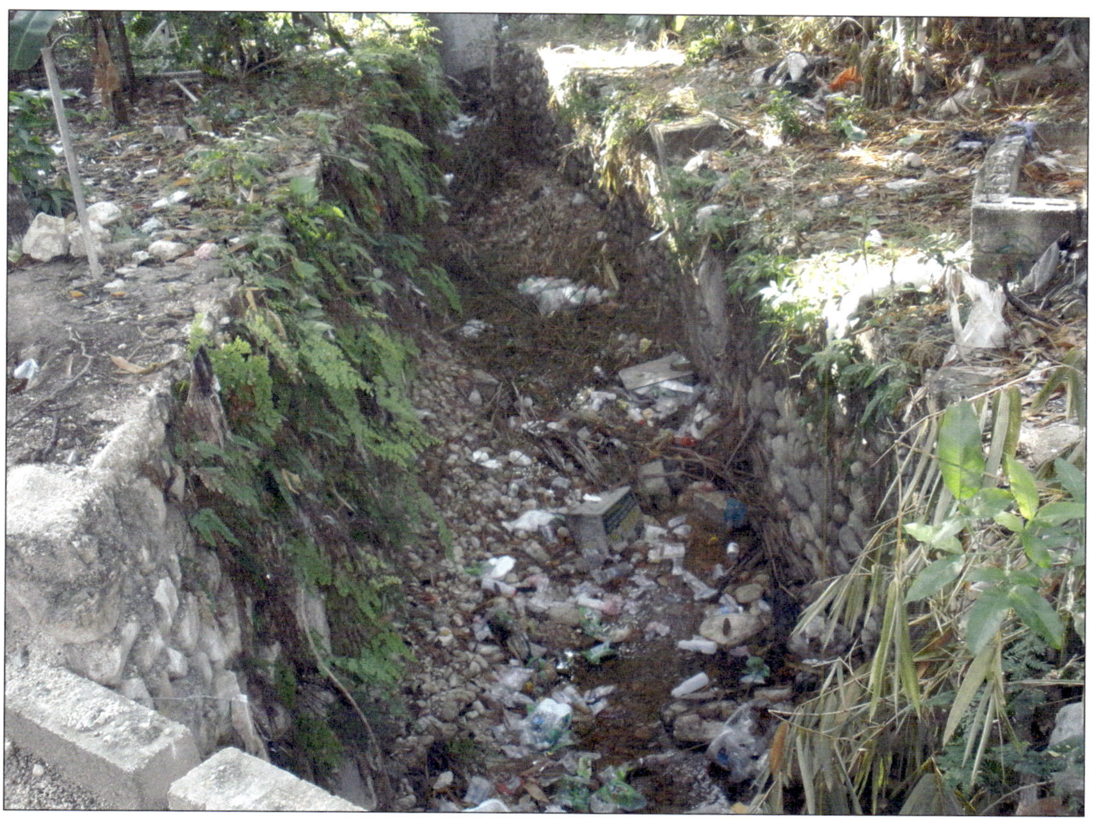

Garbage-filled ditch running through property

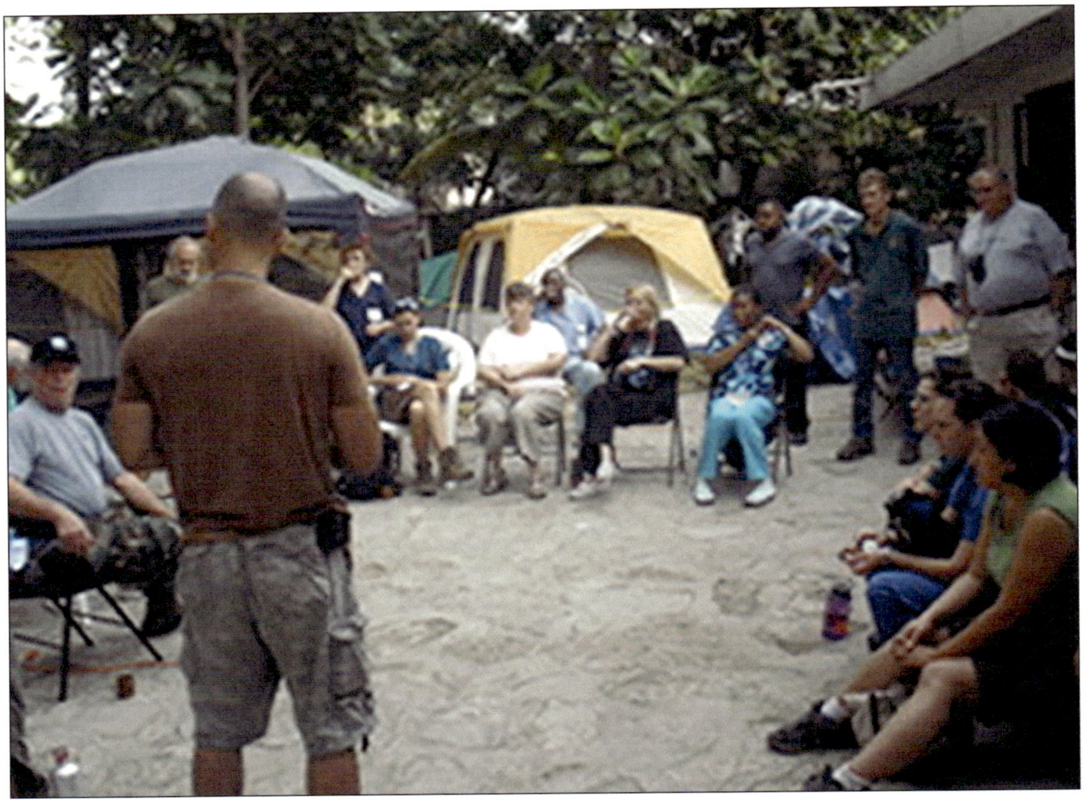

Group meeting before start of morning outpatient clinic

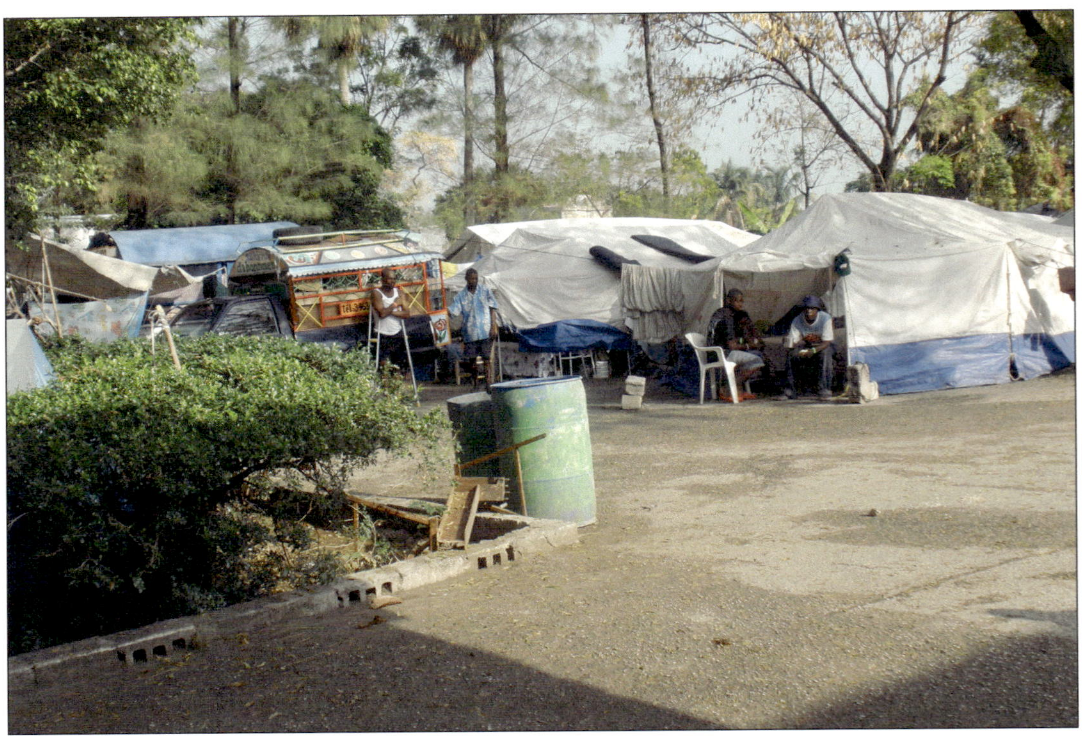

Tents on hospital grounds

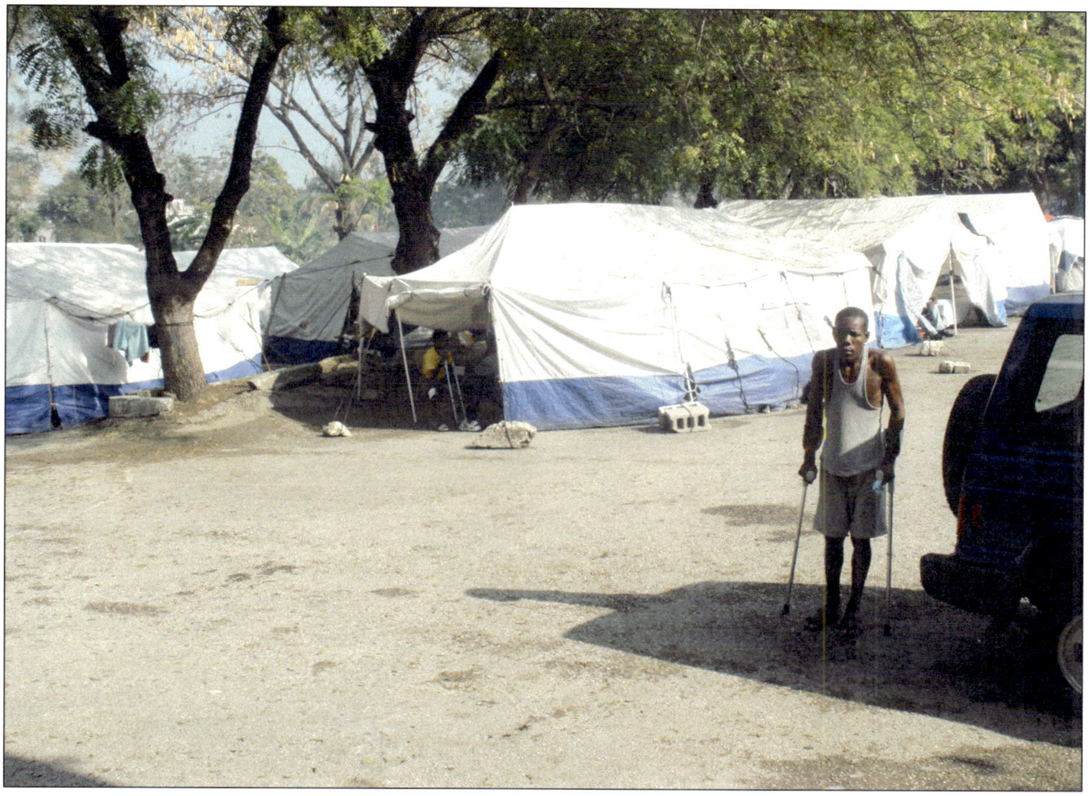

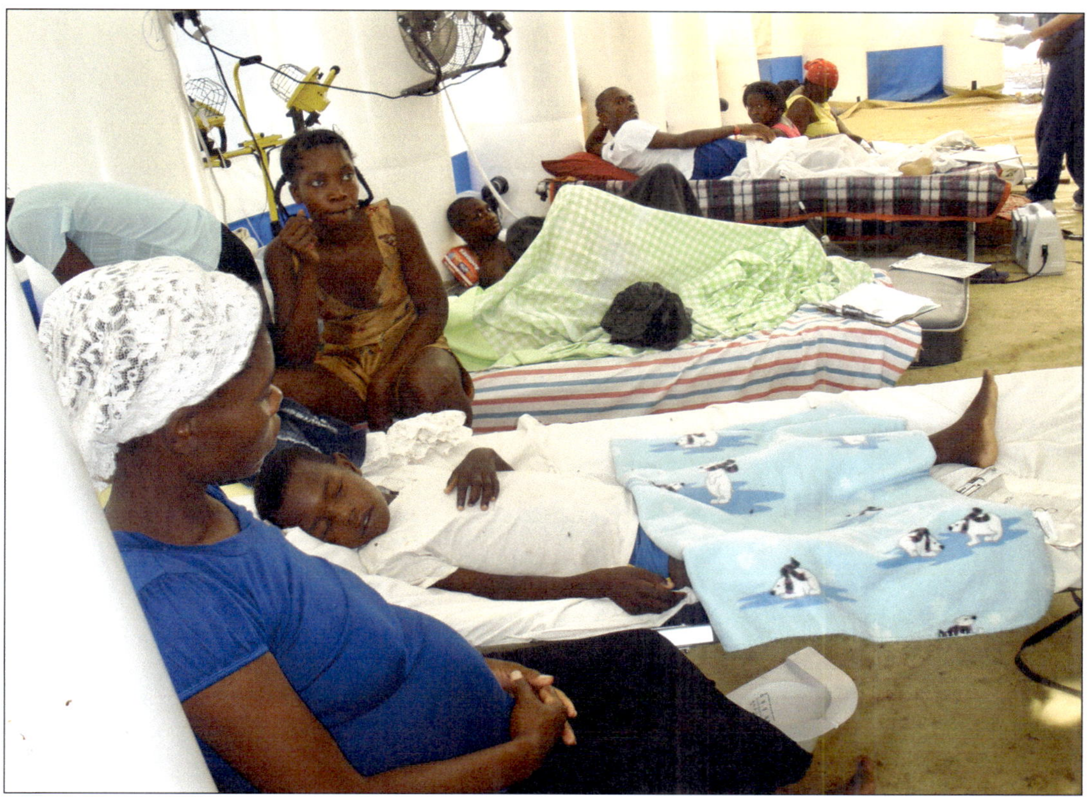

Makeshift ward outside hospital

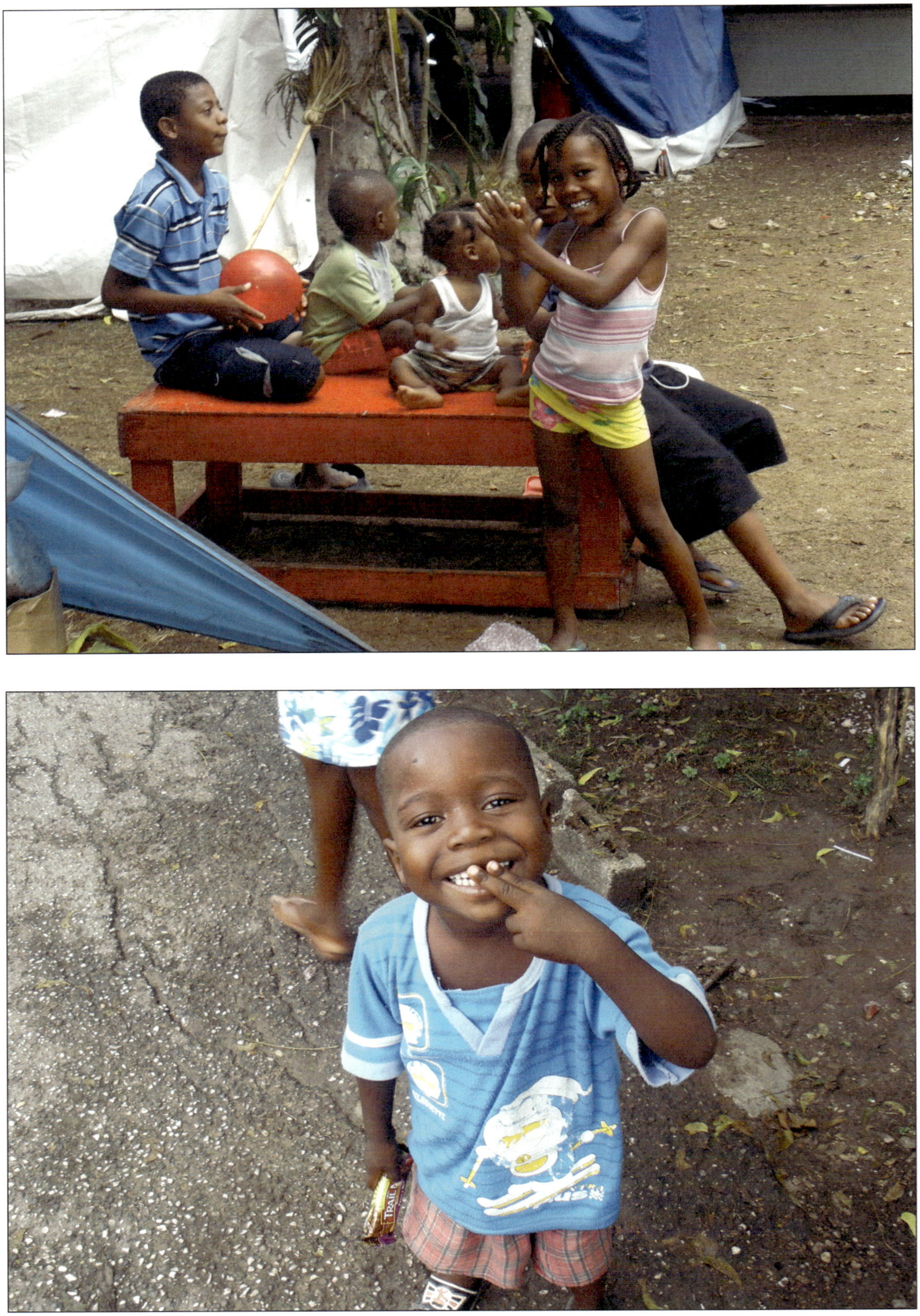

Life on the hospital grounds

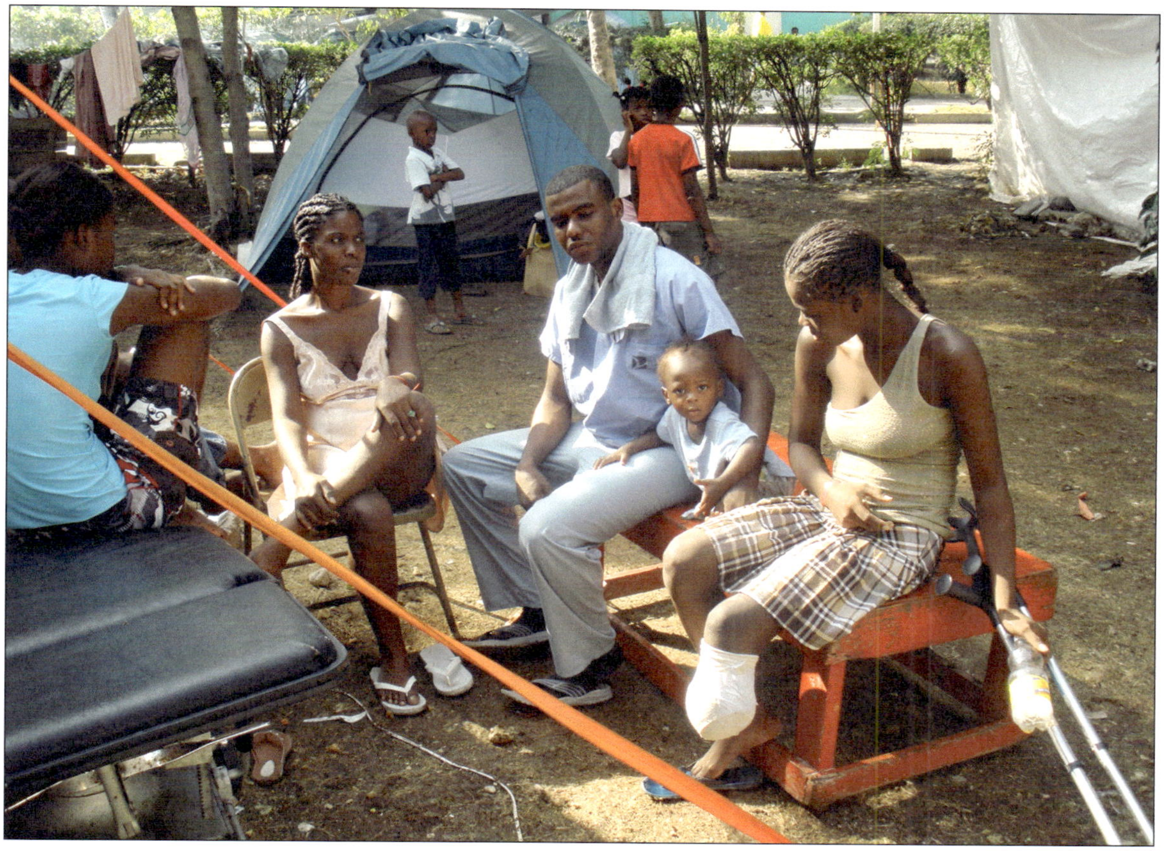

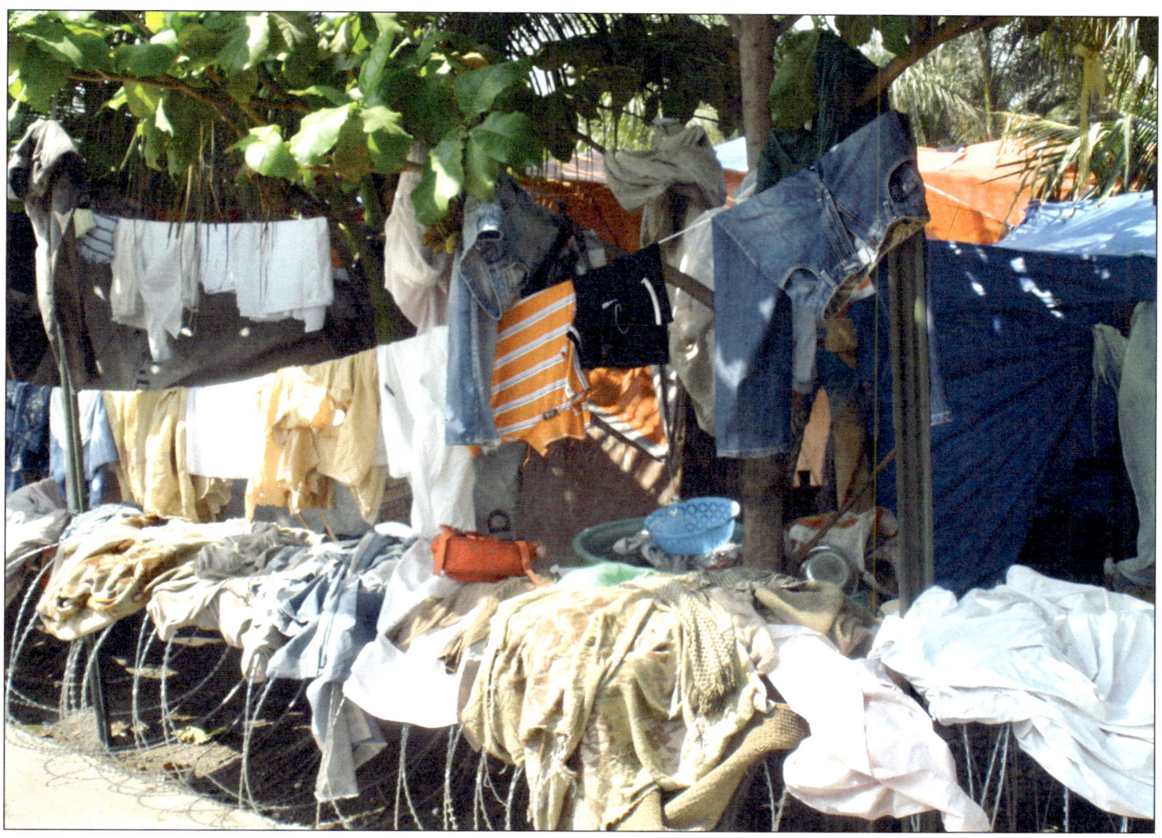

This young boy was a constant fixture in the hospital, with his great attitude and infectious smile. He and his family were caught in a collapsed building. His father and mother died, and he was trapped for three days. His grandmother bled to death on his lap. His is one of the many tragic stories of death, disfigurement, and abandonment left in the wake of the disaster.

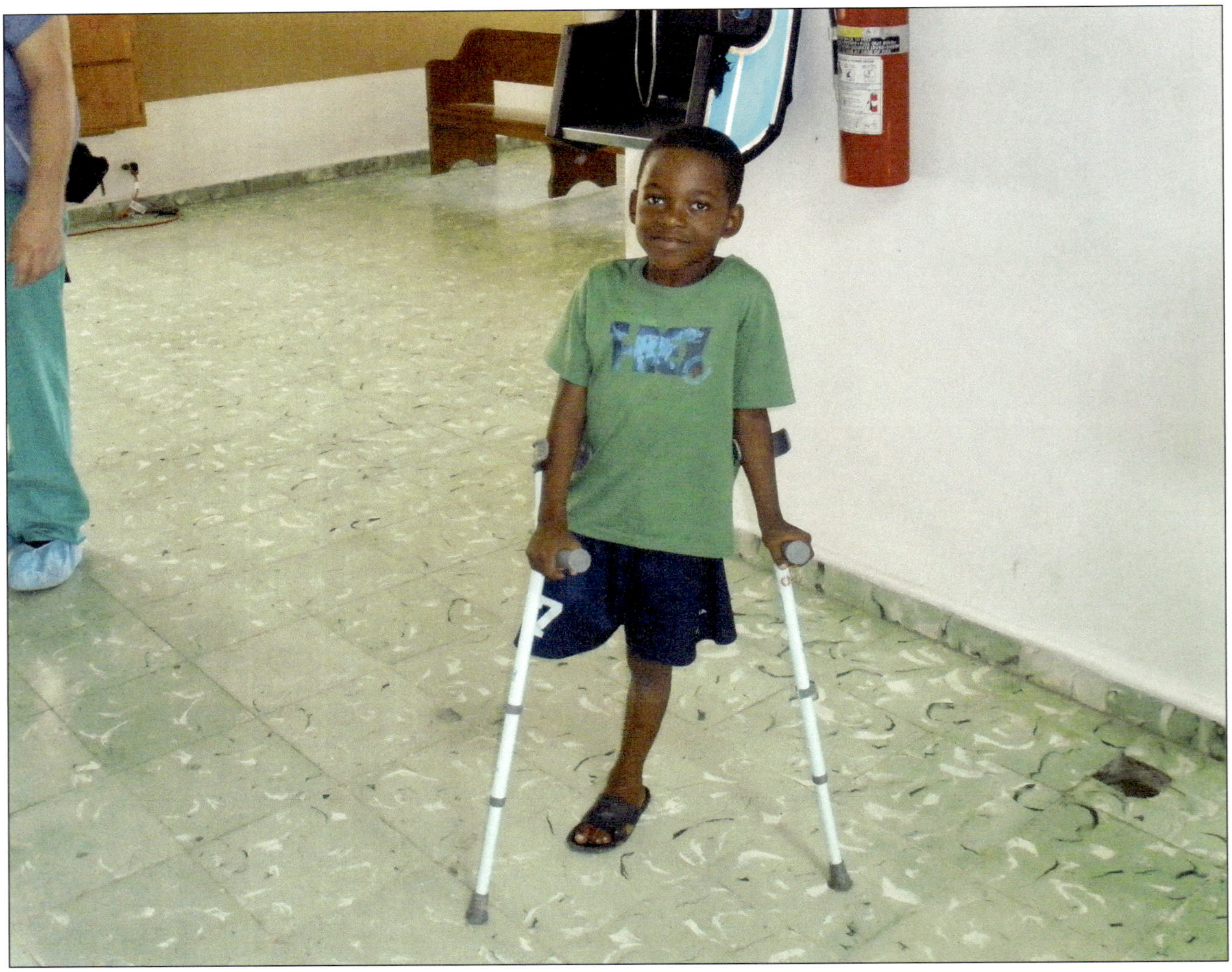

Another young boy, aged four, was transferred to our hospital with a dislocated hip he'd suffered during the quake. He was taken to a different facility, where they attempted to place the femur back into the socket, without success. They then placed his leg in traction for six weeks in an attempt to get the ball of the femur down to the level of the hip socket and then do the reduction. This also proved unsuccessful, and he was transferred to our facility. (The resident surgeon was a pediatric orthopedist from Loma Linda University.) We operated and reduced the hip after two hours of extremely difficult maneuvering. Hopefully his function will be normal, but his prognosis was guarded.

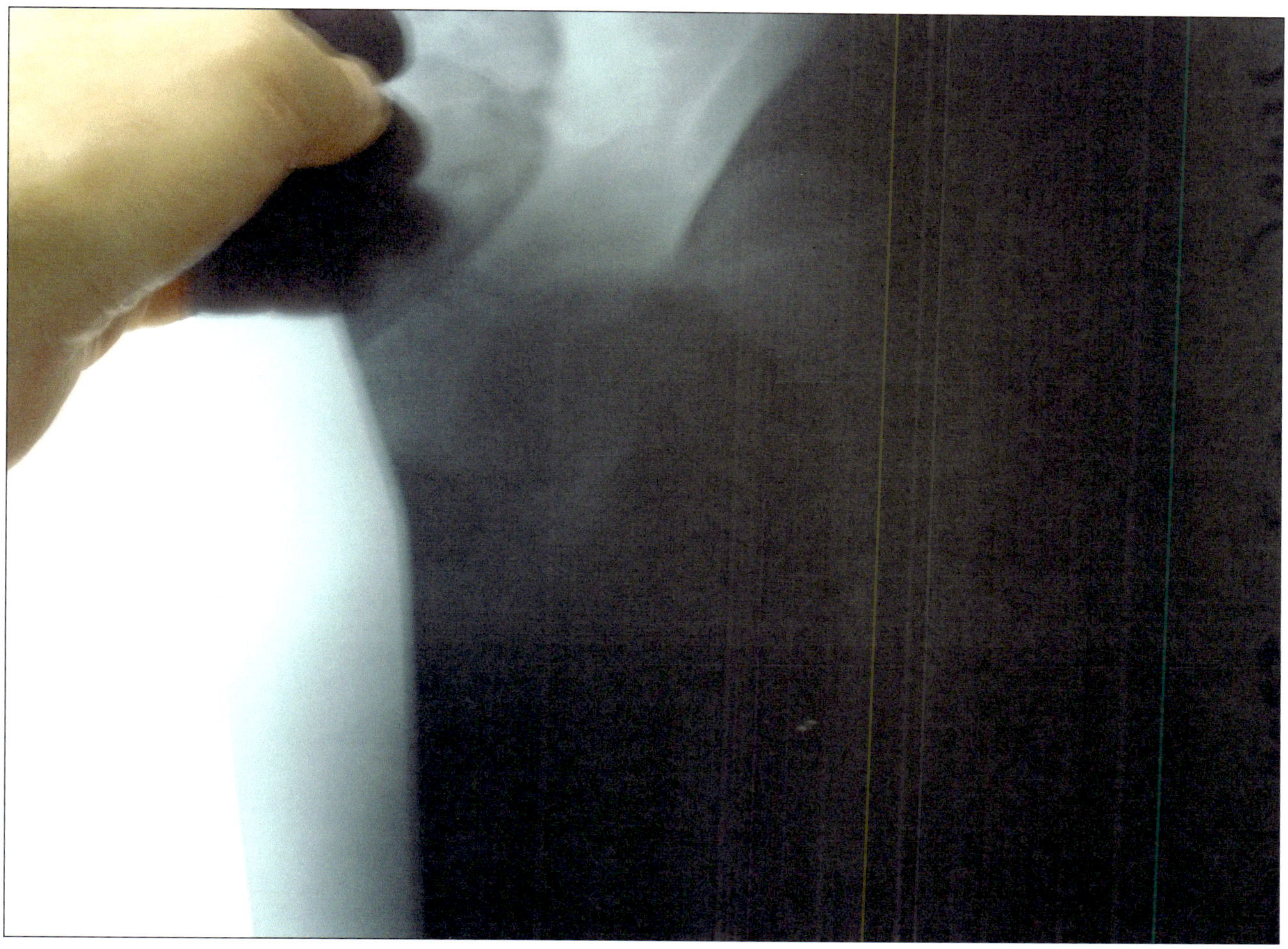

X-ray showing dislocated hip upon arrival at the hospital

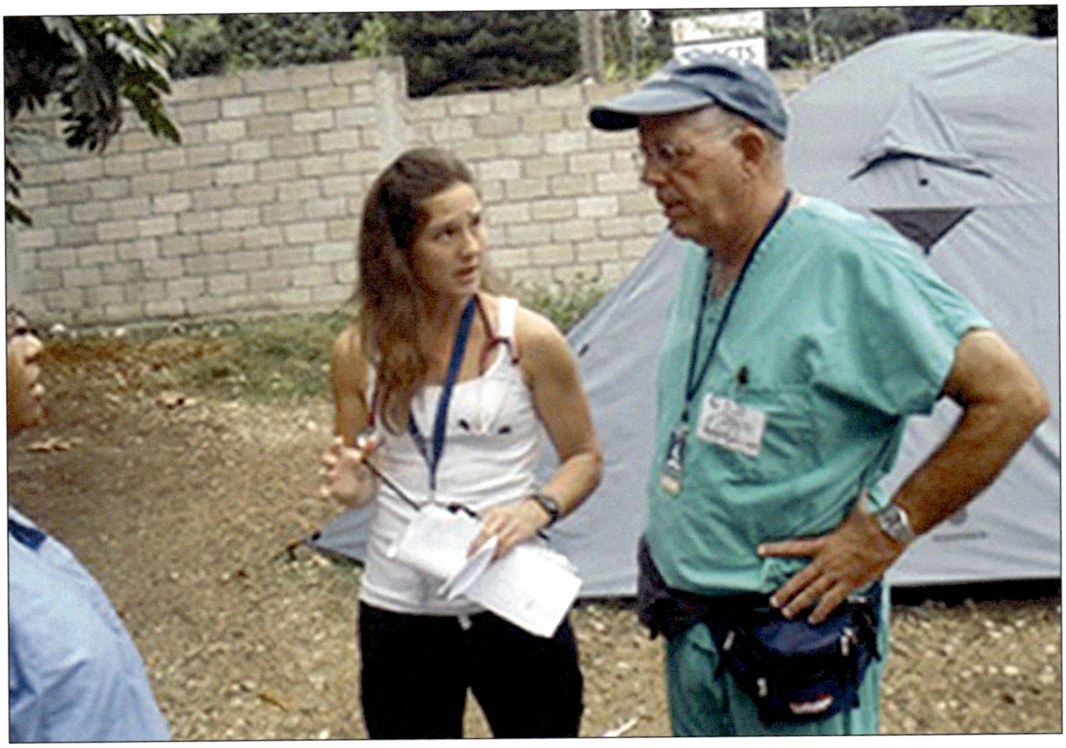

Bob Porter discussing care with nurse

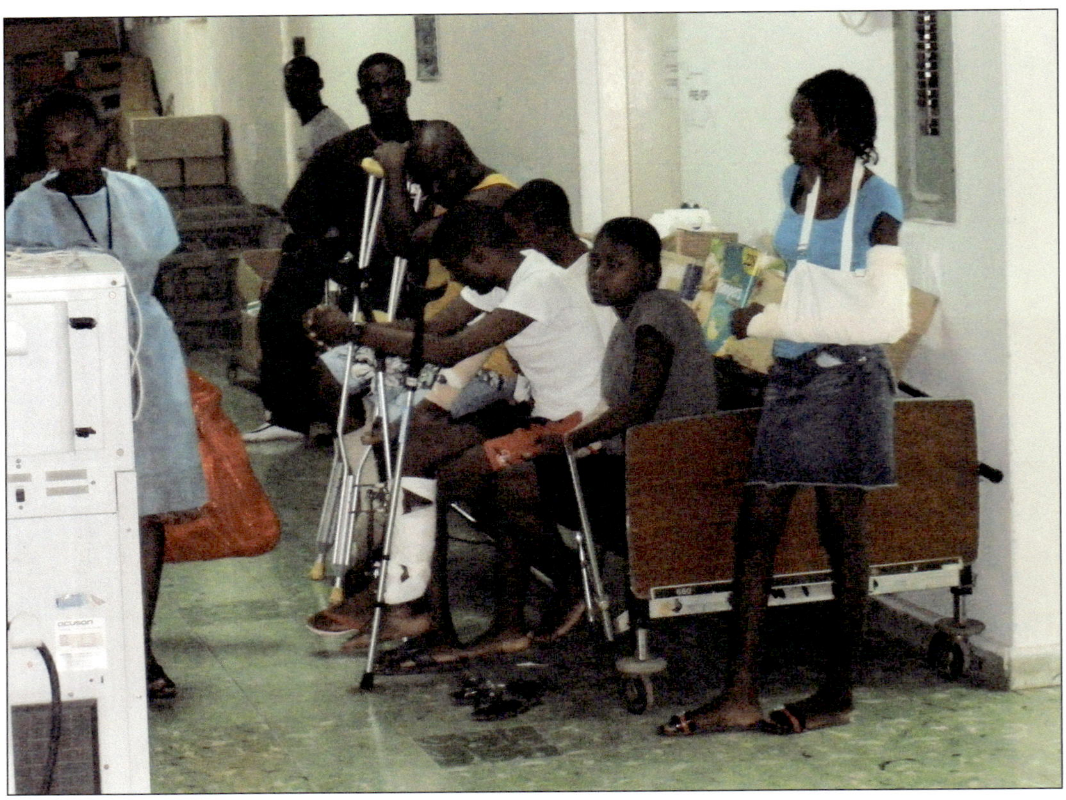

Patients waiting for X-rays

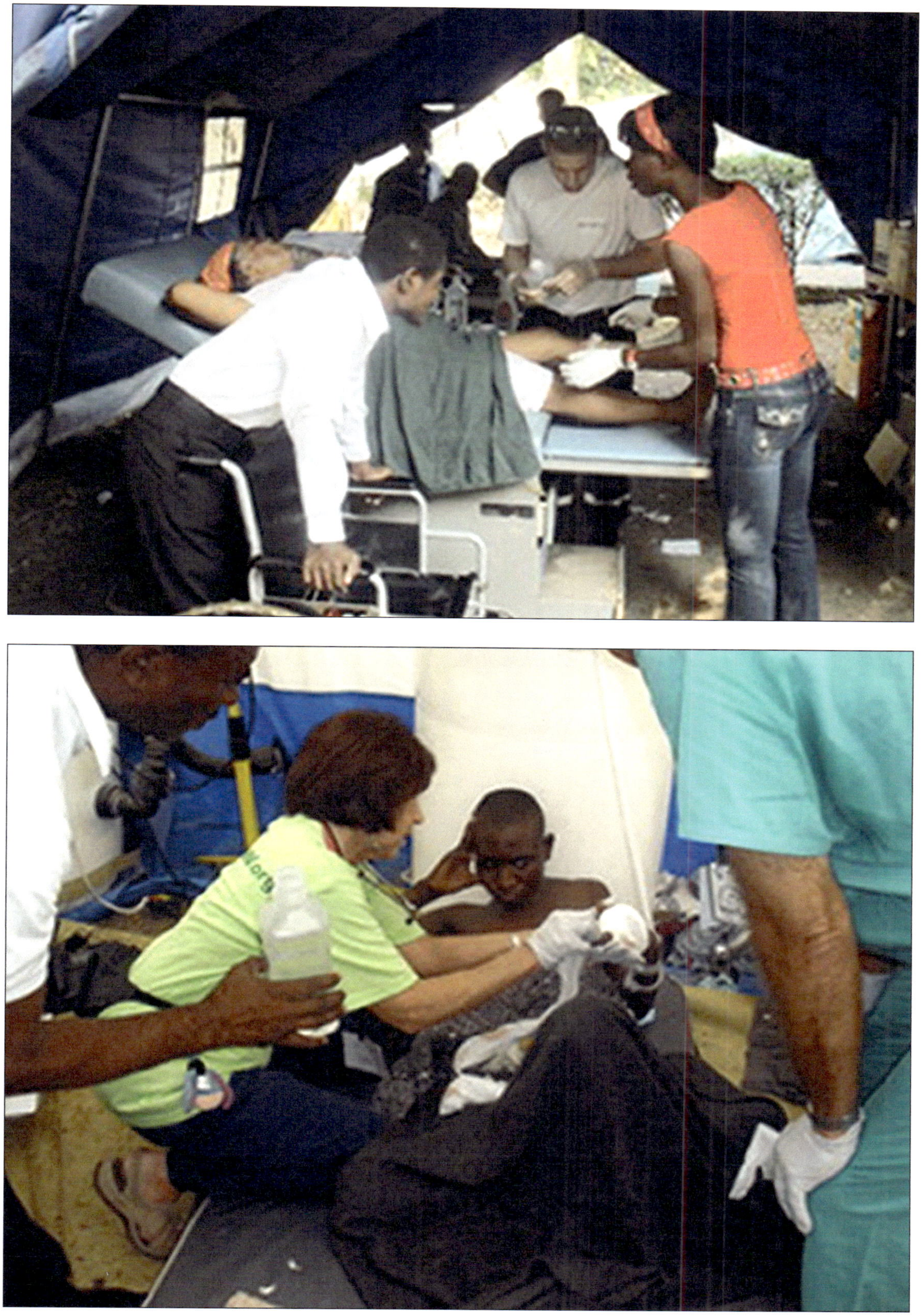

Dressing changes and wound checks

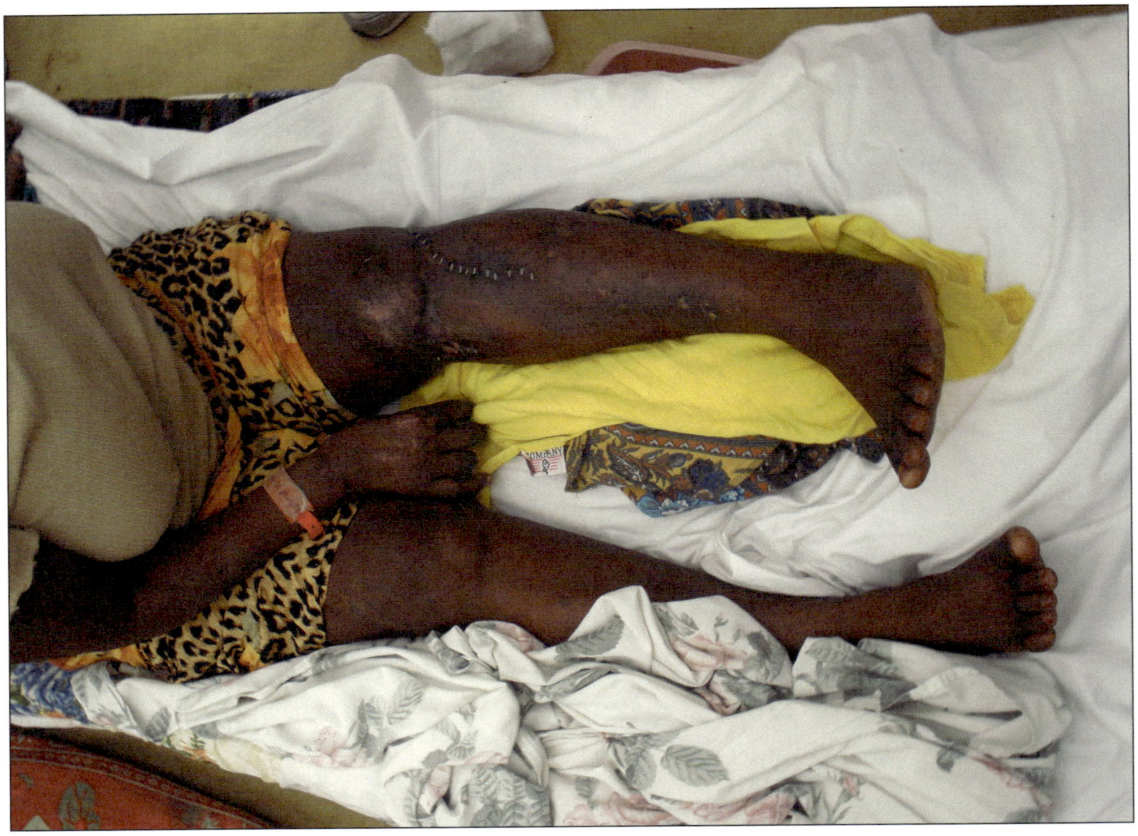

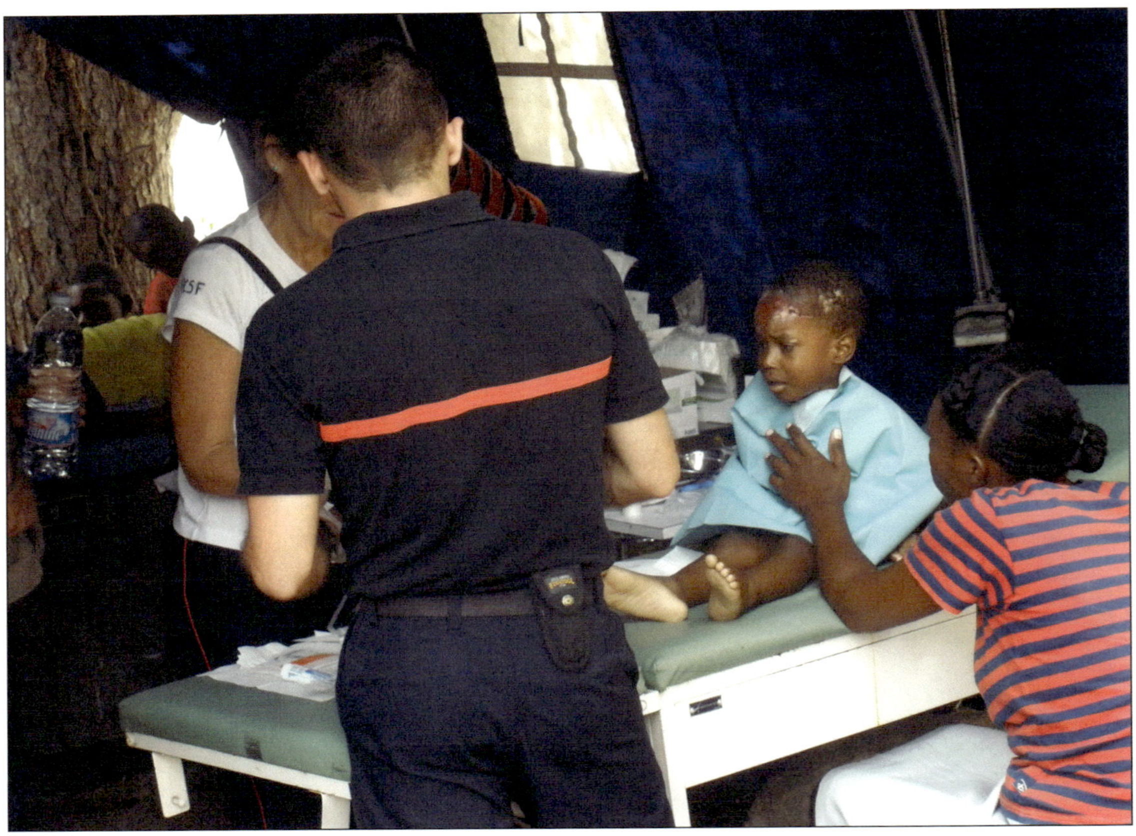

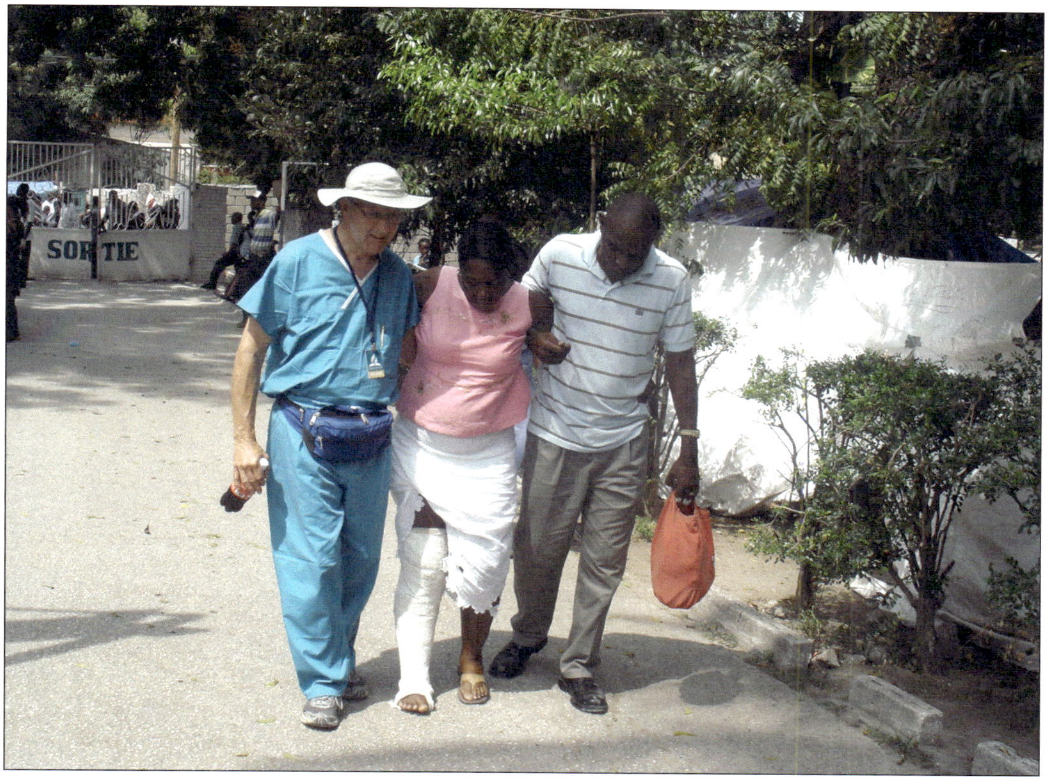

Assisting woman to cast-changing area

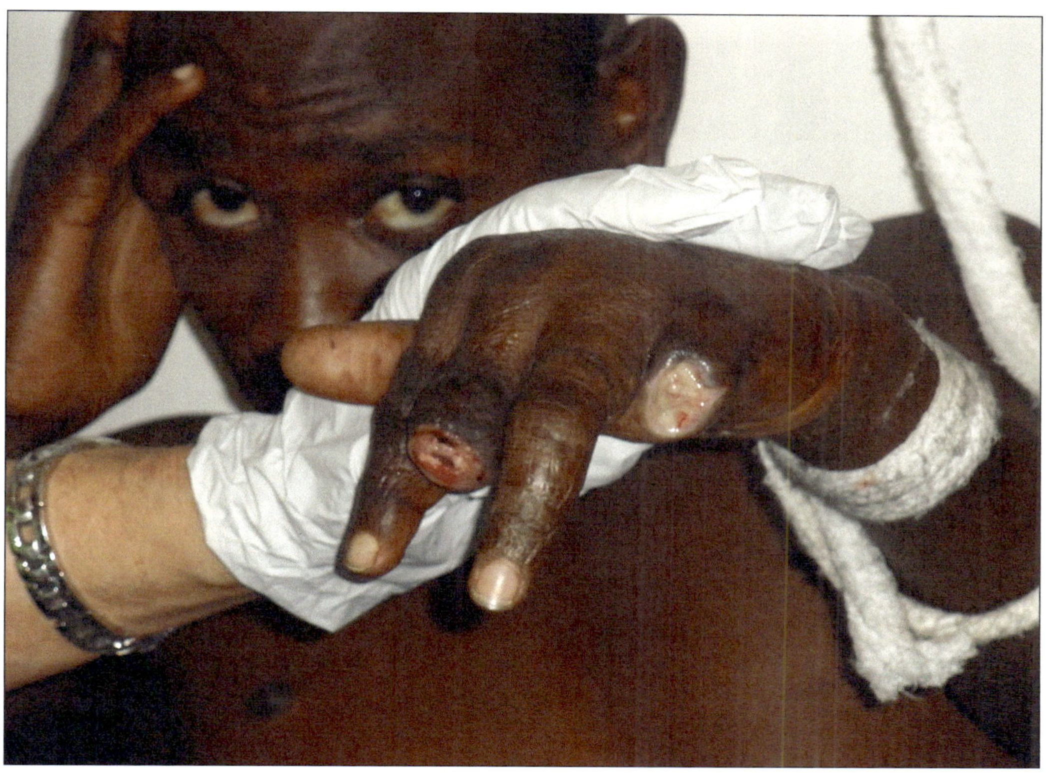

Lots of amputations from structures falling and crushing limbs

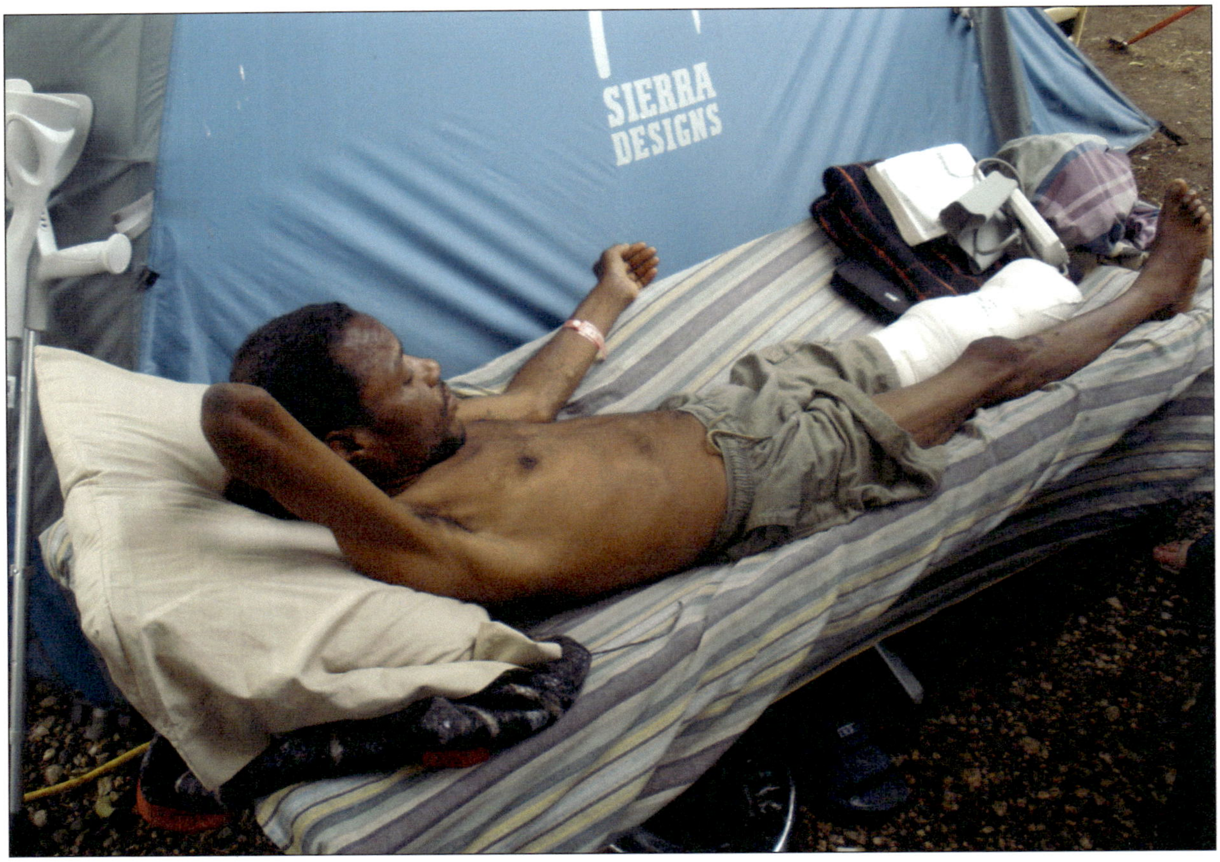
SIERRA
DESIGNS

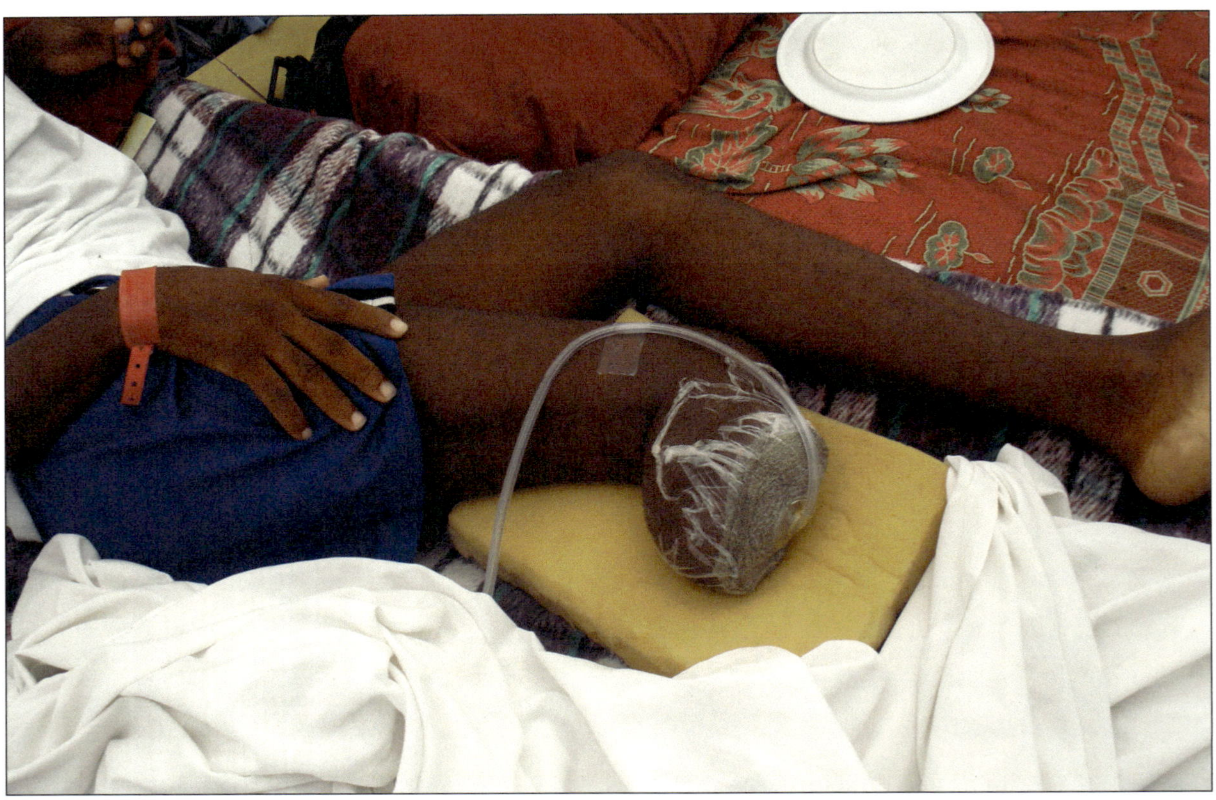

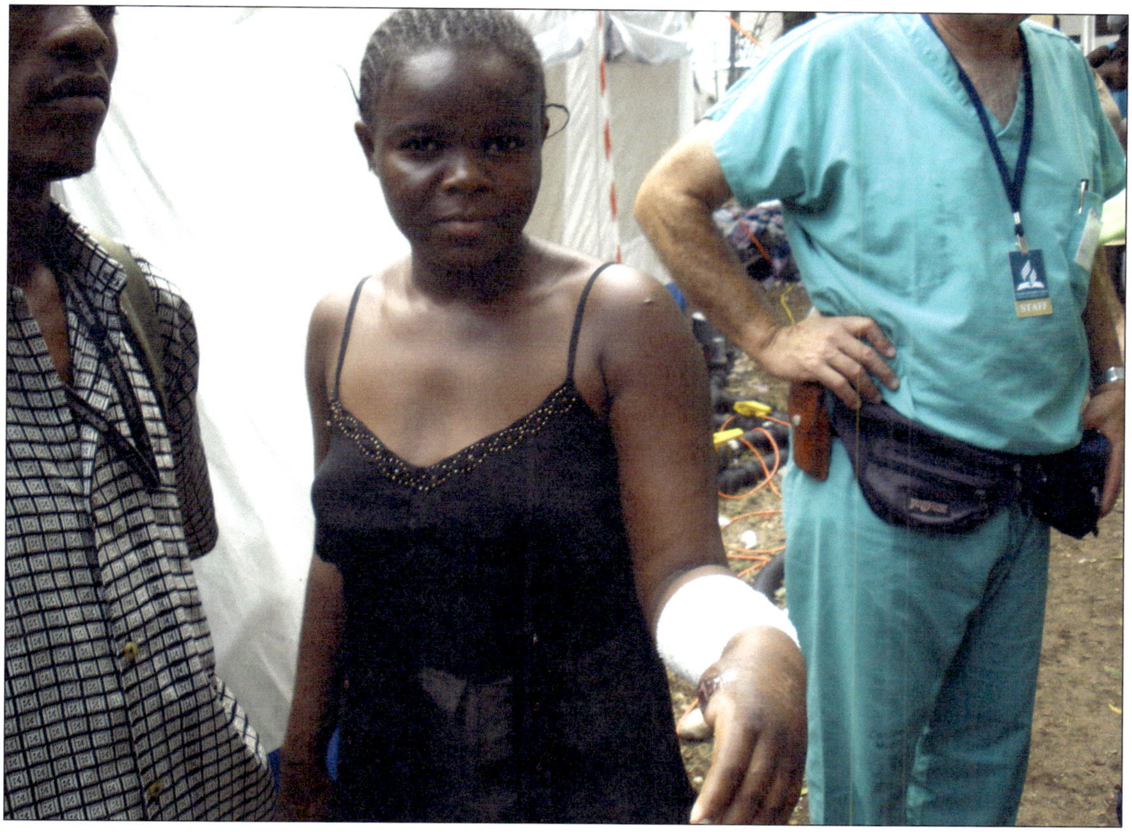

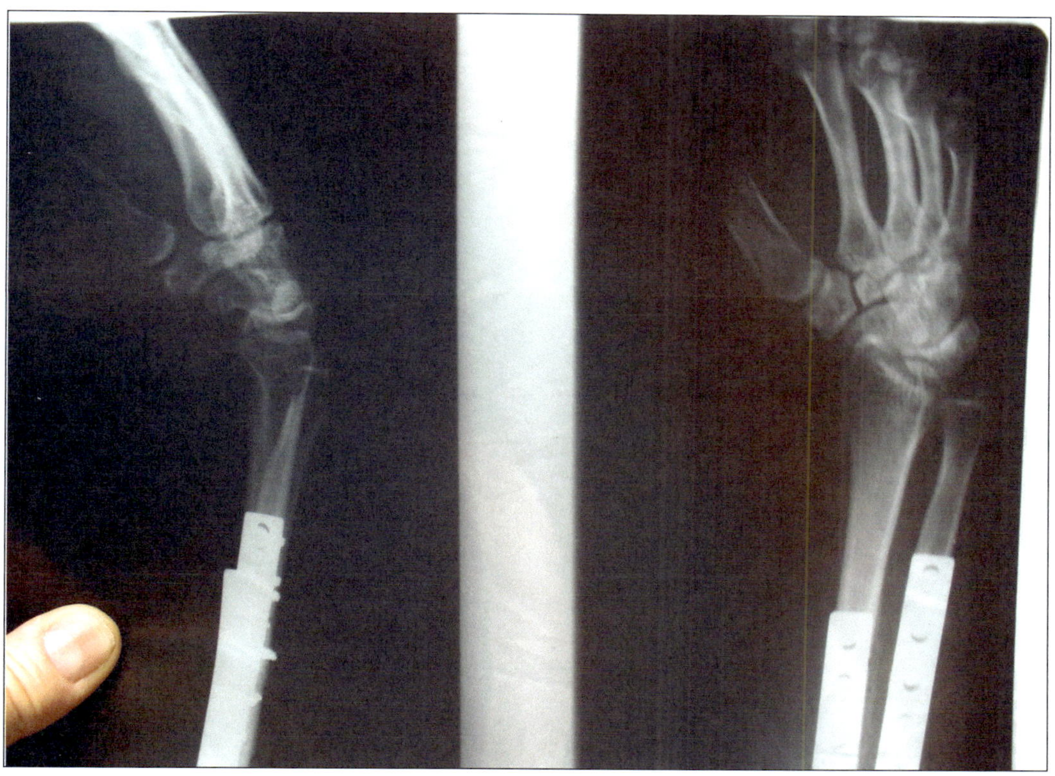

This young girl suffered loss of her thumb and fractured both bones in her forearm

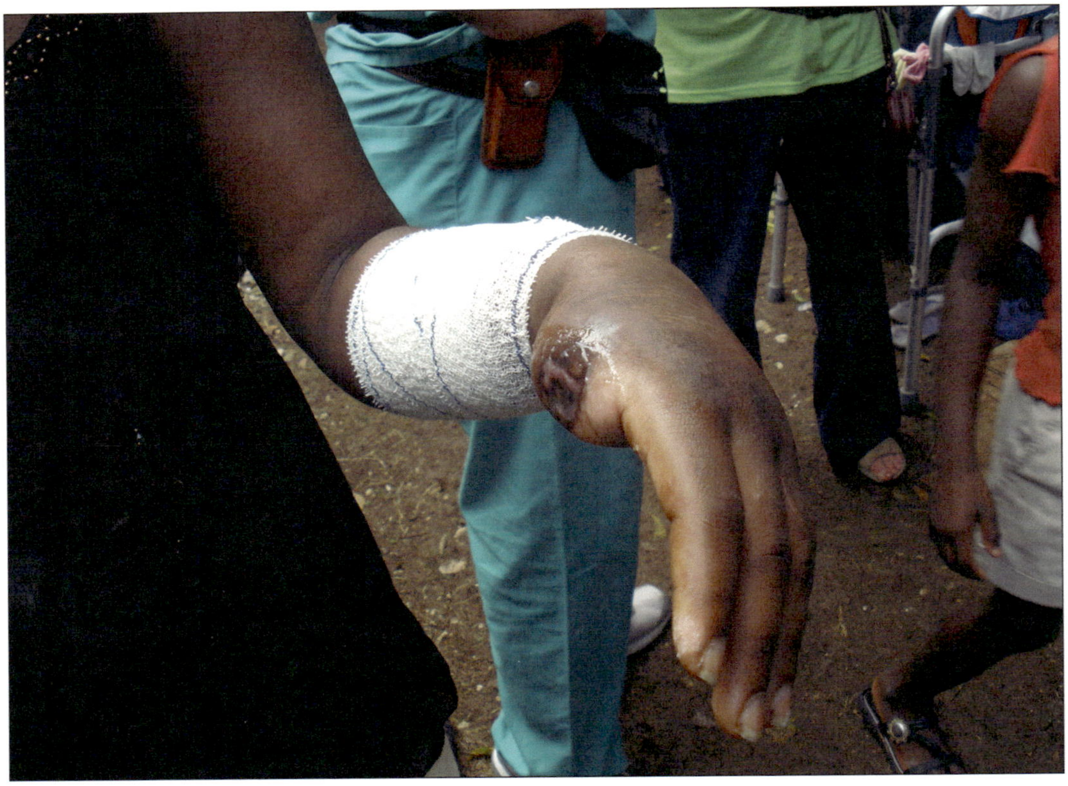

Unable to extend her wrist due to injury to her radial nerve

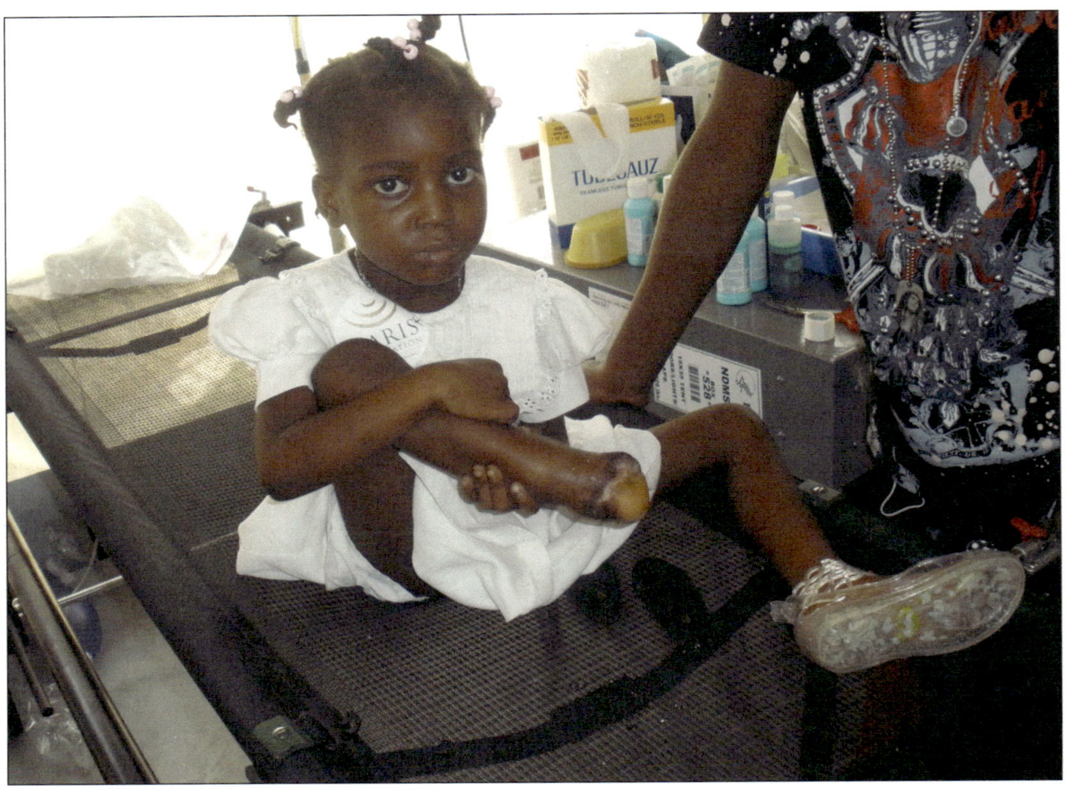

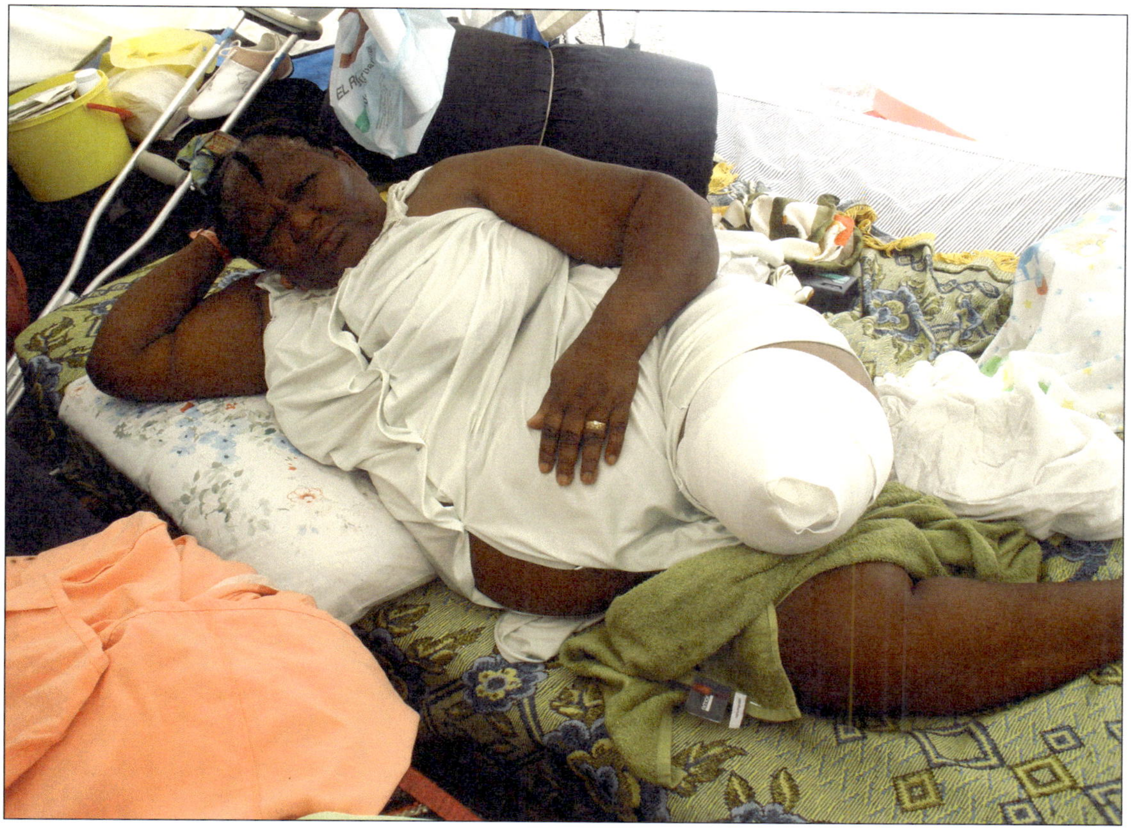

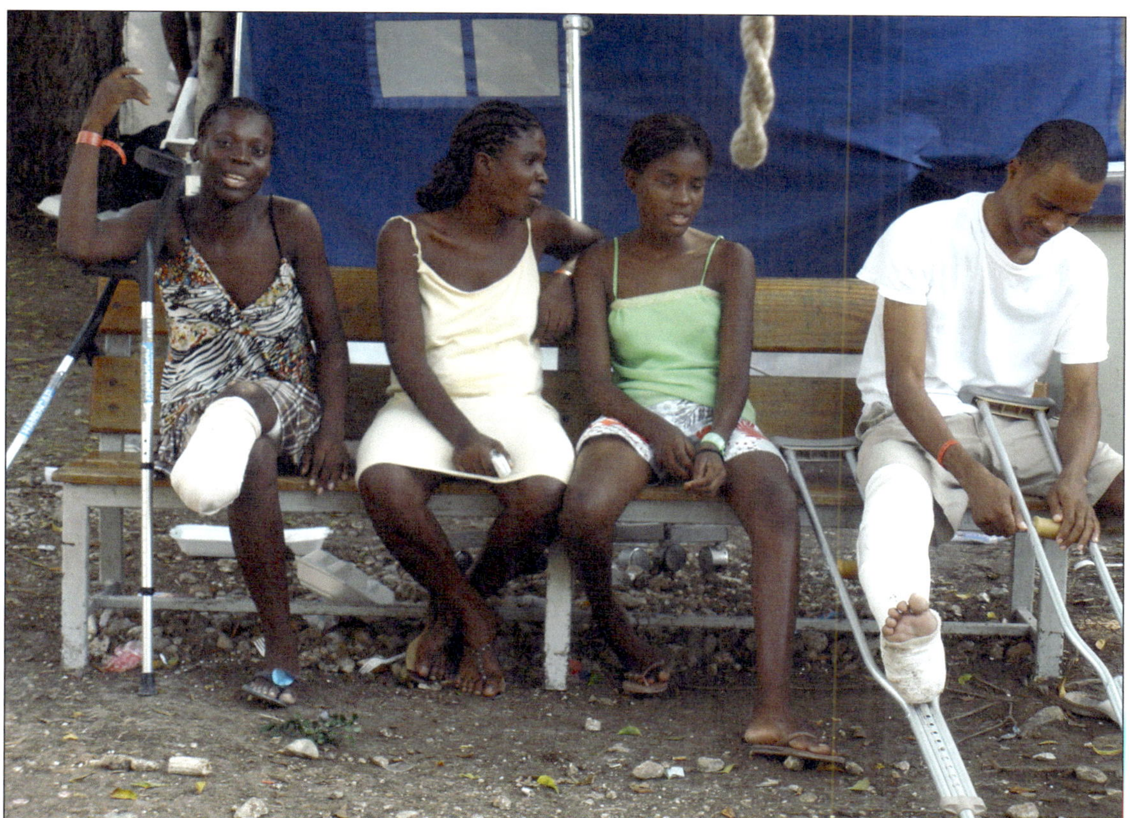

Many fractures were treated with external fixators, placing pins above and below the fracture and connecting the pins to a frame on the outside of the body. This is usually quick and effective in immobilizing the fracture site while it heals.

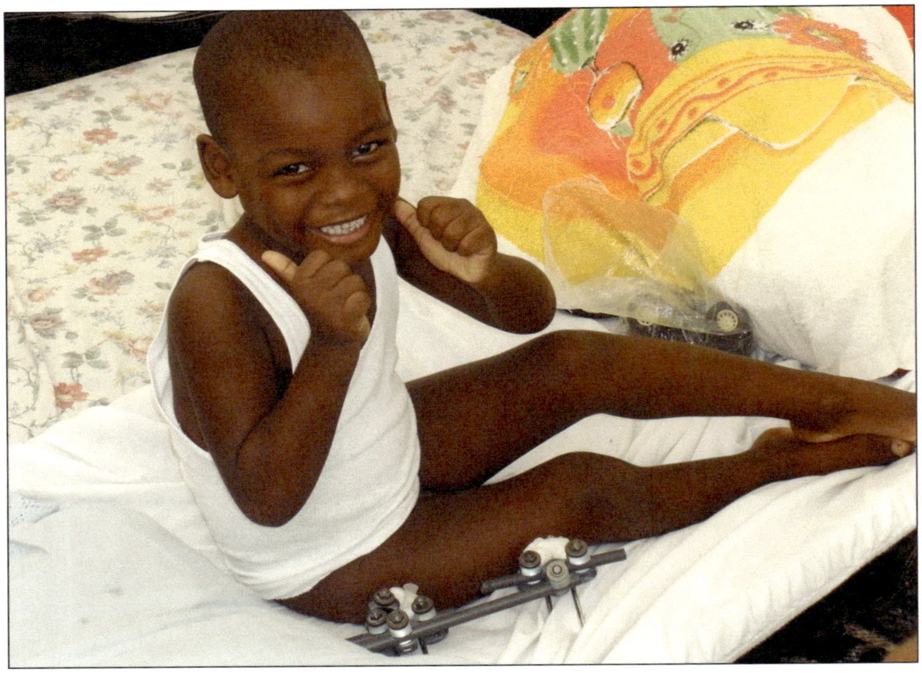

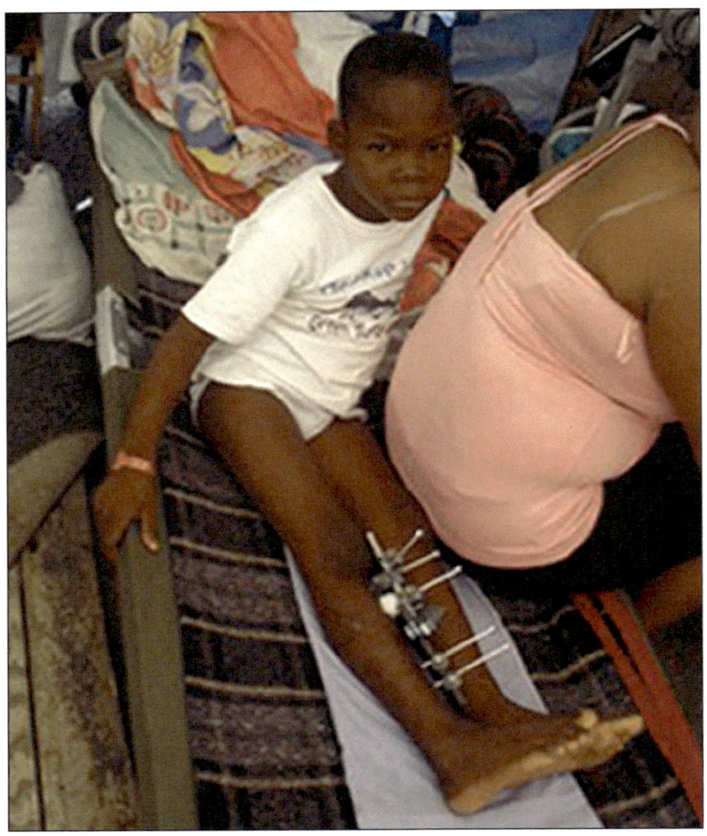

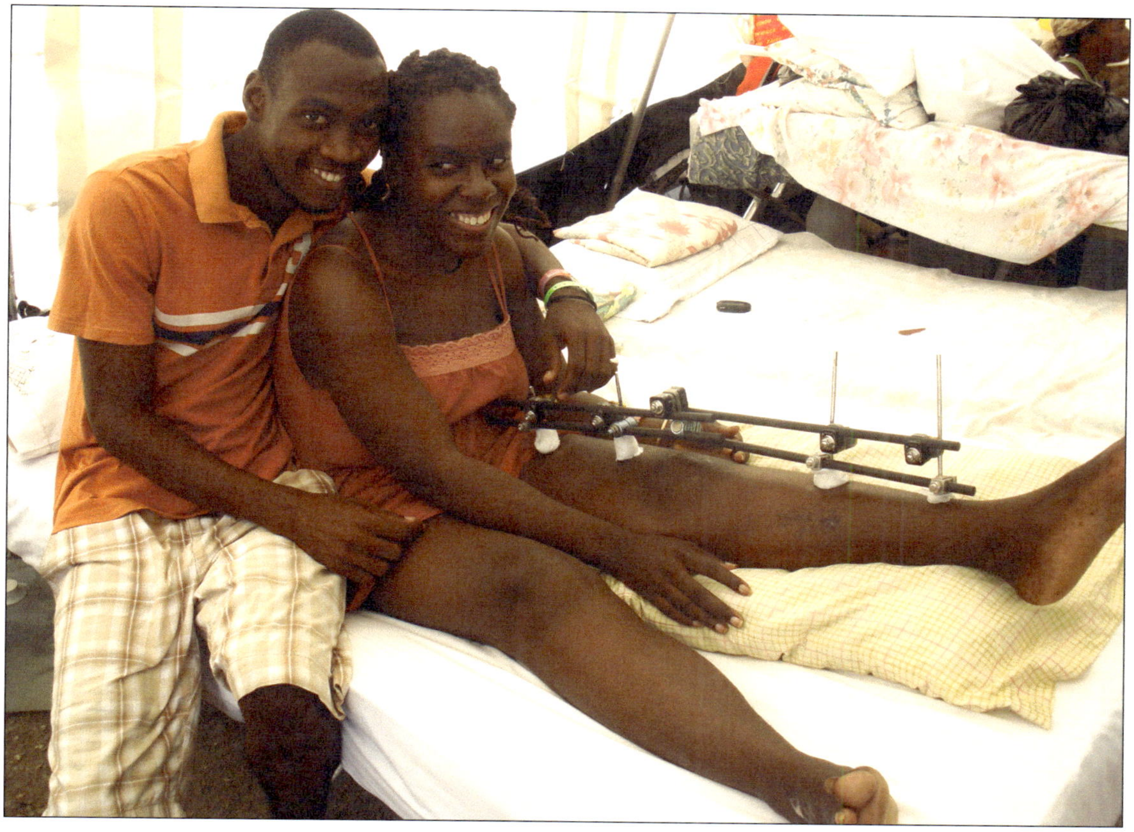

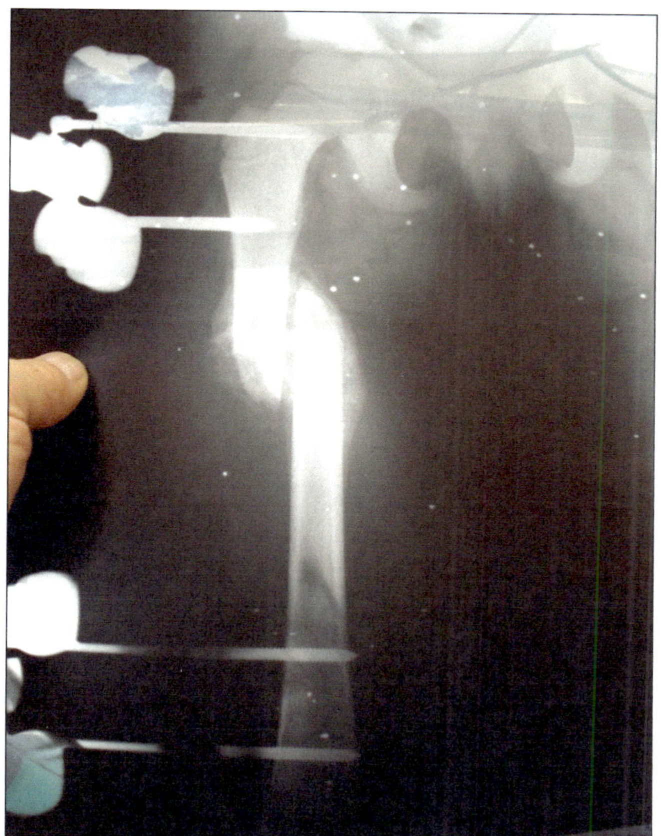

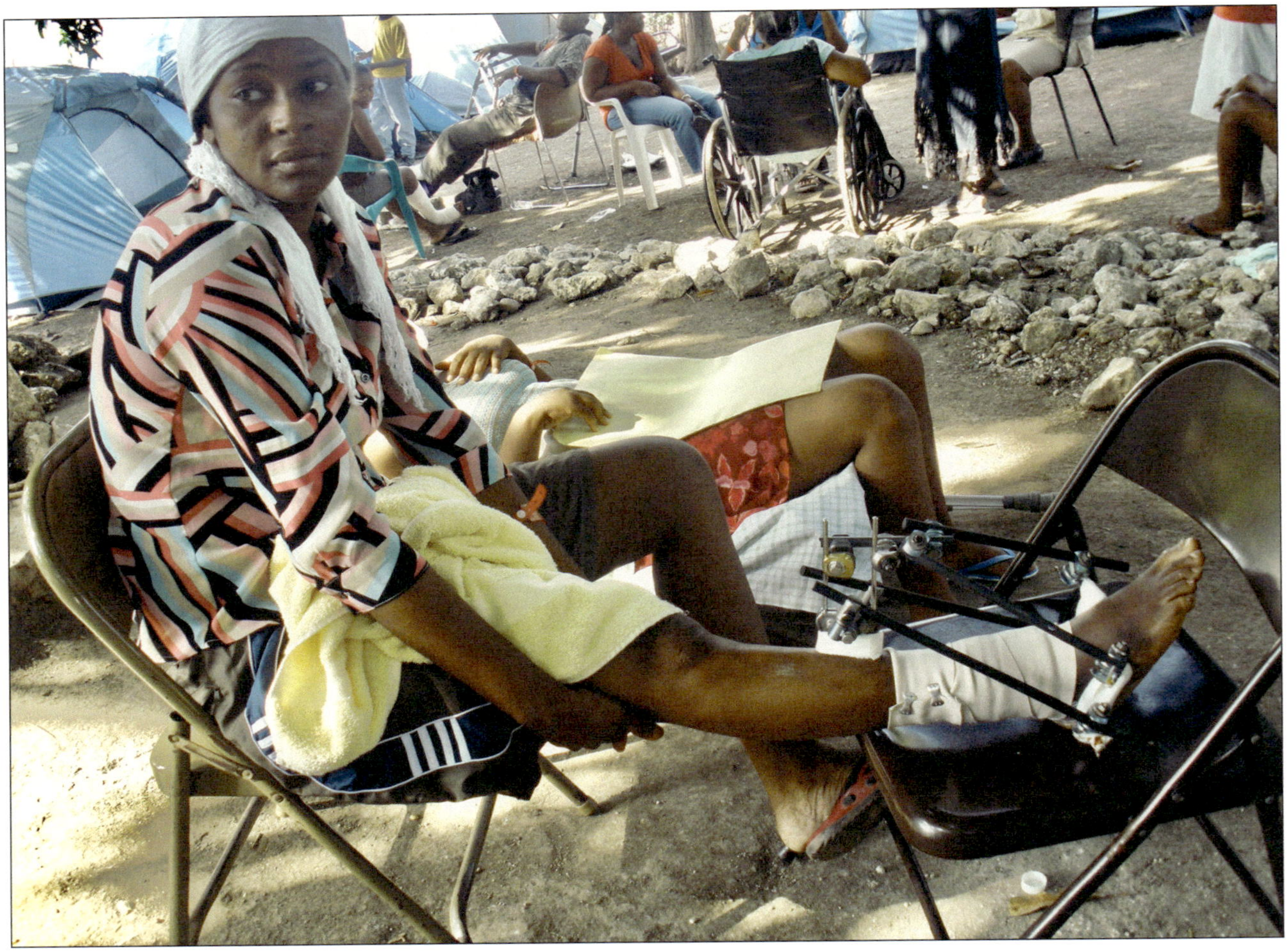

A particular sad story involved a young woman who was recuperating from surgery for a fractured ankle that was inadequately fixed and needed revision surgery. Her mother, who was with her, refused to allow any further surgery, stating she had lost her husband and another daughter to the quake and was not going to risk her remaining daughter to surgery. Unfortunately her ankle will deteriorate quickly once she begins weight bearing.

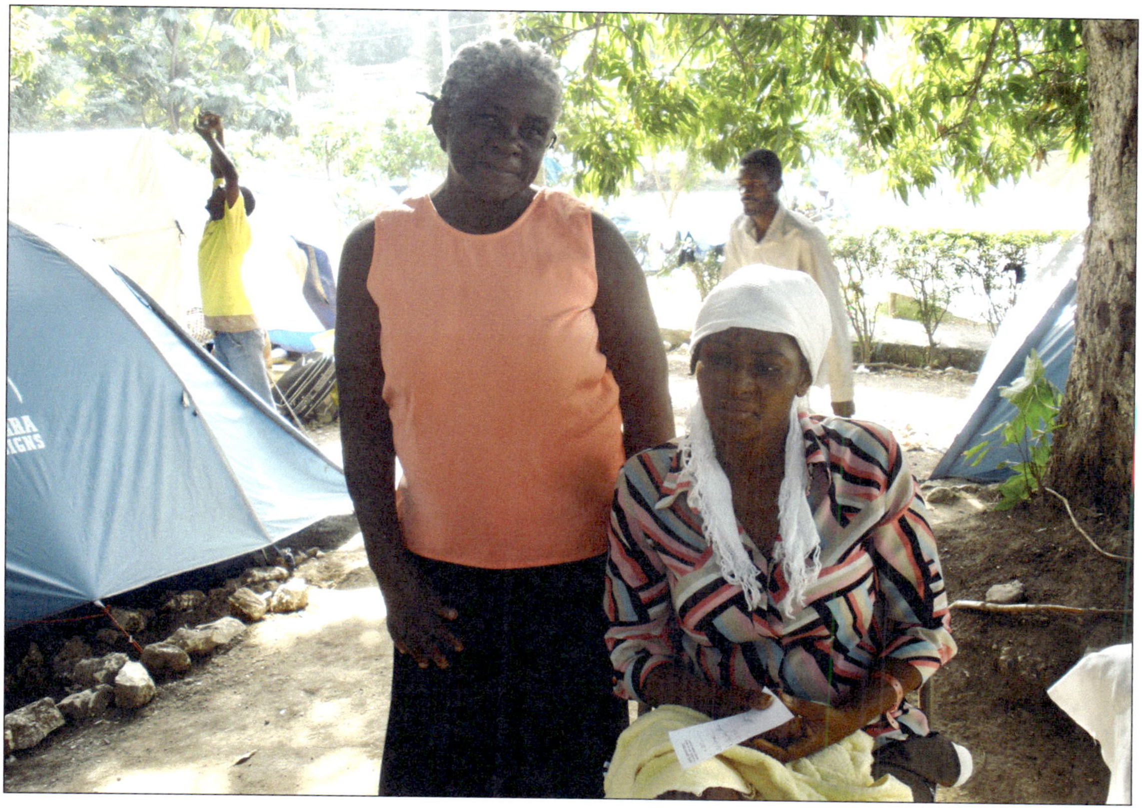

Mother and daughter. Deformed ankle X-rays below

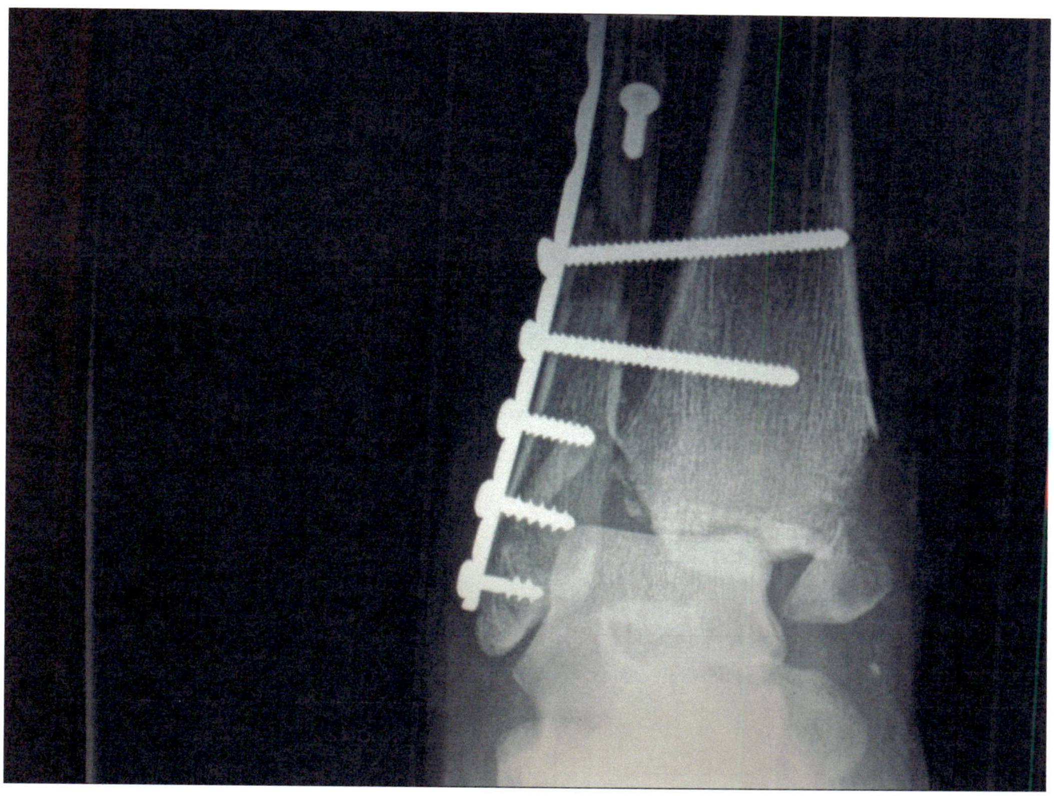

Our week went by quickly and, in retrospect, was not long enough, having taken the first two days seeking a place to work, and then, once at the hospital, taking another day to get fully oriented, which left only 3½ days to be fully engaged in the work needed to be done. It was still a rewarding experience aiding those individuals struck by tragedy to receive competent medical care and hopefully resume a normal life, but the work left to be done was staggering.

During Rita and my journeys, we encountered many different living conditions, staying in private homes, in quarters on hospital grounds, in small, one-star hotels to four-star accommodations when traveling with Operation Walk.

In Caraz, Peru, perched at 7000 feet above sea level, with temperatures in the 50s at night and no central heating, showers were almost always taken with cold water. In Bolivia, the shower water was supplied by an electronic shower head that you turned on and off once water was flowing. It always gave me pause to look up at the electric wires entering the shower head and then turning the nob to "On" with my wet hand,

A luxury in many of the hospitals in South America was a toilet seat. Most of the bathrooms had none, and toilet paper was another item rarely found.

A luxury in many of the hospitals in South America was a toilet seat. Most of the bathrooms had none, and toilet paper was another item rarely found. I always wore a fanny pack in which I kept an ample supply of TP as well as anti-diarrheal medication, as diarrhea could strike at any time. Eating was at times an adventure, but we tried to not eat anything that was not thoroughly cooked or could not be peeled. If clean water was unavailable, I brushed my teeth on many occasions with Coca Cola, as carbonation is an excellent disinfectant. Illness was not a frequent occurrence, but during our first trip to Brazil while operating on a child, our anesthesiologist was struck with sudden, severe GI distress. This was followed shortly thereafter by the circulating nurse in the OR and then my assistant. Luckily, I escaped that episode, but it was a tense period finishing that surgery.

Over a span of 29 years, Rita and I made 21 trips to 14 different countries, some multiple times. Countries not presented include St. Lucia, Guatemala, Nepal, and Taiwan. Nepal, Guatemala, and China were with Operation Walk, St. Lucia with Orthopedics Overseas, and Taiwan was an individual effort coordinated by one of our local anesthesiologists who had previously done work there.

I would be remiss if I didn't acknowledge the hard work and effort by Rita and the other support staff. While I had only to operate, Rita was often my assistant, and, after the surgery, she would be preparing the room for the next case or getting the used instruments to the sterilizer and then opening a new set of instruments for the following case. Then she'd help bring the next patient to the operating room and start surgery all over. She was often quite fatigued by the end of the day and the trip. She was not only my assistant but a wonderful companion, and I am forever grateful for her participation in these endeavors.

The experiences we gained, the people we encountered, and the camaraderie enjoyed by the operating teams were priceless, but the real thrill and feeling of accomplishment came from the patient interactions. The mother who traveled three days by boat on the Amazon to have her child's clubfoot corrected, who smiles shyly or cries when she sees the results. The gratitude of the young woman whose unsightly tumor has been removed from her knee, or the young child who is able to walk again because her severely contracted and flexed knee has been straightened, or the many men and women who are able to ambulate again without pain because their arthritic joints have been replaced. Their lives have been changed, and they are supremely grateful, expressing their gratitude in terms of gifts, hugs, or just a heartfelt "Thank you." These are the memories that will last a lifetime.

The experiences we gained, the people we encountered, and the camaraderie enjoyed by the operating teams were priceless …

Des Moines Boys

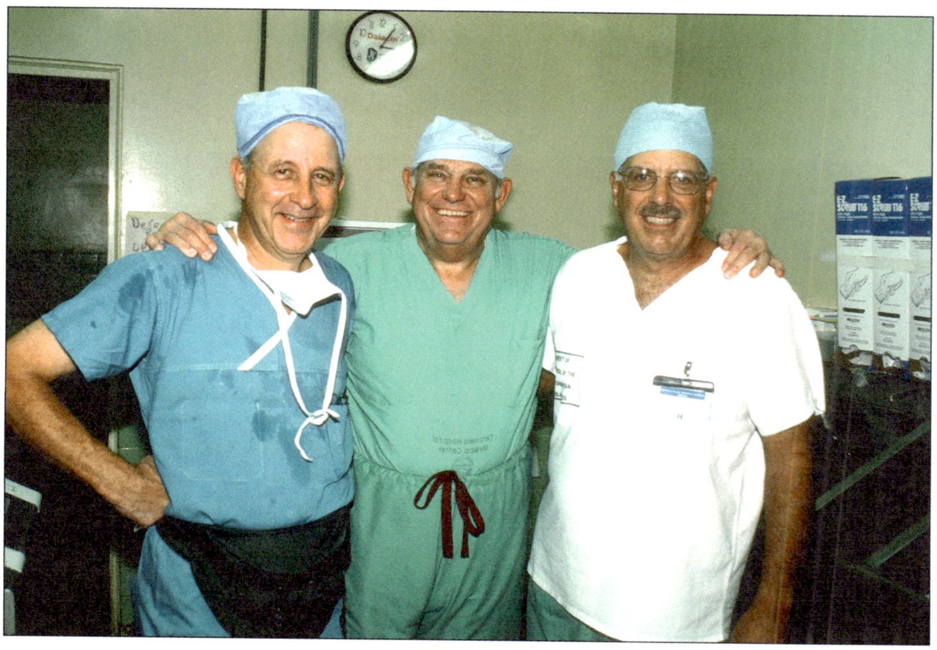

Sandler, Dorr, Porter

Made in the USA
Monee, IL
12 September 2026

62981956R00124